PENGUIN
ARKANA

THE HANDBOOK OF SELF-HEALING

Born in Lvov, Ukraine, in 1954, Meir Schneider emigrated to Israel with his parents in 1959. He underwent five cataract operations without success and at seven was declared legally blind. Years later, by means of eye exercises and movement therapy, he was able to read without glasses and began to work with other physically disabled people, receiving national attention for his work in the healing arts.

In 1975 Meir emigrated to the United States to continue his studies, gaining a BA in Liberal Arts and a PhD in the Healing Arts, and in 1977 he founded the Center for Conscious Vision in San Francisco, then establishing the Center and School for Self-Healing in 1980. In 1982 he was granted an unrestricted driver's license. Meir's pioneering work in the holistic health field is known throughout the US as well as outside it. His unique approach to health care – the empowerment of the individual – is a message of inspiration and hope as well as a practical guide to specific exercises for everyone. His book *Self Healing: My Life and Vision,* also published by Arkana, describes his own progress and the development of his therapy system during the first ten years of practice.

Maureen Larkin was born in California, in 1955, with severely limited vision. She learned to sew and embroider, however, and to play several musical instruments, and she gained her BA in Folklore from San Francisco State University. She began therapy with Meir Schneider to improve her vision in 1980 and in a very short time had doubled her measurable vision. She began her training as a Self-Healing practitioner the same year and has been teaching and practicing Self-Healing therapy ever since. She was instrumental in establishing both the Center and the School for Self-Healing and collaborated with Meir on his first book *Self-Healing: My Life and Vision.*

Dror R. Schneider (Meir Schneider's wife) is a Self-Healing practitioner/educator and a student in the Graduate Program in Biology at San Francisco State University. A native Israeli with a background in teaching, she graduated cum laude in Geology from Hebrew University in Jerusalem and began a career of translating and editing. She met Meir Schneider after translating his first book, *Self-Healing: My Life and Vision,* into Hebrew. The couple have two children. Both were born with the same vision problems that Meir Schneider has overcome. Dror Schneider has worked diligently to improve the children's eyesight, and finds the results encouraging.

MEIR SCHNEIDER, Ph.D., L.M.T.
and MAUREEN LARKIN *with* DROR SCHNEIDER

The Handbook of Self-Healing

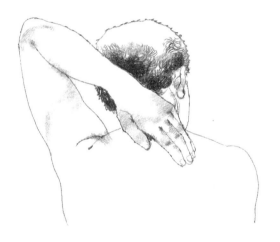

ARKANA
PENGUIN BOOKS

ARKANA

Published by the Penguin Group
Penguin Books Ltd, 27 Wrights Lane, London W8 5TZ, England
Penguin Books USA Inc., 375 Hudson Street, New York, New York 10014, USA
Penguin Books Australia Ltd, Ringwood, Victoria, Australia
Penguin Books Canada Ltd, 10 Alcorn Avenue, Toronto, Ontario, Canada M4V 3B2
Penguin Books (NZ) Ltd, 182–190 Wairau Road, Auckland 10, New Zealand

Penguin Books Ltd, Registered Offices: Harmondsworth, Middlesex, England

First published 1994
10 9 8 7 6 5 4 3 2

Illustrations by Victor Ambrus

Set in 10.5/14pt Monophoto Apollo by Selwood Systems, Midsomer Norton
Printed in England by Butler & Tanner Ltd, Frome and London

'Meir Schneider offers remarkable techniques that empower you to take charge of your own health and unlock the body's ability to heal itself. Through his innovative therapeutic movements and exercise, he has helped thousands of individuals throughout the world facilitate their own self-healing. I have personally seen functional improvement in a number of patients where the medical community had literally told them 'there was nothing further that could be done'. Meir Schneider is on the cutting edge of improving the quality of our health and well-being' – Ronald K. Takemoto, MD, Assistant Professor of Physical Medicine and Rehabilitation, University of California, Irvine

'I met Meir Schneider several years ago at a conference in West Palm Beach, Florida. During this brief but powerful meeting, Meir demonstrated to me some of the untapped power and potential that all of us as human beings have at our disposal, should we learn how to use them. Meir has learned how to use it. In this book, *The Handbook of Self-Healing,* which is clearly a labor of love, Meir is sharing his know-ow with the reader in a most straightforward and unselfish way' – John E. Upledger, osteopath, founder of the Upledger Institute, Palm Beach Gardens, Florida

'This book is "must" reading for anyone interested in the wholistic natural health movement. At a time when the healthcare system is in crisis, Meir presents many practical strategies to help people increase their vitality and well-being by replacing expense with effort, but perhaps Meir's greatest contribution with this book is his ability to teach us how to take responsibility for our health' – Paul St John, founder of the St John Method of Neuromuscular Massage Therapy, Key Largo, Florida

'Meir Schneider has written a beautiful and inspiring book. Disease is understood not as a burden to be carried but as an opportunity to get in touch with the healing powers that are within all of us. Everybody who wishes to take an active part in the healing of herself or himself will find in it valuable and practical information' – Martin Enge, MD, and Margareta Enge, MD, Austria

'Meir Schneider's second book represents a tremendous advance in our knowledge of self-healing. The exercises are easy to understand and perform. Although they are very gentle, they are the most powerful ones I have ever seen' – Beatriz Nascimento Moffat, Assistant Professor, Department of Occupational Therapy, University of San Carlos, and instructor in the School for Self-Healing, Brazil

'Meir Schneider's book is delightfully clear, easy to read, full of good solid information and a definite "must" for the ordinary human being who wants to take responsibility for his or her own health and well-being. I plan to give this book to all my patients' – Beryl Feinglass, physical therapist, mental health educator and certified Feldenkrais practitioner, San Francisco

'Meir Schneider's insight with Self-Healing is a refreshing approach for the healing professions. His techniques are a blending of easy to understand explanations with practical, thorough exercises. This book is especially useful for those interested in Natural Vision Improvement' – Samuel A. Berne, behavioral optometrist and author of *Creating Your Personal Vision,* Santa Fe, New Mexico

'Meir has a third eye and eight senses. Bridge these two with an incredible perception of the human body and you've got a genius. You *sense* Meir's ingenuity through his book. You *know* it through his work' – Yael Gottlieb, registered nurse and Self-Healing practitioner/educator, Berkeley, California

'Meir's informative, well-written *Handbook* reflects his deep understanding of how to work with the body's innate ability to heal. The clearly written exercises allow anyone, from layperson to professional, to take charge and begin their own journey of self-healing' – Daniel Dernay, chiropractor, Concord, California

'Meir's new book is an excellent source for the working knowledge of our bodies. It gives direction for choosing the most effective exercises for the appropriate time. I will be recommending Meir's new material to my students and patients. The acute- and chronic-pain patients at my practice will benefit from Meir's approach to breathing, circulation, joint, muscle, spine and nervous-system movements. This book heightened my own awareness of fine tuning the body and mind and enhanced my abilities to help others' – Gail Wetzler, physical therapist and certified instructor for Visceral Manipulation, Uppledger Institute, Santa Ana Heights, California

'I wholeheartedly endorse this book. Seventeen years ago, Meir Schneider taught me a new way to relax and move in the world. His work still impacts my life every day. Amble through the *Handbook of Self-Healing*. The exercises are easy but powerful. Do them daily and experience profound changes. Face and posture photos taken before you start will help you see the transformation. Meir's bodywork should become a part of everyone's day' – Ray Gottlieb, PhD, optometrist, Madison, New Jersey

'This is an excellent book for those who sincerely wish to take the healing of their bodies into their own hands. Meir Schneider has a great ability to demystify the physiological and pathological processes involved in common physical illnesses. Combined with his enthusiasm and years of clinical experience, this is a rare resource for those who wish to understand their bodies better – whether for healing a serious condition or enjoying greater vitality. One of the greatest testaments to his work is the warmth and love of life which shine from every page' – Judith Bradley, physical therapist, British Columbia

'Meir Schneider's innovative, yet ''common-sense'' method works easily alongside the more orthodox approaches – but, importantly, empowers individuals to help themselves. Its applications are wide ranging, with limitless potential for *anyone* – no matter their age, or how mild or severe their problems – to attain and enjoy optimal health' – Marie Askin, registered nurse, London

'*The Handbook of Self-Healing* is an excellent tool, beneficial to the patient as well as to the health-care professional. I have been actively practicing the exercises and look forward to introducing them to my patients' – Ilana Parker, physical therapist, San Francisco

Contents

Preface

This book offers a revolutionary approach to medicine, particularly to rehabilitative medicine. Many books have been written about the philosophies of alternative medicine; this one translates those philosophies, as well as our own, into practice.

It took a great deal of work to demonstrate clearly how awareness, thoughts and movement can be used effectively by virtually everyone. To achieve this clarity I needed much help, and I got it from my coauthor, Maureen Larkin. One of Maureen's greatest contributions to my life has been the clarification of how people perceive this unusual practice of mine. She has helped my communication skills with the outside world enormously.

My wife, Dror, has been my greatest help and mainstay. She worked on every detail of the book. Dror knew how to present intelligibly a whole new body of knowledge. With her background in biology and her deep understanding of my method, she was able to increase our accuracy and clarity. She worked very long hours, from 11 a.m. to 3 a. m., cross-referencing, proofreading and editing.

Each of the illustrations in this book is based on a photograph in which clients and friends are shown performing many of the exercises described here. Dror chose which exercises needed illustration, set up and managed photo sessions, and posed. I owe special thanks to our photographer, Terry Allen, who showed a rare ability to feel the motion in each exercise and reflect it in his still photographs. I am very grateful to all the people who volunteered to pose in them: Rachel Riley-Cox, Diana Stork, Micah Leideker, and especially to Jim Sharps.

I am happy that this book is complete, because the world needs it. I am looking forward to enjoying it myself with a group of friends, proceeding chapter by chapter to achieve better health.

Meir Schneider

Introduction

This book is for you. You have purchased a book with the words 'Self-Healing' in the title, so the chances are good that you are an active, self-motivated person who wants to learn how to take care of your body and maintain your health.

There are many ways to do this, and probably you are interested in a number of them. Nutrition, exercise, massage, all types of bodywork therapy: all of these fields can offer you valuable knowledge, essential to a healthy life. This holistic – meaning 'whole-person' – approach to health has become increasingly popular in the last twenty years, and is now supported by a growing number of medical doctors. The purpose of our book is to add a new dimension to your already expanding array of health-care skills. This is the dimension of kinesthetic awareness – the physical, sensory awareness of your own body. As your kinesthetic awareness develops, you will be able to feel more and more of what happens with your body, both internally and externally.

We believe that, in many people, illness is allowed to develop because kinesthetic awareness has been lost. It often begins with a small, seemingly trivial problem. Chronic eyestrain may develop into a real loss of measurable vision; contraction of the upper back and neck muscles may lead to migraines which will not respond to any painkiller; stiffness in unused joints can become an arthritic condition; shallow, infrequent breathing can even create circulatory difficulties, including high blood pressure. All of these and many other problems are preventable. All of them are preceded by very clear warning signals which, if you have learned to listen to your body and interpret its messages correctly, you can understand and act upon, remedying the situation before it becomes more serious.

It is easy to lose kinesthetic awareness when our lives are filled with all kinds of external sensory input and our minds are occupied with our everyday obligations. With so much to think about, so much to do, so many other people and things to respond to, it is no wonder that we forget about our physical selves. Often the only way the body can get our attention is by offering either great pleasure or severe pain. The only way to rediscover kinesthetic awareness is to affirm that *you* are as worthy of your own attention as anyone or anything else in your life. Does this idea make you feel guilty or self-centered for even considering it? Ask yourself this: how much good can you do in the world around you if you are not well? How much more good could you do if you had 100 percent of your resources available to work with? Obviously, your world will benefit from a healthy you as much as you will yourself.

Machines can monitor many of your body's processes, but there are things about your body which only you can really know. A reading of your pulse rate and blood pressure will not necessarily determine whether your circulation is poor; but fatigue, lack of energy, poor concentration, or cold hands and feet will make it clear that you need better circulation. No machine can really tell you whether you are stiff or loose in muscles and joints, exhausted or refreshed, energetic or slow, how much more relaxed you can be, what your nervousness is doing to your system, and whether or not you are fully functional. Only you can feel these things. They are vital clues to your health. When even you are not aware of them, your health is in danger.

This book is filled with ways – which we call exercises for want of a better word – to get more in touch with your physical self, using both your mind (consciousness) and your body (kinesthetic awareness). Whether your aim is to heal an existing condition or to make good health into terrific health, you will have the opportunity to learn much about your body. The process takes time and patience, but it gives back self-knowledge and a new enjoyment of your body.

Our emphasis in Self-Healing is upon movement, because movement is the very essence of life. In fact, the capacity for movement is one of the characteristics by which scientists define an animal life-form. An exercise is simply a movement or series of movements structured and repeated.

It is easy to see why movement, in the form of some sort of exercise, is so whole-heartedly recommended by professionals in virtually every health-care field. We would like to take that recommendation a step further and not only say that movement is good for you but invite you to fully explore how good it really can be.

'Movement' is just another way of saying 'use of the body'. Your body exists not just to be maintained but for your use and enjoyment. Beyond that, your body contains within itself just about every tool it needs to heal itself. Movement is one of the most versatile of these tools.

If you are ill, your first step should be to consult a doctor. When you do so, you will receive information, and in many cases, medication. In our opinion, the wisest and most effective doctors are those who give the most information and the least medication. The most successful patients are those who carefully follow a doctor's advice regarding healthy living and avoid drugs until every other avenue has been explored – except in emergency situations, of course. This is not because taking medicines means you are weak or self-indulgent or hypochondriac. Rather, it is because:

- most drugs have side-effects, some of which may be worse than the condition they are supposed to correct;
- drugs often mask symptoms while leaving the true cause of the problem to grow worse; and
- you can become dependent on drugs to the extent that your own natural healing mechanisms lose their ability to function.

So, it is always a good idea to find out what else might work for you. After receiving your doctor's advice and/or prescriptions, the next step of your treatment is in your own hands – and the next, and the next.

Do your own thinking – it is your own body, after all. Ask yourself what you can do for your body, besides putting it temporarily out of its misery. It is obvious that what is needed is something more than extinction of symptoms. It is time to change the way you interact with your body. It is time to learn to nurture it. Think about all the other aspects of your life and objects that you nurture – your career, your home, your car, a garden, a pet, a relationship. Creating health and well-being in your body can bring you more satisfaction than any of these.

Your first discovery will be the enormous untapped resources your body possesses. We will work with breathing throughout this book, both for its own sake and in conjunction with other body movements. Our aim will be to increase our intake of oxygen, for this is the body's most basic need and one which is fully satisfied in very few of us. Though our lungs have the capacity to take in approximately 4,000 ml of air, we normally breathe in less than 500 ml. You will appreciate the difference when you experience what full respiration really feels like. We have nearly 700 muscles, designed to perform all the body's possible functions, yet we normally use very few of them. Those few grow contracted and tired through overwork, while the rest weaken and atrophy. We do not move enough to exercise our full joint capacity; thus the joints gradually lose their mobility. We attribute this last process to aging, but there is a big difference between a person who has spent much time in the last seventy years in healthy physical activity and one who has not.

Those who have made some form of movement a part of their daily lives cannot say enough about how much it improves the way they feel — physically, emotionally, and mentally. Unfortunately, the majority of us do not seem to be getting enough movement to stay healthy. The result is that 70 million people in the United States alone suffer from frequent low-back pain and more serious spine problems; 40 million suffer from various forms of arthritis. There is no way to count how many are affected by the fatigue, depression, headaches, digestive ailments and many other problems — including just plain malaise — that can be attributed to our chronic inertia.

There is also the problem — and it is just as serious — of people who *are* physically active, but in ways which are destructive to their bodies. Sports medicine, which caters to the needs of athletes who injure themselves during sports, is one of the fastest-growing health-care fields. Most of these sports injuries could be prevented if people were more sensitive to *how* their bodies need and want to move. Vigorous movement should be done in a state of relaxation, for the sake of health and enjoyment rather than challenge or competition.

Medicine has made incredible gains in treating infectious diseases — once the primary cause of death — and in surgical techniques to correct structural problems and emergency situations. For the most part, however, the diseases which most concern us now are of the chronic type, caused not by accident or microbes but by the way we live. It has been estimated that 85 percent of all current disease is lifestyle-related. For this reason, in many, many cases, these diseases respond very well to changes in lifestyle and health habits. For the great majority of people, the key to their health is in their own hands.

Through Self-Healing we encourage people not only to work on a particular disease or disorder but to change the body's overall condition — from tense to relaxed, from rigid to mobile, from unused to fully used, from numb to fully alive. How do we know when life has left a body? When something has died it does not breathe; its blood does not circulate; it cannot move; it cannot feel; its consciousness is gone. The more we breathe and move and feel, and the more awareness we have, the more fully alive we will be.

How to Use This Book

This book is for active participants. Reading about the exercises will not change anything; doing them will. It is completely up to you to choose which exercises to try, though we do make some suggestions for specific conditions later in the book. Try a few which attract you initially; later you may add new ones and vary, alternate or combine them. Find a sequence which feels good to your body, warming up with easier movements and gradually proceeding to the more challenging exercises. Some of the exercises will work for you and some will not. There is no movement which is right for everybody; and, of course, different exercises will be helpful for you at different times. Pay attention to how you respond to an exercise at different times – it may indicate that you are making progress, or that there are specific areas which need your attention.

We encourage you to view our exercises mainly as suggestions, rather than formulas, and to use them as a basis for inventing your own forms of movement. Once you begin to move, you are likely to find that movement comes easily and spontaneously in new and varied ways. Each of the movements we describe here was 'discovered' by someone who simply happened to be paying attention to his or her body at the time, and happened to notice what effect the particular movement had at that time. This is something you can do as well as anyone else. No one is more intelligent about your body than you (potentially) are. We would be delighted to hear about your discoveries if you would like to share them.

You probably have very specific goals in mind as you begin your Self-Healing process. This is an excellent starting-point, for it provides a genuine motivation. It is also very important to care for the body as a whole. Through nurturing your body, you will find that – along with improvement in your 'target areas' – you will get sick less often, feel more energetic and get more accomplished overall. Your original goals, whether they be improving your vision, overcoming back pain, regaining mobility in joints, becoming a better runner or musician, or whatever you have in mind, will become a *part* of your healing process, rather than its sole aim. You may even revise your goals as you discover what works best for your body.

Self-Healing movement can be an excellent supplement to other physical practices. It can provide the relaxation of mind and body which is conducive to meditation (and anyone who has ever meditated knows that it is indeed a physical practice), as well as the limbering and warm-up needed for more strenuous forms of movement such as yoga, dance, martial arts or running. It can also give you a whole new approach to your body – one which may help to prevent you from injuring or stressing yourself during vigorous activity.

Practice these movements at home, before your day begins and after it ends; before work, performance or competition; during your breaks or after exertion. The effects will gradually carry over into your daily activity, until Self-Healing becomes a way of life and a state of mind. Eventually you will be able to recognize immediately what is good for your health and what is not. Learning to care for your eyes is a good example of this principle: it does not end when a session of eye exercises is finished, but extends to every moment in which you are using your eyes, which is most of your waking life. You will learn to recognize when you are tensing unnecessarily, when you are moving or reposing in a way that hurts your muscles or joints, when you need to breathe, when you need to rest, and when you need to move.

The process of reawakening awareness is rewarding and enjoyable, but it is not entirely painless. Often we find that our bodies have reacted to the stresses we impose upon them by becoming numb. In the process of revitalizing the body, we often rediscover the pain we have suppressed. This pain is part of awareness. You may be able to put in an overwhelmingly stressful fourteen-hour workday, ignoring your throbbing forehead, burning eyes, aching back and powerful urge to cry or scream – until you lie down and try to relax. Then you will feel what you have suppressed. Relaxation does not create new problems; it simply uncovers those which are already there, motivating us to deal with them. The first step in solving a problem is to know what it really is. This is awareness. Even when it is difficult or unpleasant, it is our most effective problem-solving tool.

We strongly recommend that you form a support group in which to practice Self-Healing exercises. Being part of a group often encourages an individual to keep practicing when he or she might otherwise slack off; it also gives you some objective feedback about your progress. Some of the exercises and most of the bodywork techniques are best done with a partner; you may find that not only will you improve your health through Self-Healing movement, you may become a proficient bodyworker *and* wind up getting all the relaxing bodywork you need. The ideal size for a group is from four to six members, so that you can have a variety of partners to work with without getting lost in the shuffle. If possible, meet for two or three hours or more each time, once or twice a week; if you cannot, then meet every other week. Your support group may become not just a group to work with but a social group of people who share concepts regarding health and well-being, who can help each other choose the right path of recovery from illness.

How to Get Started

Each person has special needs. You may have an illness you want to recover from, you may be suffering from 'occupational hazards' specific to your profession. Perhaps you have been nearsighted since school age and have decided it is time to do something about it. All of us share the need to communicate better with our bodies, to read the signals and respond to them. We all need to increase our bodies' function and vitality.

If you suffer from a pathology which this book addresses, such as multiple sclerosis, heart problems or arthritis, we suggest that you start with the chapter that addresses your problem specifically. Later on, return to the beginning of the book and work with the first part of it chapter by chapter in the sequence in which the chapters appear. If you have no specific ailment and you just want to enjoy more kinesthetic awareness, more mobility, better use of your resources and perfection of your health, start with the very beginning of the book and work with the whole first part, spending a few months with each chapter – spending more time on areas you feel need more attention – until you feel you have fine-tuned your body, strengthened it and perfected it. You will develop the ability to choose the right exercises for different occasions in the future.

Use this book as a friend. Our purpose is to create a dialogue with you   your body and your mind – through this book.

Remember: medicine cannot help you reverse the process of degeneration, but your mind and body can.

Part One

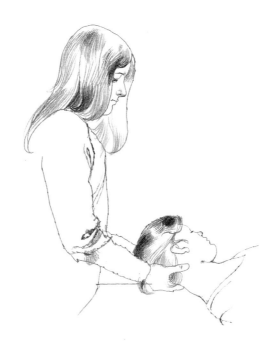

CHAPTER 1

Breathing
The key to self-exploration

This chapter is devoted to increasing your capacity for breathing. Your breathing provides your body with its most basic requirement – oxygen – and your mind and spirit with their most useful tool – dynamic relaxation. Breathing is the most vital of functions for any living creature. Improving your breathing will automatically improve all of your other body functions. This is why we have placed this chapter first.

Many people are surprised at first at the emphasis we place on breathing. They take it for granted that if they are alive they must be breathing; they soon discover that there are varying degrees of 'aliveness', and that a person who is barely breathing is, in fact, barely alive. A lack of sufficient oxygen weakens the body and slows down all of its functions, including brain function. People assume that if their bodies need more oxygen they will automatically take in more, but this is not always the case. Often the body just adapts to a lesser amount of oxygen than it really needs to enable it to function optimally and with maximum vitality. Many people breathe just enough to survive, or to function minimally, but not to function well. As we will

see, there are many factors which may keep you from breathing sufficiently.

The need for increasing our oxygen intake is a long-recognized fact. The idea of aerobic exercise was developed to meet this need. In aerobic exercise, we exert ourselves to make our heart and lungs work harder, forcing more oxygen into the lungs and bloodstream. People who do aerobics may think that, because they have done some aerobics for an hour, they are therefore breathing better all the time. That is often not the case, however. We believe that the body should enjoy a plentiful supply of oxygen all the time, not just when the muscles and heart and lungs are working at their top capacity. For one thing, it would be exhausting to keep up that kind of pace; for another, aerobic exercise simply is not available to everyone all the time. For those who are city-bound, handicapped, or pressed for time and space, aerobic exercise may be something of a luxury. Everyone should make it a priority to have some kind of vigorous exercise – swimming, walking, dancing or running – as a part of one's life. Our goal in this chapter, however, is to show you how you can breathe fully, deeply and consistently enough to supply your body's oxygen needs – even in situations that are not ideal for breathing.

Insufficient breathing ultimately affects every cell in the body, because every cell requires oxygen to function. Oxygen is carried to the cells by the flow of blood. When the blood's oxygen concentration has been lowered, our veins carry the deoxygenated blood to the heart, and the heart pumps it to the lungs, where it is re-enriched with oxygen. This oxygen-charged blood is returned to the heart, from which it is pumped to the arteries, and ultimately to the cells of the furthest periphery of the body. A pattern of deep, slow breathing improves your circulation, and therefore your blood brings oxygen and nourishment more effectively to your body's cells.

If a pattern of shallow breathing continues, circulation throughout the body decreases. Circulation to the body's periphery is especially limited, causing cold hands and feet, fatigue and the loss of mental concentration and clarity which can occur when there is not enough blood supply to the brain. Blood carries all the nutrients our cells need, and carries away all the toxic materials produced by cell metabolism. When circulation decreases, the areas which are not receiving enough blood become simultaneously starved and toxiferous. A good deep breath, however, can send oxygen-rich blood coursing through your body to feed and cleanse your cells.

There are many reasons why we might not breathe enough to meet our oxygen needs. Environmental pollution has become a major problem, and it may be that our bodies instinctively refuse to take in too much air laden with carbon monoxide, industrial chemicals, cigarette smoke or fumes from the many semi-toxic materials with which we are constantly surrounded.

However, in so many of our current health problems stress seems to be the main culprit. Stress, as we use the word here and throughout this book, means a state of emotional anxiety that is reflected in your body and is consistently affecting the way your body functions. Every thought and feeling you experience will influence your body to some degree. We all know the sense of lightness that comes with joy, the epinephrine (adrenaline) rush of rage, the dry mouth and shaky feeling that fear produces. These are dramatic physical changes produced by dramatic emotions. Less powerful, but equally influential, are the small everyday anxieties of work, family life, study and the task of simply coping with an increasingly challenging world. These difficulties are an intrinsic part of our lives, and so are their effects upon our bodies. One of the most common of these effects is a tendency to limit ourselves to shallow, infrequent, unrhythmical and completely inadequate breathing.

When we begin to work with the breath as a healing tool, we discover that breathing has an immediate calming, energizing and clarifying effect on both mind and body. It is absolutely the most helpful thing we can do in any stressful situation. So why do we so often limit our breathing when we are anxious, if this is so clearly counterproductive? The answer lies in the functioning of the sympathetic nervous system.

Breathing and the Sympathetic Nervous System

The nervous system is the messenger service between the mind and the body. The human nervous system is a complex mechanism, with several major functional divisions. The first division is between the central nervous system and the peripheral nervous system. The central nervous system consists of the brain and a dense rope of nerves called the spinal cord, which extends down to the lower back. The peripheral nervous system has spinal nerves, which branch off from the spinal cord, exiting between the vertebrae and from there continuing to branch, dividing again and again to reach every part of the body, as well as twelve pairs of cranial nerves, all but two of which serve only the head.

The peripheral nervous system is also divided into two major parts. The first is the somatic nervous system, which controls all voluntary or conscious motions such as chewing and walking. The second part of the peripheral system is the autonomic nervous system, which regulates automatic, involuntary functions such as digestion and circulation.

By this time you will not be surprised to learn that the autonomic nervous system also contains two major divisions, which are called the sympathetic and the parasympathetic. These two systems often perform opposing functions. For example, the parasympathetic nervous system acts to slow down your heart rate, while the sympathetic increases it; the parasympathetic sends blood to the surface of the skin, while the sympathetic causes it to drain from the skin. Normally, the two systems will act to balance each other, with each keeping the other from overdoing any function. Fear or stress, however, will generally activate the sympathetic nervous system and cause it to override the parasympathetic system and change the course of body function.

The sympathetic nervous system has often been described as the body's 'fight or flight' mechanism. One of its primary functions is to act as an alarm and defense system for the body during times of physical danger. When it goes on alert, it sends chemical messages throughout the body which make it possible either to escape or to overpower an aggressor, or to meet other extreme physical challenges. The pupils of the eyes dilate to admit more light and hence more visual information, blood flow is diverted away from the digestive organs and flooded into certain muscles, epinephrine release increases markedly to speed up the heart beat, and breathing becomes rapid and shallow. Your body knows instinctively that deep, slow breathing will make you relax – and this is exactly what the sympathetic nervous system is programmed to prevent.

In situations of genuine physical risk, this system functions extremely well. The problems arise because the sympathetic nervous system can interpret any mental anxiety as a sign of 'danger', and may go on full blast at inappropriate times without your even being aware of it. You may be worried about giving a speech or performing well in your job, but when your sympathetic nervous system senses your fear it will react as though trying to put several miles between yourself and a large hungry predator. *Any* form of anxiety can send the sympathetic nervous system into a state of emergency. This is very hard on the body. The blood has been flooded with epinephrine, the muscles tense up, the heart is working hard to send blood to the limbs, and yet there is no real call for action. Unless the body is vigorously used, this tension will remain in the muscles for hours, producing a nervous, jittery feeling. Your breathing will slow down but will probably remain shallow for as long as the tension persists.

Prolonged stress reinforces unhealthy breathing patterns, so that breathing becomes chronically shallow, infrequent and quick. Often a tense person will breathe through the mouth. This is a problem, because it is the nose, not the mouth, which was designed for regular breathing. The nostrils contain cilia which filter incoming air, and mucus which warms and moistens it, both of which make the air cleaner and more breathable when it reaches the lungs. However, breathing through the narrow nasal passages takes longer than breathing through the mouth. This is in fact a benefit, because it allows more time for the oxygen to diffuse into the bloodstream. The problem is that a tense person in need of air will tend to automatically gulp it in through the mouth, simply because that's quicker. Breath taken through the mouth feels like a full and satisfying breath, but it is not. Stressful breathing often consists of nervous little inhalations, never allowing for a full exhalation. A sigh of relief is a sure sign that tension has been causing you, unconsciously, to hold in your breath – for how long? Exhalation is as vital as inhalation to healthy breathing. If your respiratory system is not fully emptied of oxygen-poor air, it cannot be completely filled with oxygen-rich air.

The effects of insufficient breathing are far-reaching. In time, even the structure of the body may show the effects of poor breathing. Chronic shallow breathing hampers the expansion of chest and diaphragm, constricting the muscles there and leading ultimately to narrowing of the chest cavity, rounding forward of the shoulders, and distorting of the posture of the neck and upper back.

It may not be obvious at first that a person's problems have anything to do with breathing. Most people are not aware of how shallow their breathing is until they actually try to breathe deeply. Our experience shows, however, that almost any problem – physical, emotional or mental – will be accompanied by anxiety, tension and limited breathing. We have also found that the quickest and surest way to relax someone, to restore well-being and energy, and to get the Self-Healing process under way, is to get that person breathing deeply.

As you may already know, you can't get a tense person, including yourself, to breathe deeply just by saying 'Now breathe deeply.' It's about as effective as telling a hysterical person, 'Why don't you just relax?' In fact, it may actually aggravate their tension, by making them feel pressured to do something they can't. Someone with a long-time habit of shallow breathing – and that's most of us – has to unlearn this habit and consciously replace it with a new one. Of all the body functions we just naturally expect to be automatic, breathing is the first. The way we breathe, whether deep or shallow, is our most basic habit, and it is hard for us to believe that it can be changed. The only way to really know this is through experience. Taking charge of our breathing is a revolutionary idea. It can produce equally revolutionary changes in your body.

Learning to breathe fully is the most important thing you will ever do for your body, so it is necessary to approach it gradually, in stages. The best way to begin is by preparing your body to receive deep respiration.

1–1   Find a quiet place where you will not be disturbed and where you have room to stretch out. Lie down on your back, with your knees bent. If it helps you to relax, prop pillows under your knees to support them, and a pillow under your head. Rest your hands on your abdomen so you can feel its movement as you breathe. Now take the time to notice how you feel. Pay attention to each separate part of your body, beginning with your face and working down to your toes; see if you can sense each toe separately. At this stage, don't try to change or influence how you feel – just pay attention to it.

Some gentle movements will help to prepare your body to breathe more deeply. During the following exercises, be aware of your breathing. Remember to breathe, breathe slowly, and try to breathe fully, in and out through your nose, but do not try to influence your breathing too much yet.

1–2   Let your head roll slowly from side to side, imagining as you do so that someone else is moving it. Do the long muscles along the side of your neck feel tight, or resist the motion? If so, let your head roll to the side, and tap gently with your fingertips on the extended side of your neck, from behind the ears all the way down into the shoulder and chest. After a minute or so of this, stop and see whether you can feel a difference between the two sides of the neck. Then roll the head to the other side and tap on the other side of the neck. Roll your head from side to side once again and notice whether the movement feels different now.

1–3   With your head still moving from side to side, place your fingertips on the hinges of your jaws as you slowly open and close them. How do the jaws feel? If they feel tight, or tender to the touch, tap and massage them to help them to relax. Stop the rolling and yawn deeply, several times if you can. In addition to stretching and relaxing the muscles of the face,

throat, chest and diaphragm and moistening the eyes yawning may pull in much-needed oxygen.

1–4   Notice the muscles of your face. One of the primary functions of the facial muscles is to express emotion, and your emotions will inevitably leave their mark on your face. Sometimes the emotions your face has worked so hard to express will linger there in the form of muscular tension long after you have ceased to be aware of them. Try to feel whether there is tension in your face; if there is, try to let go of it. Imagine all the muscles around the jaw and around the eyes slackening and softening and growing warm. Then massage your face with your fingertips, using enough pressure to allow you to feel the tender places, if there are any. Pay particular attention to the areas which contain your sinuses – the cheekbones, eyebrows and bridge of the nose. Shallow breathing can lead to congestion, and massage of the sinus areas can help to drain this congestion.

1–5   Next, massage your entire chest area, using both your fingertips and your thumbs. Work from the collarbone down to the ribs, and from the armpits in toward the sternum (breastbone). You will probably find many tender spots that will need to be touched gently. These spots indicate chronic muscle contraction which has probably been caused by lack of breathing. Sometimes when the chest is massaged, suppressed emotions will surface; if this happens, try to just let the feelings flow through you and out of you, imagining that each exhalation carries away some of the negative feelings. Tap lightly on the muscles between the ribs and along the sternum. Then rub your abdomen with your whole hand, or cup your palms and clap them against the abdomen. Visualize your blood flowing into all of the areas you have touched, warming and relaxing them.

1–6   Now just lie still for a few minutes and visualize the changes you want to create in your body. By 'visualize', we mean imagine, in whatever way seems most natural to you. It is most helpful to engage as many of your senses in the visualization as possible, so try both to feel and to picture your muscles lengthening and relaxing, your blood flowing freely throughout your entire body, pure oxygen filling your lungs effortlessly, the lungs themselves expanding to their full capacity, the millions of tiny air pockets in the lungs filling like balloons as you inhale and deflating slowly as you exhale, and your whole body growing as light as a helium balloon as the oxygen expands you. Feel an ease in your breathing, a lightness, and a sense that there is no resistance to the movement of your chest, abdomen and back. Do this visualization first lying down, and then repeat it while sitting, then standing, and even while walking or exercising.

One of the muscles that tend to become chronically contracted as a result of stress is the anal sphincter. You may find that relaxing the anus promotes relaxation of other muscles in the body, and allows deeper breathing. Refer to exercise 3–10 in the Joints chapter and to exercise 6–5 in the Nervous System chapter.

Stretching Your Breathing Muscles

After warming up your breathing muscles with massage, there are a number of stretches you can do to loosen up your upper body and make it easier to expand your chest, giving your lungs more room. Trying to breathe deeply when your chest and upper back are contracted is like trying to blow up a balloon inside a test tube: your lungs can expand only as far as your muscles will allow them to. All of the tight or tender spots you discovered while massaging yourself indicate rigid muscles, and this rigidity is probably habitual. Most of our body functions are controlled and dictated by our subconscious mind, so, in trying to relax a chronic tension, you are trying, consciously, to counteract the dictates of your subconscious. This is one reason why habits are hard to change – in effect, you are fighting part of yourself. Changing habits takes time, practice and patience. The following exercises will help you to relax these muscles, making them warm, supple and loose.

1–7   Lying on your back, with knees bent and feet flat on the floor, stretch your arms straight out to the sides, at right angles to your body, with the palms of the hands facing up. Let your shoulders and arms relax completely. Imagine a gentle gravitational force pulling them toward the floor. Notice whether the two sides of your body feel the same or different. Does one shoulder feel tighter? heavier? larger? Does either hand feel lighter, or warmer? Your hands, at rest, will probably lie with the fingers curled slightly toward the palm. (Are you unconsciously clenching them? Let them relax.) Your exercise is to very slowly open the hands, extending the fingers until the back of each finger touches the floor. Imagine that the fingers stretch all the way to the opposite sides of the room, and that they are being slowly pulled toward the walls. Keep the fingers extended, inhaling slowly for a count of ten, then let them relax as you exhale to a count of fourteen. The fingers will automatically curl again – you don't need to clench the hand. Repeat this exercise several times, and each time imagine your fingertips stretching further and further in each direction and, as the arms stretch, your ribcage expanding too.

1–8 Still lying on your back, stretch your arms out behind your head, so that they are resting on the floor as flat as possible. Completely relax the right arm. Inhale. As you exhale, your left hand will clasp your right wrist and pull gently but firmly on the right arm, stretching the right shoulder (fig 1–8). The right arm should allow itself to be completely passive, neither resisting nor helping the pull of the left hand. After you have done this several times, let your arms return to your sides, and see whether you can feel a difference between the two sides. You may feel it in the shoulder, the neck, the chest or the arms.

Repeat this exercise with the left arm passive and relaxed and the right hand pulling, and again notice how the two sides feel. Then clasp the two hands with the fingers laced together and the arms stretched straight out, and swing them in as large a circle as you can comfortably make, feeling how this rotation loosens the shoulder joints and muscles.

1–9 Extend your right arm out to the side, and reach across your body with your left arm, so that your left hand is reaching toward your right hand. Without lifting your upper back off the floor – lifting only the shoulder, and that as little as possible – stretch the left hand as far toward the right as possible. Now lift your right hand up to meet the left hand, lace the fingers of the two hands, and use the right hand to pull the left hand toward the floor (fig 1–9). Feel how this stretches the left shoulder. You can also move the right hand in a rotating motion, to increase the range of the movement.

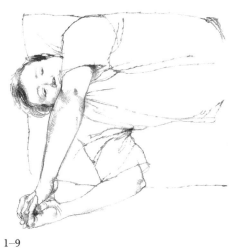

1–9

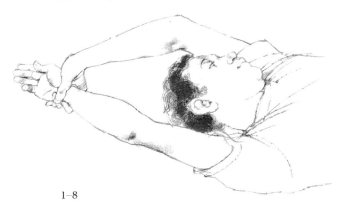

1–8

This is a great stretch for the shoulders and upper arms. As with all of these exercises, this stretch should be repeated on the other side.

As you do this stretch, you may feel a sense of compression in the chest but a wonderful opening in the upper back.

1–10   To stretch the entire upper torso — shoulders, arms, chest, neck, upper and middle back — try the windmill stretch. This helps to relieve the tension of study, reading.or work at a computer, and seems to release emotional tension as well. Lie on your back with your left knee bent and your right leg stretched out flat on the floor, then roll over toward your right, so that your bent left knee crosses your body and comes to rest on the floor to your right. Move your left foot over your right knee, and press down on your left knee with your right hand (fig 1–10A). Your left shoulder may come up off the floor a little, but try to keep it as close to the floor as possible, so that you get a nice twist and stretch to your upper spine.

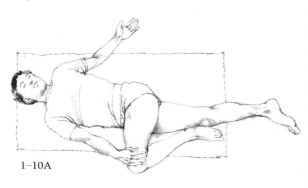

1–10A

Raise your left arm and move it in as big a circle as you can make. This means keeping the left hand touching the floor as much as possible (fig 1–10B). Imagine that you are drawing a circle on the floor with a pencil held in your left hand. If you feel more of a stretch by keeping your hand upraised when it is stretched in front, then do this, but while behind you your hand should remain as close

to the floor as possible. You should keep this movement comfortable for you — don't strain to make a huge circle, but do try to stretch your arm enough so that you really feel it. Notice how this exercise moves the ribcage and upper back. There are few movements that give the upper torso so much freedom.

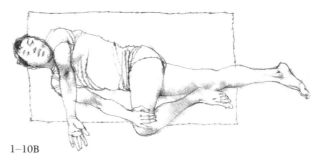

1–10B

Now stretch the left arm as far above the head as you can, your left hand touching the floor. With your right hand, grasp the ribcage area and pull it forward, toward the floor (fig 1–10C). Then rotate the left arm again. Do this both clockwise and counterclockwise, and rest on your back before you roll over and repeat this whole exercise on your other side. Again, take time between the two sides to notice whether there is a difference in sensation, and the quality of this difference. As you feel your muscles stretching, imagine that you are breathing into the stretched muscle, expanding it with the breath.

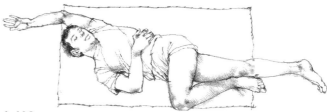

1–10C

1–11 This exercise should not be done unless your lower back is fairly relaxed. If you are unsure whether this is the case, consult your movement instructor or therapist. For a change, roll over onto your abdomen. Remember: whenever you change position, do so slowly, easily and gracefully, and especially avoid straining your neck. Lie flat on your abdomen, place your hands palms-down on either side of your chest, then slowly push yourself up until your upper body, all the way down to the pelvis, is raised up off the floor and your elbows are locked. Keep your shoulders down and your chest stretched (fig 1–11). This position is a yoga asana called the Cobra. Hold this position while you take two long deep breaths and then slowly lower yourself to the floor, and then raise yourself again. See whether you can do this without straining the muscles of your shoulders, chest, back or abdomen. Breathe deeply to relax your chest and abdomen so that they will be less likely to try to resist the lifting.

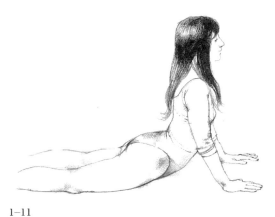

1–11

Now slowly twist to the right and then to the left, feeling how this changes the position of the chest muscles. Lower yourself slowly to the floor, and then raise yourself again. Let your arms support you, and push your weight down into the floor. Coordinate this exercise with your breathing, counting slowly to ten and inhaling deeply as you lower yourself, then exhaling slowly as you raise yourself.

1–12 Lie down on your back, pull both knees to your chest and hug them as close to the chest as you can. Now breathe deeply into your lower back. After ten deep breaths, release your hold on the knees and lie outstretched. You will probably find yourself breathing better now. Because you compressed your chest, your brain will now demand more breathing into the expanded lower back.

1–13 Standing facing a wall, stretch your arms straight up above your head and then 'climb' the wall, hand over hand, until you are on tiptoe and your arms are extended as far as possible (fig 1–13).

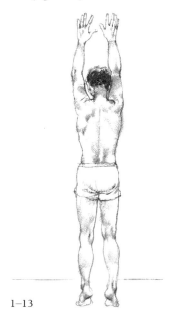

1–13

Breathe each time you move your hand higher, and feel how your elevated side is stretched, elongated and expanded. Try to make at least twenty of these climbing motions. You will probably find that your arms can stretch much further up than you imagined, and that they can continue stretching even when you think you have reached your limit. This is because not only the arms but also the shoulders, upper back and chest will relax and elongate as you continue this stretch.

1–14 Stand with your feet slightly apart and your arms stretched above your head. Inhale deeply and hold the breath in while you bend your whole body up and down from the waist several times. Exhale slowly, inhale deeply, repeat the bending and straightening, and see if you can hold the breath in a little longer each time you do this.

If these movements feel difficult or strange, it is probably because you are not used to focusing your attention on separate parts of your upper body. Many of us move as though our upper torso is carved out of one piece of wood, instead of being composed of hundreds of muscles, capable of infinite varieties of movement. But even if you have found your body stiff, painful or awkward, you have begun the work of loosening your torso. You have made the first step toward increasing your circulation and deepening your breathing – two things which will ultimately help everything in your body to function better.

With your muscles warmed and stretched, you are now ready to focus on breathing itself. There are several simple guidelines for healthy breathing which apply to all situations. The first is to breathe deeply. This instruction, 'Breathe deeply!', accompanies every exercise we teach. Many people confuse the idea of breathing deeply with breathing strenuously, but the two things are not the same at all. In fact, trying too hard will only create resistance to deep breathing, overworking the heart and lungs and, especially, the muscles. Worse, it causes us to associate deep breathing with straining. Let yourself breathe deeply but comfortably, allowing the air to flow slowly in. Give yourself a count of ten to fill your lungs completely, and don't try to overfill them. Their capacity to expand will increase naturally as you practice these exercises. Also, drawing your breath in slowly automatically creates a demand for more oxygen.

The second principle is to always breathe through the nose, both inhaling and exhaling. There are some useful disciplines which suggest inhaling through the nose and exhaling through the mouth, but we have found our way much more effective in relaxing the body. As we have mentioned, breathing through the nose warms, moistens and filters the incoming air. Without such treatment the air can irritate the lungs. The slowness of nose breathing has a relaxing effect on the body, as opposed to mouth breathing which often is associated with anxiety. It is harder to relax completely while you are breathing through the mouth. Sinus congestion is also due in part to mouth breathing. Much of the clearing of the sinuses is done by the air that passes through the nasal passages; without this constant cleansing, the sinuses can become chronically clogged.

Thirdly, breathing should be slow. Slow breathing allows full exchange between the inhaled oxygen and carbon dioxide, a waste product to be excreted by the lungs. Even more importantly, a slow breath triggers the action of the parasympathetic nervous system, with its calming, stabilizing effect on the entire body, as we shall see in the Nervous System chapter. Slow breathing is one of the techniques used by yogis to gain control over their heart rate and body temperature.

To sum up, your breathing should be slow, deep but non-strenuous, and as full as possible; you should breathe both in *and* out through your nose; and you should exhale as fully as you inhale.

1–15 Lie comfortably on your back, knees bent, with your head on a firm pillow. Close your eyes and visualize blackness, or any dark color that feels comfortable to you. Breathe slowly in and out for thirty long, deep breaths. If you lose concentration trying to get up to thirty, try counting the breaths in groups of five. Inhale each time for a count of four, hold for a moment, and then exhale for a count of six, to be sure you have exhaled all the air that you possibly can. Gradually increase the length of both your inhalation and your exhalation, until you are inhaling for a count of ten and exhaling for a count of fourteen. Remember not to try to force air into your lungs; instead, imagine a magnetic force inside your lungs pulling the air gently in.

As you inhale, the small air pockets, called alveoli, in your lungs expand. As oxygen-rich air enters your lungs, the blood vessels in the alveoli take in this oxygen, trading their carbon dioxide for the oxygen they need. The air in the lungs thus becomes poorer in oxygen and richer in carbon dioxide. The only really useful thing we can do with this carbon dioxide is to expel as much of it as possible and restock up on oxygen. Visualize that each time you inhale your entire body expands, and that each time you exhale your entire body deflates a little. Imagine that every part of you – muscles, bones, organs, even hair – is as elastic and expandable as your alveoli, and

as hungry for oxygen. Focus on each part of your body in turn, and imagine it becoming larger, lighter, warmer and more alive as it fills with oxygen. Now visualize your blood circulating to every part of your body, warming, nourishing and cleansing your cells. These processes of expansion and increased circulation are actually happening as your breathing deepens. Visualizing helps you to be more aware of them, and may also help to facilitate them, since your central nervous system is as much influenced by your thoughts as by your environment.

Creating a Demand for Oxygen

In his book, *What to Do about Your Brain-Injured Child* (Doubleday & Co., Garden City, NY, 1974), Glenn Doman describes his work with children suffering from brain injuries and other neuromuscular problems. He found that these children, without exception, suffered from insufficient respiration, and that in order to make any progress with them he had to deepen their breathing. As most of them were severely retarded, they could not learn breathing exercises. The only way to get them to breathe more deeply was to deprive them of oxygen for very short periods. Oxygen-deprivation automatically triggered their breathing mechanisms to work harder, and this increased functioning continued for some time after the oxygen-deprivation was stopped.

1–16 Take several long deep breaths to relax your body. Inhale slowly while silently counting up to seven. When you have reached seven, exhale slowly as you count to ten. Inhale

13

again, this time for a count of eight; exhale for a count of twelve. Your exhale should always be longer than your inhale. A slow and complete exhalation will both allow space for oxygen-rich air, and create a temporary oxygen-deprivation which will ensure that your body will learn to crave and to demand oxygen.

Now add the following: inhale and, while holding your breath in, move your abdominal muscles up and down six times; exhale, and do not inhale again until you have again moved the abdominal muscles up and down six times. (You will probably find your abdomen much stronger than you would have thought.) Now breathe normally for ten deep breaths, and see whether it seems easier and more natural now to breathe fully. You have created an 'appetite' for oxygen. Repeat this entire process twice more, and practice making your inhalations and exhalations last for the entire length of the counting. The more slowly you allow your lungs to fill and to empty, the more they will work to do so.

1–17 Alternate Breathing   This is an ancient technique used in yoga. Besides focusing your attention on your breathing, it helps you to make sure that you are using both nostrils when you breathe. Just as we tend to use one hand for almost everything we do – unless we make a conscious effort to use both – we can develop a tendency to be 'one-sided' in any activity. This may mean walking harder on one foot, chewing only on one side of the mouth, or breathing principally through only one nostril (or all of the above). This last may cause chronic congestion of the less-used nasal passage. It may be that this breathing pattern developed due to a blocked nasal passage in the first place, but the alternate-breathing

technique will help to clear up this condition. Some people say that there is a natural alternating cycle of use between the nostrils, where each shuts down for maintenance every 20 minutes, allowing most of the air to be shunted through the other.

Press with your forefinger on your right nostril to close it. *Inhale* slowly through the *left* nostril for a count of ten or longer, until you feel that both lungs are filled to their fullest capacity. While holding the breath in for a moment, take your fingertip off the right nostril and close the left instead, and *exhale* through the *right* nostril, again for a count of ten or longer. Let the air out as slowly as possible, keeping the left nostril pressed closed. *Inhale* through the right nostril, hold for a moment, close the right nostril and exhale slowly through the left. And so on. To put it simply, you are taking air in through one nostril, expelling it through the other, and then inhaling through the one you just exhaled from. Even if one side of your nose seems completely plugged, you can probably draw in enough air through it to fill your lungs – if you breathe slowly enough – and after several repetitions of this exercise you will probably find that the congestion is less.

Note: This exercise may not be sufficient to help a congestion. Refer also to the section on Sinus Headaches in the Headaches chapter.

Expanding the Chest and Abdomen

1–18   Lie on your back. As you inhale, push your chest out as far as you can while drawing your abdomen in. As you slowly exhale, let both chest and abdomen relax and flatten. Inhale again, and this time pull your chest in and push your abdomen out; then relax as you exhale.

When you have become fully comfortable with these two movements – and it may take several tries before you can completely control your chest and abdominal movements – then reverse the entire process. When you inhale, let the abdomen and the chest expand. Then, as you exhale, push your chest out and pull your abdomen in. Inhale to expand both, then exhale drawing your chest in, pushing your abdomen out. When you have mastered these exercises, you will have not only a deepened breathing capacity, but also unusually strong and flexible muscles in the front of your body.

Refer also to exercise 3–4 in the Joints chapter – a stretch for the chest and abdomen.

1–19 'Jug' Breathing The following is almost more of a visualization than an exercise. Its main purpose is to show you that you can control and direct the flow of your breath. Imagine yourself as an empty jug, and your breath flowing into you like water as you inhale. Remember that, when you pour water into a jug, the bottom fills up first. As you slowly inhale, imagine your breath filling you in the same way, flowing first into the abdomen and lower back and expanding them, then into the diaphragm area, and finally into the lungs, middle and upper back and chest.

When you exhale, remember that water pouring from a jug leaves the top first. Let your chest empty first, then the upper and middle back, then the diaphragm area, and last the abdomen and lower back.

Like all other breathing exercises, this should be done slowly. Practice this exercise until you genuinely feel that you can direct your breath to flow where you want it to. Then try visualizing that your inhalation fills your entire body, beginning with the soles of the feet and expanding you all the way up to the top of your head. When you exhale, try to imagine the breath leaving your skull first, and then each part of your body in succession.

Practice also exercise 6–2 in the Nervous System chapter.

Breathing and Movement

Proper breathing will help to make all of your other exercises more effective. Movement coordinated with breathing focuses your attention on your body, to increase your kinesthetic awareness and keep your movement from becoming strained or mechanical.

1–20 Begin with slow and simple movements such as turning the head from side to side while lying on the back. As your head rolls toward the left shoulder, inhale; as it rolls toward the right shoulder, exhale. After repeating this several times, let yourself inhale slowly while the head moves from left to right and back to left again, and then repeat the same movement while exhaling. Bend your knees and slowly lower the bent knees together to the floor, inhaling as you lower them to the right, exhaling as you lower them to the left. Raise and lower your arms alternately, with the right arm coming up as the left arm comes down, and coordinate your breathing with the movement so that you inhale as the left arm comes up, exhale as the right arm comes up. This can be done with any non-strenuous movement.

1–21 With more challenging exercises, it is most effective to time your breathing so that you are inhaling on the easier part of the movement and exhaling on the more difficult part. The reason for this is that your body associates exhalation with relaxation or 'letting go', so that exhaling while doing a strenuous motion will automatically eliminate some of the strain you would otherwise put into it.

Try the Cobra exercise (1–11). Inhale deeply first, then exhale while you push yourself up and inhale as you slowly lower yourself. The same exercise will be more difficult if you do not coordinate the exhalation with the effort. Try to push yourself up as you inhale, to feel the difference. Now roll over on your side, inhale, and then exhale as you raise one leg straight up as far as you can. Hold the leg raised for several seconds while you inhale, and then slowly lower it, exhaling as you do so. Try this with any movement that requires effort, and you will find the movement becoming easier.

Breathing and Affirmations

In times of emotional distress, breathing can be a powerful tranquilizer – calming, balancing and centering the mind. Your body reflects your emotions – and vice versa. If you can create a calm feeling in your body, with a steady pulse and slow deep breathing, it often helps you to quiet your emotions as well. It certainly brings oxygen to the brain to help the mind function a bit more clearly, and a calm mind is the best friend to a disturbed spirit.

1–22 Breathing can be combined with affirmations to produce an almost hypnotic calming effect, similar to the use of the mantra in transcendental meditation. An affirmation is simply a positive statement about a condition we are working to create in our lives. One potent way to combine affirmation with breathing is to imagine, and to state to yourself, that as you inhale you are drawing into your body and spirit the feelings you want to have, and that as you exhale you are expelling the feelings you want to get rid of. For example, if you are nervous about a performance, as you inhale tell yourself, 'I am breathing in confidence,' and, as you exhale, 'I breathe out self-doubt.' If you are having a hard time concentrating, affirm as you inhale, 'I breathe in clarity,' and, as you exhale, 'I breathe out confusion.' If you are plagued with general stress, try to exhale your anxiety and inhale peace.

One thing to keep in mind is not to try to force on yourself an emotion which is too far away from your present state of mind. If you are very depressed, your mind and body may not be able to inhale joy, but will probably allow contentment, or peace of mind. Begin your practice of affirmations with positive statements which seem realistic to you, and your mind will be receptive to them. The more you practice affirmations, the more power you will have to make them real.

Breathing Exercises with Friends

If you want to help someone else to breathe better, or if you are doing breathing exercises in groups or with clients, here are several techniques which can be done together to increase breathing.

1–23   Have your partner lie down on his back, arms at his sides and knees bent. Place the palm of one hand under the back of his head, and the palm of your other hand flat on his sternum. Ask him to relax his neck completely and inhale deeply while you slowly raise his head until his chin touches his chest, simultaneously pressing down on his chest with your whole hand (fig 1–23). Pressing with the whole hand will keep you from pushing too hard; if you press only with the heel of the hand you might exert an uncomfortable pressure. Ask him to exhale while you slowly lower his head again. Repeat this several times, each time more slowly, so that the length of his inhalations and exhalations gradually increases. Then have him sit up and see how it feels to breathe.

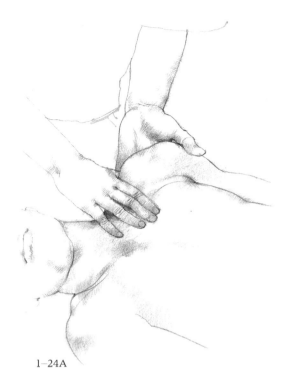

1–24A

Then take hold of that arm at the wrist and gently but firmly pull it toward you, first diagonally and then straight out from the shoulder (fig 1–24B).

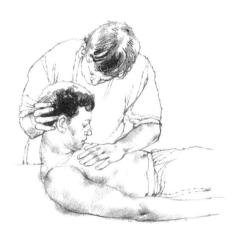

1–23

1–24   Have your partner lie down again. Slide one hand under the shoulder blade while your other hand presses firmly on the pectoral muscles, where the arm joins the chest. While pressing, lift the shoulder blade up as far as possible and rotate it, in both directions, about twenty times each way (fig 1–24A).

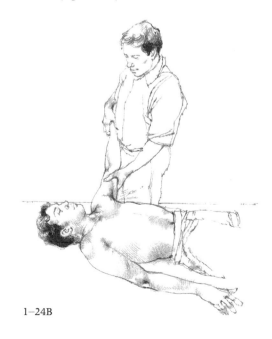

1–24B

17

Hold the wrist in one hand and with the other hand pull on each finger separately. Ask your partner to notice whether the side you have stretched feels different from the other. Then repeat this process on his other side.

1–25 The following exercise is quite demanding and is recommended only to people who know that their backs are in very good condition, as it could result in strain or injury if either person has a weak back.

Have your partner stand up. Standing at her side, with one arm outstretched across her lower back, the other across her abdomen and your hands laced together, ask her to stretch her arms up over her head and then to bend backward as far as she can. You should be supporting her weight completely (fig 1–25).

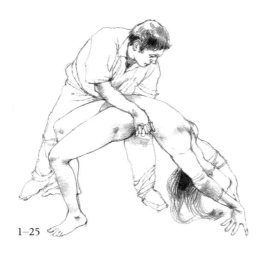

1–25

Now ask her to bring her hands up to her hips and, in this position, try to raise and lower her upper body. Her hands, her feet and your supporting arm are her points of leverage. This is the most difficult exercise we have described so far, but it gives an amazing degree

of release to the back and chest. The vertebrae which support the upper back, known as the thoracic vertebrae, are joined to the ribs and normally need more mobility than our movement allows them. This exercise gives them a chance to really move, which benefits the lungs.

Massage is perhaps the gentlest and most pleasant way to stimulate breathing. Massage of the chest, neck, shoulders and upper back is always helpful, but you may be surprised to find that massaging areas which seem totally unrelated to breathing may give the best results. If you can find the area where a person is holding their deepest tension, and release it, an increase in breathing follows immediately. That area may be anywhere in the body – it may be the lower back, the pelvis, the legs or the muscles around the eyes. Wherever it is, you will know you have found it when you hear or see a deepening in breathing. Consult the Massage chapter for ideas on massage techniques.

Any of the techniques we have described in this chapter may also be used in group situations. Breathing is the best introduction to movement, to meditation and also to study. Breathing exercises would be an excellent way to begin any class or lecture, since increased oxygen to the brain helps concentration and also improves memory. A study done with elderly patients in a nursing home proved that increasing the oxygen levels in their rooms improved their memory function by as much as 70 percent. Whatever you want to do, breathing slowly, deeply and fully will help you to do it better.

CHAPTER 2

Circulation
The body's tool to rejuvenate and heal

Circulation ranks with breathing among the body's most vital functions. Without either, we could not survive more than a couple of minutes. (There have been miraculous exceptions to this rule, but in general it is true.) Arterial blood, coming from the heart, carries to every cell of the body everything that the cell needs: oxygen from the lungs, nutrients from the digestive system and hormonal secretions from the glands. If any part of your body is not receiving enough blood circulation, you might as well be starving as far as that part is concerned. Venous blood, returning to the heart and lungs, carries away from the cells most of the waste products of the cells' life-processes. The lymph system also helps in the body's house-cleaning, supporting the veins in draining fluids from peripheral cells back to the blood, and removing micro-organisms and other foreign substances. Without this cleansing action, cells become toxiferous and, in time, so does the body as a whole. We believe that many types of cancer may have their roots in this toxic buildup. Good circulation is as vital to us as air and water. But since circulation, like respiration, is one of our body's automatic functions, we tend to take it for granted – not realizing how

much it is affected by what we do, or fail to do. Even our automatic functions, however – like breathing, digestion and blood circulation – need the support and maintenance of a healthy lifestyle and healthy attitudes.

When we think of improving circulation, we usually think of vigorous exercise, designed to get the heart pounding and the blood racing. We call this type of exercise 'aerobic', because it makes you consume more oxygen, and we picture people pumping and sweating. But here we must make a point that we will make several times throughout this book: there is much more to making a healthy body than just forcing it to work hard. There are plenty of people who do aerobic exercise every day and still suffer cold hands and feet, fatigue and many other symptoms of poor circulation. It is possible to go through an entire dance class using only a few overly strained muscles; it is also possible to jog for miles without ever breathing deeply enough. Increased pulse rate does not guarantee better blood-flow; it increases the output of blood from the heart, but it does not guarantee that the blood will reach each part of your body that needs it. If, during aerobic exercise, the muscles are demanding more blood and the heart is sending more, but at the same time your muscles are so contracted that their blood vessels cannot fully receive the increased blood output, what is the result? Your heart works too hard, and for nothing. Only if the muscles that are not needed to produce the movement are relaxed is such a workout beneficial. Conversely, it is possible to create a strong, steady blood-flow that reaches every part of your body, without straining a muscle. We are not trying to discourage anyone from vigorous exercise – far from it: a relaxed and healthy body enjoys vigorous movement. We are saying that, before vigorous exercise can truly benefit your circulation, there are many factors to be considered.

If you, like so many other people, are stressed out, mostly sedentary and suffering from physical tension or pain, you should consider easing your way into the world of exercise *gradually*. A tense body is injured more easily than a relaxed one, especially if that body is suddenly subjected to unusual demands. The fast-growing field of sports medicine caters less to professional athletes than it does to 'weekend athletes', who try to force unprepared muscles into heroic performances once a week. In movement, muscles must contract and relax. If you are inactive, most of your muscles don't do much contracting. This is no guarantee that you are relaxed. The chances are more that your body will be, in a sense, 'frozen'. If you are suffering from stress on top of all of this, a number of your muscles will become chronically contracted into tight, hard knots. With some of your muscles unable to relax and others unwilling to contract, movement can become difficult, and strains, sprains and back and joint injuries are predictable results.

And yet, the person we have described needs aerobic, breath-deepening, circulation-stimulating exercise as much as anyone else. The question is, how to get it without wasting your efforts, or risking injury. Our aim is to get blood flowing into the smallest capillaries in the farthest periphery (that is, farthest from your heart) in your body. To do this, it will help if you understand how your circulatory system works.

The sole function of your heart is to keep blood flowing constantly throughout your body. The beat of your heart is the sound of it contracting to push the blood into the arteries. The heart is a little larger than your fist, and is a hollow structure with strong thick walls. It is located between the second and fifth ribs, just between the lungs, each of which has a notch at the top (called the cardiac impression) into which the heart fits. It is encased in a membrane sac called the pericardium, filled with a watery fluid which helps to decrease the friction of the heart's continuous pumping.

The heart has four sections or chambers: the right and left atrium and the right and left ventricle. The right atrium receives your body's deoxygenated blood from three large veins and passes it into the right ventricle. From there it goes into the lungs, where it exchanges carbon dioxide for a new supply of oxygen. From the lungs it flows into the left atrium, and then is pumped out through the left ventricle into the aorta, a massive arterial tube which feeds all the other arteries. The path that your blood follows is as follows: large arteries, arterioles, capillaries, venules, larger veins and, finally, into the right atrium through the three large veins which feed the heart. It is within the capillaries – the smallest and thinnest-walled blood vessels – that fluids are exchanged between the blood and other body cells.

The action of the heart is involuntary, which means that the heart does not require a direct conscious command from the brain to keep pumping. If the heart received no other messages from the rest of the body, it would beat, on its own, at the rate of about forty beats per minute. Normally, however, the heart is responding to messages from various parts of the body, slowing down if blood pressure becomes too high, increasing its rate if pressure becomes too low or if too little oxygen or too much carbon dioxide is detected in the blood. To some extent, the autonomic nervous system, discussed in the Nervous System chapter, directs heart action. When the parasympathetic nervous system exerts its generally calming influence, heart rate will slow down; when the excitatory sympathetic nervous system takes over, heart rate is accelerated. Hormones also affect heart rate.

The size of the heart changes according to how much blood it receives from the veins and how much it is required to send into the arteries. This amount can vary from two liters per minute, to as much as twenty-five liters from the heart of a highly-trained male athlete during exertion. Five liters is about normal for a healthy person at rest. If the circulation is strong, the heart will have to expand more during the intake of blood and to contract more during the expelling of blood. If the circulation is weak, the heart motion is decreased. Like any other muscle, the heart benefits from plentiful healthy exercise, as long as it is not worked beyond its capacity. As with other muscles, the heart must be exercised steadily and regularly. This will make it easier for the heart to respond to a sudden

increase in circulation or heart activity. During vigorous exercise, some people find it best to take frequent breaks to cool down, relax and allow your heart rate to return to normal and your body to enjoy the benefits of the increased circulation before you return to more strenuous efforts. For others, including Meir, aerobic exercise is sustained for a longer period of time, without breaks, moving in a variable way at a more moderate pace. No matter what model of aerobic exercise you follow, it should not be speeded through heedlessly, sacrificing awareness of bodily sensation to 'improved' performance for example, ignoring initial sensations of fatigue or illness and launching oneself into vigorous exercise. You need to continually monitor the changes in your body before, during and after your workout. Meir likes to sit on a hilltop after running, breathing deeply and noticing the changes that running has brought about. He recommends that you take a few minutes after exercise to notice the changes in your heartbeat and breathing, identifying sore areas that may need massage or stretches and stiff areas that need to be loosened with gentle movement.

The causes of poor circulation vary from person to person. Of course your physical make-up can play a role in determining how efficient your blood flow will be. There are people who can break all the rules of good health – eat the wrong foods, take little or no exercise, exhibit the full range of Type-A behavior – being very competitive, impatient, always in a hurry and trying to do different things at once – and still have strong hearts and healthy circulation, simply because they were blessed with the powerful constitution you need to survive such abuse. There are also people who follow every health dictum but, while they do show improvement, still have circulation problems due to hereditary weaknesses. These people are very interesting to study and discuss, but in our experience they don't constitute a majority. Most of the people we have seen who have circulatory problems have them because of the way they treat their bodies. Either they are completely inactive, or they are active in ways which hurt the body more than they help it.

Respiration is very closely linked to circulation. As we explained in the chapter on Breathing, a pattern of shallow breathing is a major cause of poor circulation.

Emotion also influences our respiration. Depression, anxiety and sadness almost always reduce our breathing, which in turn reduces our circulation. Therefore, the best way to begin to improve your circulation is, of course, to improve your breathing. Not only does deep breathing provide the oxygen your blood needs, but the movement of breathing also gives a stimulating massage to the heart itself, as the lungs expand and contract against the pericardium. The heart appreciates massage as much as any other muscle! If you have not read the Breathing chapter yet, our first suggestion is that you turn to it and begin with the exercises described there. It will be helpful for you to return to those exercises on an ongoing basis as you move through this book, because they will help you to benefit fully from all the other exercises we will be describing.

The next step along the path-of-least-resistance to promoting circulation is massage, which is just about guaranteed to improve both breathing and blood flow. Just by lying down on a table and surrendering yourself to someone else's touch – preferably that of a qualified bodyworker or a member of your Self-Healing support group – you will allow more circulation to every part of your body.

While doing bodywork, we have often noticed that an area particularly in need of blood supply will grow warmer and redder than the surrounding areas when it is massaged, as though the touch had drawn blood to that area like a magnet. During massage, you increase blood flow without raising the heart rate, which is especially helpful for people suffering from high stress or hypertension. You don't even need a partner for massage – there are many areas of your body where self-massage is very useful – but for total relaxation it's best to just lie down and let someone else straighten you out. The Massage chapter is entirely devoted to techniques for self-massage and massage of partners, both of which promote circulation. We will also describe some massage techniques specifically related to increasing circulation in this chapter.

The third step toward improving blood flow is movement. Even if you are not interested in learning or practicing exercises, keep in mind the one word 'move'. Most of the suggested 'exercises' in this chapter will combine the three elements of breathing, massage and movement, but keep in mind that all of them are designed to produce some movement – either the internal movement of organs and blood vessels or the external movement of the muscles. External movement serves the double purpose of strengthening the muscles themselves and of increasing vital internal movement of blood, lymph and digestion and nerve function.

The Chest

In this chapter, we are dealing with a function which is largely automatically controlled, and of which we are unaware most of the time. As in all Self-Healing work, awareness is the key to creating change. So we will first get to know intimately, on a kinesthetic level, our base of circulation, the home of the heart, our chest. The chest, also known in anatomy as the thoracic cavity, is braced at front and sides by the ribs, and in the back by the twelve thoracic vertebrae, which attach to the ribs to form the strong protective structure known as the rib-cage. While the neck and lower-back vertebrae are designed to move and twist easily, your thoracic vertebrae are intended to protect your heart, lungs and liver, as well as to allow your lungs the maximum room for expansion, and therefore they are held more rigidly in place – your lungs might be in trouble if they were in danger of being suddenly poked by a rotating rib. Because the chest area is not a naturally flexible part of the torso, we tend not to move much in this area, particularly if we lead an inactive life that doesn't include reaching, turning, sideways or backward motions of the upper body. Sitting bent or slumped over a pile of papers on a desk doesn't do much toward freeing the torso. Freeing the chest and upper back of this rigidity, whether inherited or acquired, is very important for the health of your heart.

At the floor of the ribcage is the diaphragm muscle, which separates the lungs from the abdomen. This muscle pulls downward when you breathe in, making more space for your lungs to expand with air. The ribs are lined by two sets of muscles called intercostals. The outer intercostals raise the ribs to expand the ribcage when you breathe in, while the inner intercostals lower the ribs to slightly compress the ribcage, forcing more air out when you exhale. The muscles of the upper chest, which connect to the muscles of the shoulders, sides and arms, are called the pectoral muscles. We

believe that breathing and circulation would have to be related functions, if only because the heart and the lungs are surrounded and affected by many of the same sets of muscles.

It is interesting that the muscles of the chest (and also of the arms) may often be extremely tender to the touch even when they do not hurt or ache otherwise. Many of our clients, when touched in these areas, are very surprised to find the extent of the soreness there. The intercostals, in particular, may be so sensitive as a result of their tightness that even a light touch will be painful or very ticklish. Another very important feature of this region is the extent to which emotions appear to be 'stored' there. It is still not possible to state scientifically how, or even if, this process occurs. We feel that depression or grief may lead to shallow breathing, which tends to contract chest muscles. Many bodyworkers have observed that massage of the chest, and often of the arms, can produce a great uprush of emotional expression and release, and that a person with very tense and tender chest muscles will often prove to have been carrying a burden of unexpressed emotion which the massage can do much to relieve. It is no coincidence that the heart has been named as the seat of emotion. It is possible to speculate that much heart disease may also have an emotional basis.

The muscles of the chest directly affect the expansion of the lungs during breathing. The external chest muscles affect the posture, size and shape of the chest, and will determine whether the chest can be fully mobile, able to expand to its fullest capacity, or will be immobile and 'shrunken'. When the chest cavity is compressed, there is less room for both the heart and the lungs to expand to their natural capacity. A state of chronic, unrelieved contraction in the chest muscles can be dangerous. This section is devoted to stretching and expanding these muscles and promoting movement in the upper torso. If you have any doubts that this is important, we offer an interesting statistic. The professionals with the lowest rate of heart trouble are symphony conductors. They also have a life expectancy which is much longer than average. If more of us had the opportunity to wave our arms in joyous emotional expression for a living, we are convinced that heart disease would decrease.

We would like to recommend that anyone with serious heart or circulatory problems consult with his or her doctor before proceeding with these exercises. When these areas have been overstrained, it is extremely important to avoid stressing them further. If your doctor feels that any of these exercises could be too strenuous, please do only those which are approved for you.

Can you feel whether your chest is tight? Some people first discover the tightness in the chest only when they have their first heart attack, for this is an area that sometimes will delay sending real pain signals until it may be too late – an area where body awareness may truly spell the difference between life and death. Other people may discover tightness in the chest when they first attempt to take a full breath and discover that something is holding them back. That something is often the chest muscles refusing to allow full expansion in the lungs.

2–1   Try to take a deep breath. If this is easy for you, pay attention to how your chest muscles feel when you inhale. Enjoy the smooth and elastic feeling of their expansion, and the buoyant sensation as the lungs fill with oxygen. Notice how your breathing affects your shoulders, arms, back and abdomen. If you do not feel you are taking a full breath, try to feel what is stopping you. Where does the holding or blockage occur? Does trying to expand the lungs make you aware of tension or pain in any other area? Be aware that your greatest obstacle to relaxing may be a lifelong habit of tensing your abdomen to hold it in. You may actually be encouraging a potbelly by constricting your muscles this way, and it certainly limits breathing. Let it go.

2–2   Take another deep breath and, as you inhale, lay your palm on your breastbone and shake your chest vigorously. Do you tighten anywhere to inhibit this motion? Exhale, then again shake your chest as you inhale, trying to let go of any holding in the shoulders, spine or chest cavity. Repeat this exercise ten times, until you can feel that you have become looser. This is a good exercise to release nervous tension.

2–3   Inhale deeply again, this time rubbing and warming your chest muscles with one hand, in a rotating motion, while the other hand rubs and warms the upper abdomen.

2–4   Look at yourself in the mirror to see how your posture affects your chest. Does your chest jut forward? If so, you probably have great rigidity in your upper back and abdomen. Is your chest caved in, with the shoulders rounded forward? If so, you probably have tension in your shoulders and neck, as well as weakness in the abdomen. Look at yourself and think about how you would like the picture to change, and then look at yourself after each exercise to see whether you can see a difference.

2–5 See if you can feel your pulse. If you are dedicated to improving your cardiovascular health, it would be a wonderful idea to buy a stethoscope from a medical supply store, to enable you to listen to your heartbeat. If you don't have a stethoscope, you may be able to feel your pulse by simply laying your hands over your heart, or by feeling with your fingers (don't use the thumb) the pulse points at your wrist (fig 2–5) or throat.

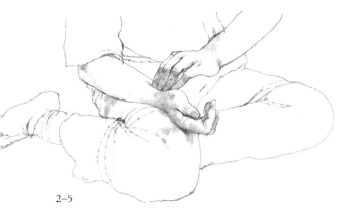

2–5

With the aid of a clock or watch, count the number of beats per minute. Then leave your hand on your pulse point and feel it as you visualize that the pulse becomes slower. Most of us find ourselves often under stress, at which times typically the sympathetic nervous system speeds up the heart. A too-rapid heart-beat is often associated with cardiac problems. The opposing nervous system, known as the parasympathetic, has the job of slowing the heart rate. When you visualize your heart rate slowing, you are aiding the parasympathetic nervous system in its work, and helping to prevent the sympathetic from going into overdrive.

2–6 Lie down on your back, with your arms and legs comfortably outstretched. Inhale deeply and, before you exhale, while your lungs are still filled with air, raise and lower your chest several times. Exhale, and notice how the chest feels. Remember that every sensation has meaning, and any change in sensation means an actual change in the functioning of your body. Often, when you touch, move or breathe into a part of your body, that area will feel warmer; this is the result of increased sensory awareness, and sometimes an actual raising of skin temperature caused by increased blood-flow. The area may feel larger; this is due to actual, measurable lengthening of the muscle fibers as they relax. Paying attention to these changes helps you, ultimately, to create them at will.

2–7 Inhale, hold in the air and move the entire abdomen up and down, expanding it upward as far as possible and pulling it down toward your back as far as you can. This is a great exercise for strengthening the abdominal muscles, which have an unfortunate tendency to slacken in adults. Repeat this several times, and then do the same with your lower back, pushing it down against the floor as you expand it, pulling it in toward the abdomen as you contract it.

2–8 Inhale again, hold the air in your lungs as before, and this time try to expand your diaphragm. The movement will not exactly be up-and-down as before; rather, the diaphragm pulls downward toward the abdomen when you breathe in, and moves upward toward the chest when you breathe out. The movement of the diaphragm may feel jerky at first. Move it four or five times before you exhale, and then repeat this part of the exercise until it feels smoother and easier.

2–9 So far, you have been moving each part only after you inhale, while the lungs are inflated. Now do the same after you exhale. The pattern of the exercise will be as follows.

Inhale. Move the chest up and down several times before exhaling. Exhale. Move the chest up and down several times before inhaling. Now do the same with the abdomen, lower back and diaphragm. Notice where your difficulties lie in doing this. Is it harder to hold the air in or to hold it out? Spend more time with the more difficult parts of the exercise.

Refer to exercise 6–2 in the Nervous System chapter, which is important for your chest and heart. Try once again to take a deep breath. Does it feel any different to breathe now? You are becoming aware of the inward sensations of your chest.

2–10 Now, to fully open your breathing, get acquainted with the outward sensations of the chest muscles. Still lying on your back, touch your sternum with all your fingertips. The sternum, or breastbone, is attached to your first seven pairs of ribs by strips of cartilage; it runs from your collarbone to about where your heart is. Pressing on the lower third of the sternum also massages your heart and is the basis of cardiopulmonary resuscitation. Applying a firm pressure, begin at the base of the sternum and work your way up, massaging along the bone with circular motions of the fingertips. Notice any sore places, and massage them a little more gently and breathe into them, visualizing that they expand with your breath – as indeed they do.

When you have reached the top of the sternum, massage outward toward your shoulders, in the space between your clavicle (collarbone) and first rib. It may be easier for you to do this sitting up. Tapping is as effective as massage for bringing blood into the area you are touching, so use both techniques. Your touch, whether you are massaging or tapping, should always be firm enough to stimulate and to detect the sore spots, but not deep enough to inflict pain.

Touching your chest may turn out to be a real voyage of discovery for you, especially since very few of us make a habit of touching this area. See whether you can feel each individual rib, and massage the spaces between each rib and the next, where the taut intercostals lie. Beat gently with your fist on the pectoral muscles where they stretch from the sternum to the armpits. With one hand, gently pull the pectoral toward the side while the other hand taps on the muscle and shakes it (fig 2–10); do the same with the serratus anterior muscles, just below the armpit. Do this with the pulling hand in several different positions, so that each part of the muscle gets stretched.

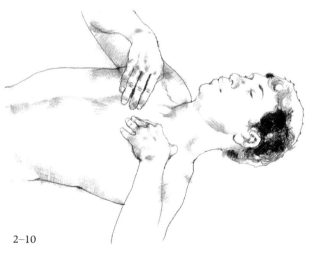

2–10

Bend your elbows, and use your thumbs to massage your sides between the ribs just below the armpit. Women should not massage the

breast, but just below or beside it. Make loose fists with your hands and pound on your chest muscles, just hard enough so that you can feel some release from the impact. You can usually create a little more impact by beating with the right fist on the left side of the chest, and vice versa. Remember to breathe deeply and continuously as you release the chest.

Creating Movement in the Chest and Shoulders

2–11 Standing, slowly twist your upper body from side to side, from the waist up, letting your arms swing with the movement as you turn (fig 2–11). They will feel almost as though they are floating, as if the air is supporting them. As you swing to the right, allow your left foot to follow the motion by lifting the heel from the floor and twisting the ankle. As you swing to the left, your right foot follows.

2–12 Slowly lift one arm to the side to shoulder level, feeling as you lift it all of the muscles which are involved in lifting it – then let it drop to your side. Now lift it again, imagining that someone else is lifting it, pulling it. Stretch it as far up and out as possible, and then let it drop again. Can you let it drop, or do you try to control its fall? This will give you some clue as to the level of tension you maintain in your arms, which directly affects the tension in your chest.

2–13 Clasp your hands behind your hips and move your chest back and forward. Are you using your chest or your shoulders to do this? Most people will have a tendency to move the shoulders, letting the chest be moved with them. See if you can actually feel your chest leading the motion, with the shoulders following behind.

2–14 Extend your arms above your head, clasp your hands, and swing your arms in a

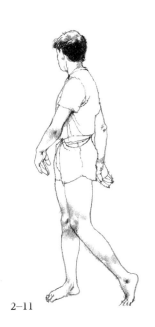

2–11

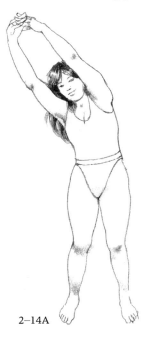

2–14A

27

rotating motion, keeping your back straight but not freezing it (fig 2–14A). Be aware of how this motion moves your chest. When you bring your arms up, let the chest lift and expand upward; when you pull the arms to the sides, feel how the chest muscles stretch to allow the motion.

Now lift your arms above your head, grasp each elbow with the opposite hand, pull your arms behind your head (fig 2–14B) and move your upper body in rotation, bending slightly from the waist as you move forward and backward, and visualizing that your hands on your elbows are really pulling the body in whatever direction you want them to go. Feel how this pulling stretches the muscles between the ribs, creating more space for the lungs to expand.

2–15 The following exercise is one of the most helpful for the heart itself. Stand facing a wall, and extend your arms so that the palms of your hands are flat against the wall. Move your feet back until you are leaning some of your weight on the wall, with your body at an angle to the wall and your elbows firmly locked. Now move your chest backward and forward, without bending the elbows. Don't let your shoulders or your abdomen do the work; they will follow the motion, but the chest should lead it. During this exercise, your back will be in three distinct postures. Take the time to feel each one separately. When your chest moves forward, your upper back is in a concave posture; stay in that posture for a few moments and move your head slowly from side to side three times (fig 2–15A).

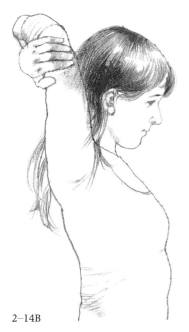

2–14B

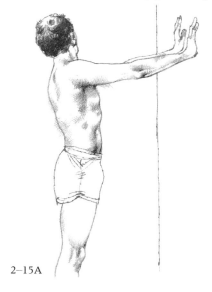

2–15A

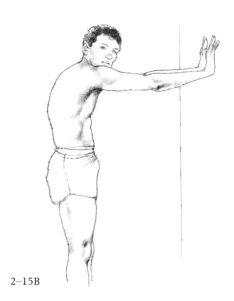

2–15B

Return to your starting posture, with your back straight, and repeat the head movement. Last, when you pull the chest backward, the upper back becomes convex; repeat the head movement in this position as well (fig 2–15B). After doing this several times, take your hands from the wall and stand straight; place one thumb on the sternum and one on the upper spine, and move the chest back and forward

(fig 2–15C). Now return your palms to the wall and visualize the points you have just touched with the thumbs pulling you backward and forward. Be aware of the sensations in your upper back as well as in your chest. Feel how much this moves your upper back as well as your chest. This movement relaxes shoulder and upper-back tension as much as chest tension. Now inhale as you move the chest forward, exhale as you hold it there, and inhale again as you move it backward, and feel how the combination of breathing and movement fully expands the chest muscles. In our opinion, movements such as this, which move the sternum, are also providing massage to the heart itself. Do this exercise thirty times daily until your chest and upper back are loose enough to do it easily and fluidly.

2–16   Stand or sit, and move one arm, from the shoulder, in a very large circle, while tapping on the chest muscles with the other hand (fig 2–16). Do this at least fifty times in both directions, stopping to rest if your arm becomes tired. Then do the same with the other arm.

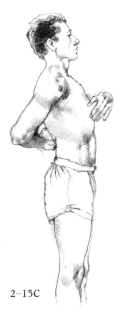

2–15C

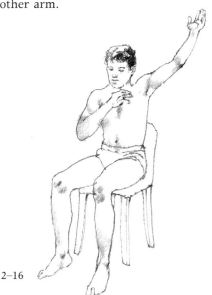

2–16

2–17 Standing, swing one arm up above and behind your head; as you swing it back down, swing the other arm up. Try not to strain your shoulders as you alternate between your arms – imagine that the fingertips are creating the motion effortlessly. This exercise helps relieve high blood pressure by drawing blood to your hands and thus easing the work of your heart.

Throughout all of these exercises, you should stay constantly aware of how your chest feels. If it begins to feel tight, stop the movement and concentrate on relaxing and deepening your breathing. If your chest is constricted or your breathing shallow, you will not enjoy the full benefits of movement. This is also true of your diaphragm and abdomen, since tightness in these areas will also interfere with the full expansion of the lungs and the easy flow of circulation.

Tense abdominal muscles may also hamper the functioning of the digestive system. The abdominal muscles are known as 'red muscles', since under ideal conditions they are bathed in a constant rich supply of blood. Unlike the muscles of our back or limbs, the abdominal area is in almost constant activity, with some stage of digestion taking place. Digestion, the breaking down of food, has three major aspects: breaking the food down, sending the useful parts of our food to the areas that can use them, and sending the useless or harmful parts out of our bodies. The blood plays a crucial role in each of these processes, so digestion cannot proceed efficiently if circulation is hampered by contracted muscles. Strong and relaxed abdominal muscles will promote abdominal circulation, and thus improve diges-

tion. Spasm (i.e. involuntary contraction), cramps and tension of the abdominal muscles adversely affect digestion.

Sitting

The typical Western adult (and very often, lately, the child as well) has a daily life which may include several hours at a desk, perhaps several more at table, maybe an hour or more in a car, and how many hours in front of a television or a computer screen? All this sitting tightens the chest, distorts the posture and limits the circulation. Is it any wonder that heart disease is the major cause of premature death in the West? So, if you never do anything else for your heart, at least you can walk. We don't mean jogging, we don't mean 'power walking', we don't mean anything exhausting or intimidating. We just mean putting on your shoes (though walking barefoot is even better, if possible) and getting out of the house and not coming back until you feel like you've actually had a little exercise. This is movement at its most basic – movement for the sake of knowing you still can.

A person who never moves will become weakened and stiffened to the point where the idea of movement is naturally unappealing. This is very dangerous, since movement is essential to circulation. One of the ways your blood gets back to your heart from the rest of your body is by way of muscle contractions which help to push the blood on its way. Only movement produces these kinds of contractions. If you are out of the exercise habit, begin the work of reactivating your body with leisurely walks. From there, you can expand your movement repertoire into infinity.

However, we don't mean to suggest that only the time you spend in exercise should be valuable, with the time you spend sitting being written off as a total loss. Since we do inevitably spend so much time sitting, it's as important to maintain good circulation while sitting as it is to get up and move. The idea behind our exercises is to help the body to function at its best under all circumstances. A sedentary lifestyle, per se, is not the main problem. The stiffness of underused joints and muscles and the problems caused by poor posture – such as slumping the lower back, rounding the shoulders forward and sticking the neck out, all of which depress the chest cavity – are serious problems, and these can be minimized even if the time you have to spend sitting cannot.

Sitting in chairs is more of a challenge than most of us realize. It is well-documented that countries which traditionally embrace floor-sitting, such as Japan and India, have far fewer back problems statistically. It's a good idea to substitute floor-sitting for chair-sitting whenever you can (unless of course you find it very uncomfortable, in which case we refer you to the exercises in the Spine chapter). Many people find that sitting cross-legged or in the lotus position (each foot resting on the opposite thigh) on the floor gives them a better feeling of support than sitting in most chairs. Changing your position as often as possible will help to prevent stiff muscles and joints.

2–18 Get used to the idea of relaxing while you sit. Sit comfortably on a couch or chair with armrests, and rest your elbows on the armrests. (If on a couch, prop pillows under the arm which does not have an armrest.) Breathe deeply and relax your shoulders, feeling them drop as low as they can. Let your forearms and elbows sink all their weight into the armrests, and feel as though your arms are dropping away from your shoulders. Turn your head from side to side, then move it in a slow rotation; slowly open and close your jaws, and relax your spine. Most of all, let the shoulders drop. If the shoulders are held high and tight, they compress the chest cavity, putting pressure on the heart and lungs; they tighten the neck, interfering with blood flow to the head; and they make it impossible to really relax the arms.

When you sit down to work, take a few minutes to orient your body to sitting. Place your feet flat on the floor; do not cross your knees for long periods of time. The urge to cross your knees comes from pelvic tension and lower-back weakness. It may feel more comfortable, but it twists your spine into a distorted position, interfering with the spinal cord, and drastically reduces the circulation in your legs. Use the exercises in the Spine chapter to reduce tension and increase strength in the back.

Relax your pelvis and thighs, and make sure that your back is as fully supported as possible, which may mean drawing your chair closer to your table or desk. Rest your hands on the desk, and relax your shoulders, your elbows and your wrists. Breathe deeply and feel the blood flowing to your fingers and toes. Breathe into each hand and each foot separately, for the space of five long, deep breaths each time. Drop your shoulders, let go of your abdomen if you are holding it in, let your back fully accept the support of the chair back. With the elbows resting on the desk, draw circles with your hands on the desk. Completely relax your arms and shoulders and visualize that your fingertips are moving your hands. Lean your elbows on the table and rotate your forearms, again visualizing that the fingertips are leading the motion. Everything above and below the elbow is at rest. Your wrists are loose. Extend your legs in front of you and rotate your ankles, relaxing the hips and legs and visualizing that all of the movement comes from your toes. You may be surprised to find how much tension you have been maintaining just to keep yourself upright in your chair. These relaxation exercises are to show you that it is not necessary.

2–19 Let your hands rest on the desk in front of you and your feet rest flat on the floor; visualize your blood flowing to your fingertips and your toes. Take five slow, deep breaths – one for each finger – while you imagine the blood flowing to the hands, and another five – one for each toe – while you imagine the blood flowing to your feet. Then imagine that the breath itself flows into your hands and into your feet. Whether or not this is actually physically possible is not important – the visualization will give you a sense of energy in the area that you have imagined. Your central nervous system in some ways treats a thought and an action the same way, so thought can be very powerful. Just as thought can produce quickened pulse, sweating, nausea, goosebumps and other physical reactions, so imagining a condition in your body can help to create that condition in reality.

Even after learning to sit so that you are comfortable and relaxed, and to maintain maximum circulation while sitting, you must still remember to incorporate some movement into a sedentary day. Think of how good it feels to get out and stretch after driving a car for a couple of hours. Even a few minutes of

standing, stretching and moving the muscles does wonders for the circulation. A two-minute walk up and down a flight of stairs, or even outside if you can make the time; a couple of minutes of back exercises such as hip rotations (exercises 4–5 to 4–7) or the spinal arch (exercise 4–2); a few minutes of floor stretches (such as exercise 4–13) – whatever seems feasible according to your work setup – repeated at intervals throughout the day will make a world of difference in the efficient and comfortable functioning of both your body and your mind.

It is especially important to get up and move around a little when you are under stress. The reason for this is that your nervous system, when it senses anxiety, reacts in a rather primitive fashion by flooding your muscles with chemicals which are supposed to make movement easier and faster, or to help you win in a physical fight. If you are being threatened by a bloodthirsty predator, this reaction will help you either to run away from it or to hit back. If you are being threatened by your tax office, the chances are that you will not have the opportunity to respond to these chemical impulses by actually running, hitting or any other useful movement. The chemicals remain in your bloodstream, concentrated in your muscles, making you feel extremely uncomfortable, as you may have noticed in the shaky aftermath of anger or fear. This is why so many people find physical activity a relief during times of stressful emotion, though it may take the form of throwing things or punching people. You may not want to do either of these in your place of work, however, and you will probably not have to if you remember to continually use movement to drain off stress before it can build to a dangerous point.

Getting Blood to the Periphery

Your extremities – hands, feet and head – will usually be the first places to manifest a lack of circulation. If your hands or feet are chronically cold, or if you often feel fatigued, confused or spacy, you probably need to improve your blood flow. Exercises for the hands and feet will attract blood to these areas. They will also benefit the rest of the body, since if the blood reaches the extremities it will also have to have reached every point along the way. Thus, hand exercises also nourish the chest, shoulders, upper back and arms as they draw blood toward the hands; exercises for the feet bring blood through the lower back, gastrointestinal tract, pelvis and legs.

Hands

If your hands tend to be cold – even if they feel warm to the touch but cold on the inside – you will find the following exercises helpful.

Note: Though all the exercises for the hands are described as being done lying down, they can also be done in a sitting position. Sitting, you can either support your forearm on your thigh or lean your elbows on a table and support one forearm with the opposite hand while exercising the supported arm.

2–20 Lie on your back, extend your arms to either side, with the backs of the hands against the floor, and completely relax the arms; then slowly open and close both hands. Focus your attention on the many small muscles of the hands themselves as you do this, and don't

allow your upper arms or shoulders to work for the hands. If you feel your arm muscles working hard, tap on the muscles of one arm, lightly, with the fingertips of the other hand, to relax the muscles of that arm while the hand is moving. Inevitably, some of your arm muscles must work, no matter how you try to focus the motion in the hands. Try to feel which muscles these are. Breathe deeply and imagine the breath and your blood flowing freely through the arm muscles into the fingertips. Open the hands until the fingers are straight, then let them curl up again.

2–21 Turn your arms so that now the palms are against the floor, and tap your fingertips against the floor by lifting the hands from the wrist and dropping them, twenty or thirty times. Once again, try to use only the muscles of the wrists and hands to do this. If you feel muscles in your arms and shoulders tensing, relax them by visualizing that the fingertips alone are doing the motion. Notice how your chest, your abdomen and your back react to this motion. Let your whole body sink into the floor and become completely motionless, except for the hands.

Now move your wrists in a rotating motion, first one at a time and then together, imagining as always that no muscles above the wrists are doing any work at all. Of course, this is not and never can be true. Just about any body movement requires that one group of muscles will move to act and another group to support them, and still another group will resist the motion to prevent it from being overdone – for example, if you reach forward, several muscles will pull you slightly backward to prevent you from falling on your face. However, our experience is that most people tire themselves by using muscles which are simply not needed at all, as well as tightening more intensely than is really necessary. This is why we encourage both creating and imagining more independent, economical muscle movement.

2–22 In the same position, rotate each finger separately, beginning with the thumb. Imagine that the motion begins at the tip of each finger, relaxing the rest of the hand; feel the base of each finger following the movement of the fingertip; the wrist should be completely at rest. Do this with the palms turned down, and then with the palms turned up. Does either way feel more comfortable than the other? Most people find that either pronating (palms down) or supinating (palms up) is noticeably more comfortable, due to differing patterns of tension in the arms and shoulders. Doing this exercise in both positions may help to alleviate some of these tensions.

2–23 With the hand hanging limp and relaxed and the upper arm resting on the floor, move the forearms, from the elbows, in rotation. Make this rotation as large as you can; your fingertips should sweep across the floor and across your shoulder as they move. Imagine that the fingertips are leading this motion, with the rest of the forearm passively following.

2–24 Now massage the chest as we described earlier in the chapter (exercise 2–10), this time focusing on the sensations in your fingertips as you do so. Let the fingertips do all the work. You may find your entire upper body trying to work hard, but don't let it. Imagine that your fingers are moving with a completely independent life of their own as they explore the chest muscles. If you are interested in

massage, either of yourself or of others, this is a great exercise to develop sensitivity and relaxation in your hands.

Think of all the things you do with your hands – probably more than you do with any other part of your body. Now imagine how it affects your body if you are tensing your hands, forearms, upper arms, shoulders, chest, upper back and neck every time you use your hands. Imagine this tension being created every time you write, cook, drive or touch something – and remember how blood-flow is hampered when muscles are tense. Is it easier now to understand why you have cold hands? These exercises, by relaxing all the muscle pathways, will ensure better circulation to your hands.

Feet

The feet are farther from the heart than any other part of the body, and so they suffer most of all from poor circulation. Injuries to ankles or feet often take longer to heal than any others, for the same reason. Pelvic and hip tension is often the cause of decreased circulation to the feet, since many of the largest veins and arteries in the body run through the pelvis. If this area becomes contracted, circulation to and from the entire lower body is slowed. If you suffer from icy feet, try these hip exercises first, then go on to the exercises specifically for the feet.

2–25 Lie on your back and pull your knees as close to your chest as possible, holding one knee in each hand. Pull your knees as far apart as you can and move the knees in a rotating motion (fig 2–25).

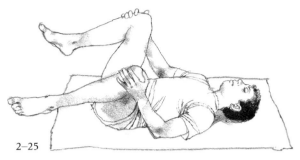

2–25

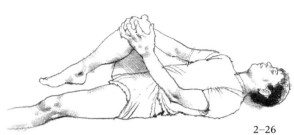

2–26

You will create the maximum movement in the hips by moving one knee clockwise and the other counterclockwise (most people do this instinctively anyway). Rotate the knees slowly, making the circles as large as you can, imagining your whole back, down to the tail-bone, sinking heavily into the floor. Relax your legs until they feel completely passive, allowing your guiding hands to do all the work. After about twenty rotations, change the direction and notice whether it feels different when you do so.

Visualize your hip joints, where your pelvis and thigh bone come together. These are among the most heavily used joints in your body. If you are tense while walking, standing or sitting, you will eventually feel the effects of this tension in your hips. Keeping the hip joints lubricated and the muscles surrounding them limber will make your active movement much easier – as well as increasing the flow of blood to the groin, legs and feet.

2–26 With one leg stretched out flat on the floor, pull one knee up to your chest, holding it with both hands (fig 2–26).
If this seems to place a strain on your back, you can bend the knee of the outstretched leg until the back feels comfortable. Move the knee

in a rotating motion, both clockwise and counterclockwise. This is one of the quickest ways to relieve low-back pain. Now stretch out both legs on the floor, and see whether the one you have been rotating feels any different. Many people find that the leg will feel longer, due to the slight gentle stretching of the muscles, and many report a sensation they describe as 'warmth', 'tingling' or simply 'more aliveness'. They often feel that that side of the back has become straighter, with more of the back touching the floor. This is a sure sign of increased blood-flow into the legs.

2–27 Pull both knees to your chest, hugging them close with your arms crossed over them. Breathe deeply and feel your lower back expanding. As before, relax your back into the floor and your legs into your arms. Now hold your knees with your hands and use the hands to move the knees, together, in rotation. Where the other two movements have focused on the joint where the thigh bone meets the pelvis, this one concentrates on the sacral region – an area of great tension and pain for many people. It may be difficult for people with lower-back problems to do this motion, so don't push it, but if it feels comfortable you can rotate the knees as many as 100 times in each direction.

35

2–28 Lying on your back, knees bent, feet flat and legs together, slowly lower both knees to the right, until the right knee rests on the floor (fig 2–28).

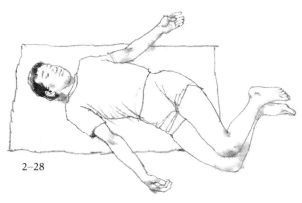

2–28

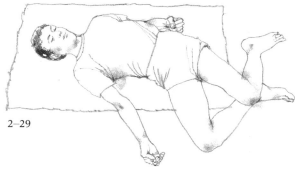

2–29

Bring them upright again, then lower them to the left until the left knee rests on the floor. Alternate to the right and the left at least twenty times, visualizing that the knees are leading the motion, as though someone else's hands are guiding them. Let go of all the tension in your thighs, hips and back, and breathe deeply and slowly. The main stretch is in the side of the hip and the outer thigh muscles. Do you feel restriction to the movement? Is it in your hips, your thighs, the knees themselves? Stop and take a few minutes to massage the area that seems stiff or unyielding, or pound the area lightly with a loose fist (don't pound the knees!). Then try the exercise again and see whether it feels easier.

2–29 Lie on your back with your knees bent and your feet flat. Separate the feet until they are hip-width apart. In this position, lower both knees to the floor, alternating the movement to the right and to the left. This time you may feel the stretch in the groin. If you feel tension in the outer side of the hip, you can release it by tapping gently on the hip with your fist while the hip moves (fig 2–29).

Repeat this motion at least thirty times to each side, remembering to breathe and to completely relax your torso. If your hips and pelvis are tight, as most people's are, you will have great difficulty improving the circulation to your feet. You may want to refer to the Hips section of the Joints chapter at this time.

2–30 Still lying on the floor, knees bent and feet flat, straighten one leg until it is stretched out flat, allowing the ball of the foot to lift off the floor as the leg straightens. Then slowly bend it again and, as you do so, straighten the other leg, keeping both feet on the floor. Continue alternately to bend and straighten the legs, bending one as the other straightens, and vice versa, as you do when riding a bicycle. Visualize that your feet are leading this motion – don't tense your abdomen or pelvis to produce it.

When you feel comfortable with the motion, begin to focus on your feet. Become aware of how they feel as they move against the floor. First imagine that they are getting a massage from the floor, with the slight pressure stimulating each part of the foot as it moves. Then imagine that your feet are giving the floor a massage. See whether you can feel different textures on the floor as you move your feet, and let the heels, balls of the feet and toes explore those textures. Now gradually increase

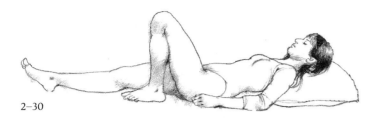

2–30

your speed, without tightening your hips, and repeat the motion 100 times, till your feet and legs feel loose and alive.

You may choose to do this exercise in a semi-reclining position (fig 2–30), supporting your back with pillows.

2–31 Do the above exercise with your knees turned out, each to its own side, and the soles of the feet facing toward each other, so that only the outer side of each leg rests on the floor (fig 2–31). Again, bend each leg as far as it will go, but do not strain.

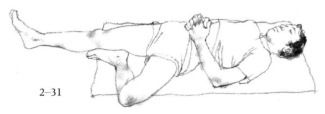

2–31

2–32 Lying with your legs stretched out flat, rotate your ankles, making small circles with your toes. Imagine that your toes are leading this motion, and try not to tense the ankles themselves. Feel how this motion uses muscles up and down the length of your leg. Many people walk very stiffly, with their feet held as rigidly as slabs of wood, their ankles frozen and the whole leg moving as if it were one piece, instead of a collection of bones, joints, muscles and tendons. When you walk in this way, the entire impact of each step shoots directly into the hip, instead of being absorbed by the various joints and muscles along the

way. Loosening your ankles is the first step in improving the way you walk. It will also allow more blood-flow into the feet themselves.

2–33 Now bend your knees so the feet are flat on the floor, and move your feet in circles. This limbers the knee joints and stimulates the feet. Gradually move your feet faster and press them harder against the floor, to create a warming friction.

2–34 Straighten one leg and massage it with the opposite foot, from the ankle as far up the thigh as you can reach (fig 2–34A).

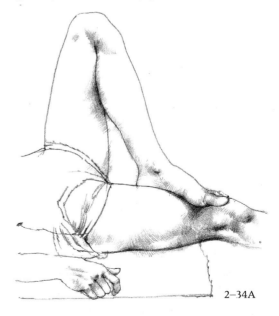

2–34A

Try to give your leg a genuine massage. You may be surprised to find how sensitive and dexterous your foot really is. See whether your foot can feel the tight or hard places on the leg; use the ball and heel to stroke hard and the toes to palpate various areas. Now switch and massage the other leg with the other foot.

You can complete your 'foot massage' by rubbing the soles of the feet together, and then the toes. This will be easiest to do sitting up. Grasp your ankles (fig 2–34B) and rub the soles of the feet briskly together (fig 2–34C).

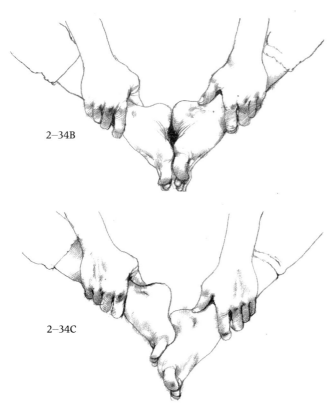

2–34B

2–34C

Don't strain! If you find your back, hips or abdomen tightening while you do this, return to the hip exercises at the beginning of this section, and remember always to breathe deeply and relax any part of the body you are not actively using.

You may not be able to make your feet warm and glowing after just one session of doing these exercises, although many people have. With practice, however, these exercises will increase the circulation into your feet, and also the way you move your lower body.

Meditation

Meditation means something different to everyone who practices it, yet there is a basic understanding of the meditative process which is shared by all who experience it – and which can be achieved only by practicing it. Meditation is a unique experience, combining perfect focus with complete letting-go, an inner searching with a sense of becoming part of everything that is. Its greatest value to our physical health is its ability to redirect our thoughts. Thoughts can be our greatest source of stress if they are uncontrolled. Much of the emotional pain caused by our thoughts, with its resulting physical tension, may be completely unnecessary. You may spend days worrying about things which never come to pass, or being angry about situations you have completely misunderstood. You may waste your energy being upset about situations you cannot change. You may concentrate obsessively on one negative aspect of a situation, shutting out the possibility of a positive side. Even if your perceptions are completely accurate and there is real reason for pain, you may allow your pain to grow to a point where it can harm you. No matter how you struggle to control your thoughts, it may seem next to impossible.

This is where meditation can help. Meditation can defuse your thoughts by diffusing them. In meditation, you concentrate for a given period of time on something other than your problems, whether that something be breathing, a mantra, affirmations or God. When you return to your thoughts after this brief vacation from them, they often look quite different. Meditation breaks the cycle of endless rationalization, obsession or blame. It takes you into a world greater than yourself, giving you a perspective wherein your problems look smaller and therefore more manageable.

A process we often use in our sessions and workshops is guided meditation. The group leader will suggest affirmations, visualizations or simply images, while the other participants quietly focus on these things if they seem helpful and on their own visualizations if not. We would like to offer a guided meditation for the health of your heart. You may want to tape this meditation so that you can listen to your own voice making these suggestions to your body as you relax and breathe.

2–35 Sit cross-legged or lie on your back, relax your body, breathe deeply and focus on your heart. Your heart is the life of your physical and emotional self. How does it feel? Sense its location, place your hand over it, feel your pulse points, sense your chest, your diaphragm, your abdomen, your back and shoulders moving with your breath, and feel how the rhythm of your breath affects the rhythm of your heart. Imagine the movement

of your heart as it sends blood rich with oxygen coursing into your body. Imagine the heart moving gently within the pericardial sac, massaged by the movement of the liquids within the sac and by the movements of the lungs and chest muscles. Imagine your heart growing and shrinking, expanding and contracting. Reflect on the strength of the heart which allows it to continue its motion throughout your entire life.

Visualize the movement of the blood through your body, flowing from the aorta to the smaller arteries as they branch and branch again, reaching at last the capillary beds within the tissues, bringing nutrients, oxygen, warmth and energy to the farthest periphery of your body. Imagine the blood coursing back toward your heart, returning there for fresh oxygen. Breathe slowly and deeply, visualizing that your inhale sends the blood into the arteries, and that your exhale returns the blood to the heart. Visualize each part of your body expanding, relaxing and glowing as it receives blood, and then gently pushing the blood through the veins toward the heart. Imagine that the movement of your heart and blood vessels is as effortless as the rippling of water in a stream.

With new awareness of your breathing and blood flow, you are now prepared for a fuller, more active range of movements.

CHAPTER 3

Joints
The more you move, the easier you move

There are people who seldom think about their joints, and people who seldom think about anything else. The first category consists mainly of people who have never experienced any problems with their joints. The second category includes anyone who suffers from joint trouble. This chapter is for both groups.

If you have never been troubled by your joints, we would like to show you how to keep it that way, and to demonstrate how vital joint flexibility is to your total health. It is worthwhile to work on your joints, even if you have never experienced joint pain. You will be surprised to find how much more flexibility and mobility your body can have, and how good this ease of motion can make you feel. The exercises in this chapter will help you to increase your joint flexibility, which is extremely important for everyone. Most of us use only a fraction of our capacity for joint movement, just as we do not use our potential for muscle movement. Our range of motion in general is limited, confined to narrow and repetitive movements; this narrow range ultimately stiffens muscles and joints alike. Working to free up your joints will give you another experience of how working on one body system improves body function as a

whole: strengthening muscles and improving circulation, respiration and nerve function.

Arthritis – the catch-all name for over 100 types of joint disorder – is almost never a killing disease, but it can cause so much pain as to seriously interfere with the quality of life. One in seven people in the world suffers from some form of arthritis. Many people speak of 'arthritis' as though it were a specific disease, which it is not. The word 'arthritis' is literally translated as 'inflammation of a joint', but no inflammation at all is involved in most conditions which people think of as arthritis. For simplicity's sake, however, we will use the word 'arthritis' to refer to any condition which affects the health and functioning of joints.

To understand how joints work, we need to understand how they are constructed.

A joint is a joining-place, the space where movable body parts connect to each other. Joints are hinges and, like hinges, must allow for smooth, gliding movement. If two bone-ends – say, for example, the bottom of the humerus (the upper-arm bone) and the top of the ulna (a forearm bone) – were constantly to rub against each other whenever you moved your arm, they would eventually grind each other down — an extremely painful and destructive process.

Joints are beautifully designed to prevent this. The majority of the joints are of a type called synovial joints. In these joints, the bone-ends are capped, or faced, with a protective layer of cartilage. The cartilage may be compared to a fluid-saturated sponge. It is smooth, strong and elastic, and it can absorb and expel fluid.

The joint is enclosed by a fibrous joint capsule which helps to hold the bones together and at the same time allows for movement. The inner lining of the capsule is the synovial membrane, which secretes synovial fluid. This fluid lubricates and nourishes the cartilage and cushions the joint. Its internal pressure allows joints to withstand the often huge compressive forces that come with some activities. By moving more, you increase the circulation of the synovial fluid in the joint space — or, to put it another way, the more you move, the better you move.

Ligaments, a form of connective tissue, hold the bones to each other at the joint, while the muscles are anchored to the bones just above or just below the joint by tendons, which are actually the long tapering ends of the muscles themselves. Sometimes there are small fluid-filled sacs called bursae lying between layers of muscles, or between muscles and tendons, close to a joint, to provide further cushioning and lubrication for movement.

A problem with a joint can arise from damage or malfunction involving any of the various parts of the joint: the cartilage, the synovial membrane, the joint fluid, and the connective tissues and muscles which hold the joint in place.

Osteoarthritis, or degenerative joint disease, is by far the most common type of joint problem, since it affects nearly everyone at some time in life. It would be nearly impossible to find an older adult skeleton which showed no signs of cartilage deterioration. At least 30 percent of the total population, and at least 60 percent of people over sixty, have noticeable osteoarthritis. The problem occurs most commonly in the hips, knees, fingers and spine, but may attack any joint or any combination of joints. Unlike rheumatoid arthritis, which is a systemic condition that can be detected by blood tests, osteoarthritis is a local condition, even though it may be found in more than one area at a time.

It is important to remember that not everyone who has cartilage or disk degeneration is bothered by it; it does not always cause pain in the areas where it is found. Many patients with back pain have agreed to have surgery after X-rays have shown signs of spinal deterioration; however, they have often been disappointed in the results, since their pain actually had a source other than arthritis. If you have a back problem, it is very important to explore every possible cause and every possible remedy before agreeing to undergo surgery; even if your X-ray shows degeneration in the spine, this may not be the source of your pain, which may instead be a result of muscle spasm and may be resolved by relieving the muscle spasm. An operation, in that case, may not help at all. The same is true of bone spurs in other joints: a person may have degeneration or spurs without pain, and vice versa. An area where cartilage has degenerated is by no means doomed to pain and stiffness for the rest of its life.

As osteoarthritis is often described as 'wear and tear' arthritis, many people mistakenly assume that this condition results from overuse of the joint. This is not the case. 'Wear and tear' is created as a result of repeatedly using a small portion of the joint, and not using the joint to its full range of motion. Virtually the only time overuse is the culprit is when a joint has been badly injured and is later subjected to overvigorous use, as is the case in a great many sports injuries. A repeated series of heavy impacts or shocks to the joint may also cause damage, and again this is a problem that most concerns athletes, dancers, and carpenters and other laborers. Proper, frequent use of the joints actually promotes the health of the cartilage.

Overstrenuous, tense repetition of the same action or motion, which is involved in many people's work, may also irritate the muscles, tendons and connective tissue which surround a joint, producing arthritis-like symptoms but without damaging the actual cartilage.

Active joints have, if anything, healthier cartilage than inactive joints. A wonderful example of this was the pianist Artur Rubinstein, who gave concerts well into old age. He developed arthritis in many parts of his body, but none in his hands, which had been in constant motion for most of his life. Why did his hands escape when arthritis developed? As a pianist, he would have been using every finger and every joint frequently, fluidly and flexibly. Playing well would depend on the performance of each finger; each would have to be strong and supple, capable of quick, precise and subtle movement. Piano-playing itself fosters exactly these abilities in the fingers, but it may at the same time encourage stiffness in the back, shoulders, neck, hips and knees. Rubinstein gave his fingers exactly what they needed to prevent the development of arthritis: lots of balanced, fluid, low-impact movement. The rest of his body, lacking the same care, became the victim

of the disease. Use of the joints is not the problem — improper use is.

The traditional medical belief has been that cartilage, once destroyed, cannot repair itself. However, some doctors now believe that cartilage, like most other body tissues, usually can and does repair itself, and that arthritis happens only when something prevents this normal repair process. Much research is being done into what may cause this breakdown. We believe that the answer, to a great extent, lies in how we use or abuse our bodies, and that movement is a key to the cure. What most doctors now agree on is that some forms of exercise may be beneficial to joint problems.

Why should movement be so beneficial to the health of the joints, and in particular to the cartilage? There are many reasons. One of these has to do with the synovial fluid. This fluid is to the cartilage as blood is to the rest of the body. There is no direct blood supply to the cartilage: unlike other body tissues, it must receive its oxygen and nutrients from, and expel its waste products into, the fluid in the joint space. It can do this only during movement, when the pressure of the two bones against each other actually forces the fluid into and out of the cartilage. Using the joint — i.e. moving — keeps the joint fluid flowing in and out of the cartilage, so it seems clear that more movement, not less, is needed to prevent cartilage degeneration.

Again, we have to stress that we are talking about proper movement — movement which is balanced, as relaxed as possible, and respectful toward the part of the body being used. Movement which is performed through tension, movement which uses the body in an unbalanced way, movement which places more stress on one side of the body, movement which places undue demands on some muscles while allowing others to atrophy – all of these may have as bad an effect on the joints as on the muscles. Such movement may cause numerous muscles to tighten, thus limiting their capacity to perform their full range of motion – and, as we have seen, this will reduce the circulation of synovial fluid. It may also distort the posture, so that pressure is not evenly distributed on every part of the joint. If only a part of the joint must absorb all the impact of a movement, this will have the same effect as the repeated-shock treatment of the joint that occurs in sports injuries, creating genuine wear and tear of the cartilage. Combined with long periods of non-movement, these destructive movement patterns all contribute to cartilage degeneration.

Often an arthritic condition will develop in just one knee or hip or hand. A patient who is told that her arthritis is due to age may wonder how her arthritic right knee managed to get older than her unaffected left knee. The problem in osteoarthritis is not age: it is abuse. If you are taking good care of your body, it can actually improve with age. If you are not, then it simply suffers that many more years of being neglected, and of course will be worse at seventy than at thirty. The seventy-year-old woman with one arthritic knee and one good one simply has one knee which has been abused and one which has not. Normally this abuse comes in the form of walking and postural patterns which place unbalanced stresses on her body. She may walk more heavily on one foot, causing her leg muscles to stiffen and thus reducing the movement-potential in the ankle, hip and thigh. Or she may habitually sit with her legs crossed at the knees, creating a similar effect. She may have had a job which required her to stand for hours at a time, and may have spent those hours leaning on one

leg with the other more or less dangling; the person who actually stands evenly balanced on both feet is very rare. The effect of this would be to throw the hip socket out of alignment, which would cause pressure on the joint to be unevenly distributed. She may have been sedentary, leading to stiffness in the hips which could affect her walking and standing. Her movement patterns may have originated in a hereditary weakness or in an injury, but they will be reinforced every day by how she moves her body.

Paying attention to how and how much we move can prevent arthritic conditions from developing in the first place, and changing the way we move can do much to alleviate them and prevent them from worsening.

For a discussion of other forms of joint ailments, and exercises which can help, please turn to the chapter on Arthritis.

Promoting Joint Flexibility

When a part of the body begins to function badly, this usually happens because of circumstances which have interfered with its function. The way to restore lost function is to provide circumstances which support it. Often, this means doing exactly the opposite of what we have been doing. Different behavior leads to different conditions. This is one of the first principles in Self-Healing.

The Self-Healing exercises require equal participation of body and mind. You must first become aware of your tensions, and then allow yourself to release them. Many of our tensions go unnoticed: we may tighten our abdomens, wear our shoulders up around our ears, tense our thighs, forget to breathe deeply for hours at a time, clench our fists and grind our teeth, and never be aware of doing so. This is partly because tension is so unpleasant to feel that our conscious minds learn to block it out and we discover its presence only when it has done real damage to our bodies. A major part of learning to relax is acknowledging the tension we have, so that we can work specifically on releasing it.

Much of our muscle tension comes from spasms in our largest, strongest muscles, such as the trapezius muscle which spans the shoulders and upper back, the gluteal muscles of the buttocks, and the quadriceps muscles in the front of the thighs. These muscles are designed to be used, and when the human race was more physically active these muscles had nothing to complain about. Our gluteals, for example, were not meant to provide cushions for our endless sitting. Unfortunately, the only use these muscles get from many people nowadays is to be held rigidly in a fixed position for hours at a time. They protest at this treatment vigorously by going into spasm – a deep, chronic contraction – and staying there. Because these muscles are very strong, and connected to many other muscles, their tension exerts a powerful pull on the surrounding muscles. This in turn affects the ability of the joint to move freely. A contracted trapezius muscle can freeze a shoulder so completely that movement of the elbow and wrist will also be limited. The remedy for this is to give the trapezius the full range of motion which it craves.

Virtually everyone who has ever worked with problem joints agrees that gentle exercises which take a joint through its full range of motion are the ones which help the most. For example, your wrist can be flexed, extended and partially rotated, and has some

limited movement to the right and the left. Taking your joint through all of these motions can promote the health of the joint cartilage, strengthen the muscles and tendons of the wrist, and help to disperse the fluid buildup that often accompanies joint problems. It can do this effectively, however, only if you engage the muscles which are meant to assist in these motions. Most people who try these motions will tighten their shoulders and work hard with every muscle in their arms, rather than engaging the few muscles of the forearm and wrist which are actually needed for these movements. The exercise becomes less concentrated and less effective; you cannot strengthen the wrist by tightening the upper arm. It may seem hard to accept that we very often choose the least functional way of performing a motion, but it is unfortunately so.

The idea of using only the appropriate muscle or muscles for a motion is repeated in this book several times, since it is central to our movement therapy. It is a tribute to the wonderful design of the human body to recognize that certain muscles are ideally suited to certain tasks, and others to completely different tasks – just as we design tools for very specific purposes. The principle of isolated muscle movement is really a principle of relaxation, as it allows unneeded muscles to rest while the few which are needed do the work. Some movement disciplines have taken this concept a step further, into the realm of micro-movement. Micro-movement uses not groups of muscles like regular movement, nor individual muscles like isometric movement, but specific groups of fibers within a muscle. We will encounter exercises for micro-movement within this chapter. In the meantime, we would like you to keep this image in mind as you do each of the exercises: that your motions should be as close to micro-movement as you can make them. Focus your attention closely on the specific area you are working with, and let the rest of your body rest. This will give you maximum flexibility.

In the following pages we will describe movements for promoting flexibility in various joints. Joints vary greatly in structure and function, and so may demand completely different types of movement. You may be particularly interested in working with just one set of joints or just one part of the body, especially if you have had arthritic problems. We strongly recommend, however, that you try all of the exercises, since flexibility and ease of movement in any part of your body can only enhance the functioning of your body as a whole.

Hips

The hip and shoulder joints are similar in structure. They are called ball-and-socket joints, since both the femur (the thigh bone) and the humerus (the upper-arm bone) have a large ball of bone at the top which fits comfortably into, respectively, the pelvis and the scapular bone. This type of joint allows for all categories of movement – moving the limb sideways, away from the body or toward it; moving the limb backward and forward, and rotating it. Not every joint can do that. The knee, for example, is a hinge joint, capable only of straightening and bending.

With such a wonderful potential range of movement, one might wonder why the hips are so often tight, allowing very little actual movement. Part of this is because as adults we do not often take advantage of the hip joint's

movement potential. As children, we kicked, squatted and leapfrogged a lot more than we do as adults. Sitting – one of our favorite grown-up activities – places even more stress on the pelvis than does standing, especially if we sit for long periods in the same position.

If you must sit for long periods, try to vary the angle at which you are sitting. An ordinary chair places your hips and your knees at the same level. On the other hand, a cushion placed on a chair keeps your knees lower than your hips, while sitting in an ordinary chair with your feet on a small stool will bring your knees higher than your hips. Having your knees at the same level or lower than your hips will tend to make your lower back concave, while having the knees higher than the hips will make the back more convex. The more variety you have in your sitting position, the less your back muscles are likely to stiffen; varying your position also varies the amount and location of pressure placed on the hip joints. Make sure that the pressure is evenly distributed on both sides of your body. Sit on both buttocks, with both feet on the floor. Leaning harder on just one hip will stress that joint. Sitting on the floor allows for a wider variety of positions, which may help to explain why people in floor-sitting societies, as for example in the Far East, have less back trouble than Westerners do. We recommend sitting on the floor when possible if it is comfortable for you.

The hip joint is stabilized by very strong, and often very contracted muscles. If the gluteals, abdominals, psoas (connecting the middle and lower spine to the thigh bone) and lower-back muscles are in chronic contraction, the hip will not be free to perform its full range of motion. Its stability will decrease, except within a limited range of motion. In order to loosen the hip, we need to loosen the muscles which hold it.

The gluteal muscles, especially the maximus and medius, are among the body's most powerful muscles. They take part in keeping us upright when we stand or walk. Precisely because they are such strong muscles, they react strongly to stress. In times of stress, those muscles which are involved in either defending ourselves or escaping from danger are contracted to be ready for action. If we do not actually use the muscles then, the contraction can remain in them for a long time. A lot of stress-related lower-back pain actually begins with this tightening of the buttock muscles, pulling downward on the lower-back muscles. Needless to say, it also affects the mobility of the hip. The gluteus maximus and medius are only the top layer of buttock muscles. Beneath them lie the gluteus minimus and the deep lateral rotators, which, as the name suggests, aid in rotating the hip. When the gluteals are contracted, they prevent the underlying muscles from doing their work.

3–1   To relieve tightness in the gluteals, you can sit in a chair or cross-legged on the floor. Shift your weight onto one buttock, and then move your torso in rotation around that hip joint, shifting the pressure of your weight onto each part of the buttock. Move as far forward, backward and to each side as you can while keeping all your weight on that hip. Make twenty or thirty full circles in each direction, then just sit and feel whether there is a difference between the two hips. Do you sit more fully, flatter or more comfortably on the side that you worked with? Do you sense any difference in how your back supports you on that side? Now repeat the exercise on the other side, and notice whether it feels any different

to do the exercise with this hip. Is it more relaxed than the other, or tighter?

3–2   A variation of exercise 3–1 is to sit on the floor, with your back against the wall or a sofa, pull your right knee up to your chest and move as we have described above, around your left hip. This allows less movement of the spine, but strengthens the pressure on the gluteals. Do the same on the other side.

3–3   The effect of exercises 3–1 and 3–2 can be intensified by placing a tennis ball under the buttock, and rotating so that different parts of the buttock are pressed against the ball. You can move the ball around to hit various tight spots. Do not tense against the pressure of the ball, but try to relax into it. If you feel a sharp pain or twinges, you may be pressing the ball against a nerve, in which case you should move it until it presses against a tougher, less sensitive part of the muscle.

3–4   Another way to release tension in a strong muscle is to tighten it even further, then release it, tighten it and release again. To do this with the buttocks, lie face-downward on the floor, place your hands palm-down on the floor in front of you, and raise both legs behind you, knees bent and lifted slightly off the floor, toes pointed toward your hips, as high as you can. Now push yourself up with your arms until your torso down to the pelvis is lifted up off the floor; this motion will bring your legs down to touch the floor (fig 3–4A). Continue alternately raising your legs (fig 3–4B), then your body, then your legs, until you are rocking back and forth like a cradle and using the impetus of one motion to push you into the next.

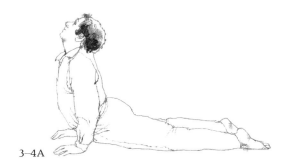

3–4A

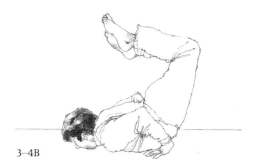

3–4B

This will release buttock tension while it stretches and relaxes the abdominal muscles, including the psoas. (Note: this exercise is also referred to as 'yoga-sex'. It increases circulation to the pelvis, and may help to overcome impotence.)

After you have practiced the exercise several times, lie on your back, bend one knee to your chest, hold it with your hand and move it in rotating motion. Repeat with the other knee.

3–5 Lying on your abdomen, reach back and grasp one ankle with your hand and pull it back toward your buttock (fig 3–5A).

Hold it for several seconds, then release it and tap, squeeze and pound with your fist around the upper buttock, at the top of the pelvic crest. Repeat with your other ankle.

Roll over on one side, and pull your knee up to your chest, then – holding the ankle – pull the foot back as far as you comfortably can (fig 3–5B). Repeat this several times with each leg.

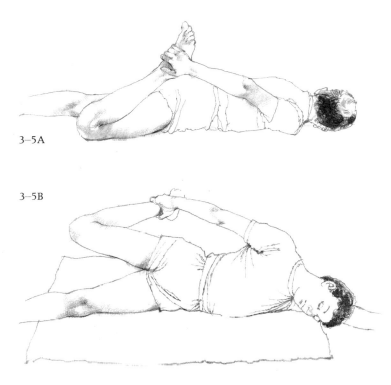

3–5A

3–5B

3–6 Lie on your back with your knees bent and feet flat and lift your pelvis up as high as you can, pressing your shoulders and upper back into the floor to support the weight (see fig 4–8 in the Spine chapter). Hold this position for a count of seven, then slowly lower your hips to the floor. Repeat this several times.

3–7 To release lower back and leg muscles, stand with your back to a wall and touching the wall down to about the middle back, with your feet hip-width apart and about a foot in front of the wall. Begin to move your entire pelvis in a large circle, leaning slightly on the part of your back which is supported by the wall. This takes the burden of supporting you *off* the lower back and outer thigh muscles, which normally tend to work very hard to help you stand. If you do this exercise correctly, the only muscles working will be those which are making the hips rotate. Now slide down a little on the wall, until your feet are about three feet away from the wall, your knees are half-bent and only your shoulders are pressing against the wall, and repeat the pelvic rotations. Next, turn and face the wall, extend your arms and press your palms against the wall, and lean forward so that some of your weight is supported by your palms; in this position, rotate the pelvis as before. This will give you a larger range of motion and let the lower-back and abdominal muscles stretch a little. Now you are ready to focus on the hip joint itself.

3–8 The next exercise is done standing, with one leg raised and resting on something so that it is completely, comfortably supported. This could be a stair, a table-top, the arm of a sofa, a shelf, a counter-top or a ballet bar — anything that will not give way if you push against it. It should be able to support at least half of your weight, and should be just high enough for you to feel a *comfortable* stretch in your hip and thigh muscles. If you are a flexible person, it could be at waist height; if you are less flexible, you will need to make it lower. You may also want to have a chair to hold onto for extra support. Lift your right leg and extend it sideways and up until the arch of the foot is firmly planted against the counter-top, sofa arm or whatever. Take a minute to feel that your left leg is comfortably aligned and firmly planted on the floor, with your weight evenly distributed on each part of your foot. The elevated foot should also be bearing half of your weight. This position leaves the right hip free to move, without having to tense to hold you up.

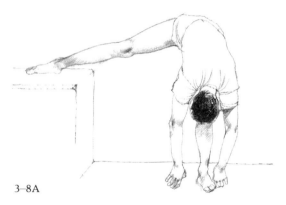

3–8A

Bend your body forward toward the floor (fig 3–8A). Bend your body as far to the left as you can, holding onto a chair for support if necessary. See how far you can extend your head toward the floor, and feel the stretch in the right-hip muscles. Do this facing forward (fig 3–8B) and facing toward the left (fig 3–8C). Now bend toward the right, extending your head toward your right knee. Do this facing forward and facing the right (fig 3–8D). This will stretch your left hip as well as the inner muscles of the right thigh.

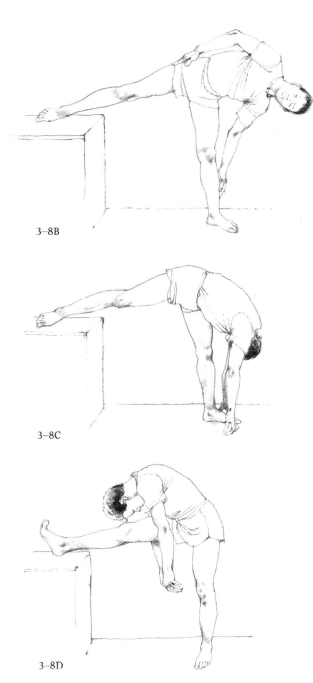

3–8B

3–8C

3–8D

Next, slowly and carefully twist your whole torso sideways, first toward your left shoulder and then toward your right, turning as far to each side as you comfortably can. Continue this twisting motion slowly ten or fifteen times from one side to the other until the motion

feels fluid and smooth, and make sure that your gluteal muscles do not tense as you move. If your feet are solidly bearing your weight, the gluteals do not need to work in this position.

Repeat the exercise with your left leg raised.

3–9 With your right leg raised again, slowly bend and straighten the right knee. Do not allow the left knee to buckle or you will lose the support of your left foot. Meanwhile, both hips are free to relax, and expand. Last, with the knee in its bent position, lower it toward the front (fig 3–9), which will turn your body slightly toward the left; then bring it up and lower it toward the back, which will turn your body toward the right. This last position, especially, opens up your hip joint into a position which normal movement does not often place it in, and so is very freeing for the joint.

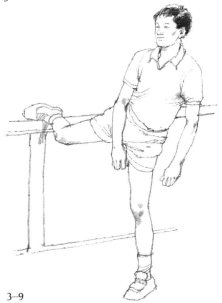

3–9

Repeat this exercise ten times forward and back, pounding lightly with your fist on the extended thigh and on the buttocks as you do so. Now stand on both feet and see if one side differs from the other in sensation. You may feel the difference all the way down to your feet, and up to your shoulders. Repeat all the above exercises with your left leg raised.

See whether you can discover some other ways to move in this position, concentrating on movement which will mobilize the hip.

3–10 Sit on a carpeted floor or a mat, bend each knee out to its own side and bring the soles of the feet together, being careful to keep your weight evenly distributed on your buttocks. Place one hand on each knee and gently press downward, first alternating the pressure from the right knee to the left about ten times and then pressing down on both knees simultaneously (fig 3–10). This motion expands the hip joints and stretches your inner thigh muscles. Feel where there is resistance to the stretch. Is it in the thigh muscles? The groin? The knees? If it is in the knees, proceed slowly and carefully. Do not push on your knees to an extent that causes pain.

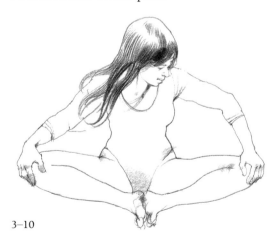

3–10

Lean forward and grasp your ankles, so that your elbows are resting on your knees, and again press the knees down – if you pull upward on your ankles, this will automatically

press the elbows down, and the knees with them. This gives an even greater stretch to the muscles that surround the hip joints.

Now do the same without pressing on your knees – just pulling them down with your leg muscles. Inhale deeply, and lower your knees toward the floor as you exhale.

Last, sit with the soles of the feet together, with your back completely supported against a wall (you can lean against a pillow), and again press down on both knees simultaneously, twenty or thirty times.

3–11 Still sitting on the floor (with your back supported if you feel the need), bend your knees, place your feet flat on the floor and pull your knees up toward your chest (fig 3–11A).

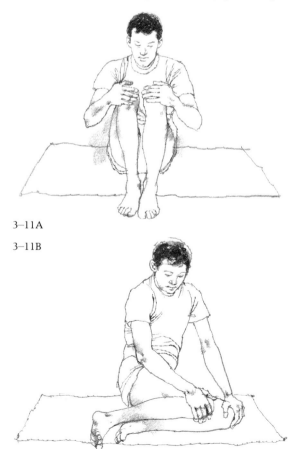

3–11A

3–11B

Grasp one knee in each hand and push the knees down toward the floor on your left (fig 3–11B). Let your legs, back, abdomen and especially your gluteals relax as you do this motion, using only the power of your hands to move your knees up and downward, first to the left, then to the right, five or six times in each direction.

You may feel a strong resistance to this simple motion, especially when it comes to letting your muscles relax when they are so used to controlling the hip motions. Stop and visualize doing this motion, imagining every muscle in your lower body relaxing completely to allow a fluid, unhampered swing from side to side.

With both knees lowered to the right, pound lightly with your fist along the outer left thigh, from hip to knee, going up and down the thigh several times. Then lower the knees to the left and pound along the right thigh. After this visualization and 'massage' (which should leave the thigh tingling and feeling invigorated), try the exercise again, and see whether it feels any easier now.

3–12   Lie on your back with your left leg outstretched, your right knee bent and your right foot resting on your left thigh just above the knee. Keep your foot there as you hold the right knee in both hands and pull it down toward the floor, first to the right (fig 3–12A),

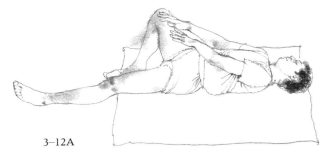

3–12A

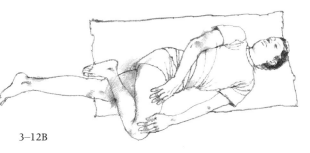

3–12B

then to the left (fig 3–12B). Notice where you feel resistance to this movement – which muscles try to help or to hamper the motion. After you have repeated the exercise several times, stop and massage the areas where you felt resistance.

Massage the lower abdomen, just above the pubic area – massage with both hands, in long deep strokes. Next, massage the groin area and the area all around the pelvic bone. Then try the motion again and see whether it feels any easier. Concentrate on letting all of your muscles relax while just your hands pull the knee from side to side.

Before you reverse your position to repeat the exercise with your right leg straight and your left knee bent, lie on your back with both legs stretched out and see whether you feel a difference between the two sides.

3–13   Still on your back, stretch both legs out flat, then slide them simultaneously out to the sides and then toward each other ten or twelve times, rapidly, without lifting them off the floor. This motion activates and stretches the side muscles of your thighs. As you do this, make sure that your back muscles and abdomen are relaxed, letting the legs do all the work.

3–14   Lying on your left side with your head on a firm pillow, lift your right leg as high as you can, until you feel a slight stretch in the muscles of the inner thigh, then quickly lower

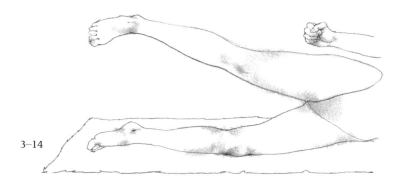

3–14

it so that your back does not have time to become strained. Do this about five times, then lie on your right side and repeat the exercise raising your left leg.

Then, back on your left side, lift your right leg about half as high as it will easily go and rotate it about five times in each direction, swinging the leg in as wide a circle as you can. Imagine that the foot is leading the motion. Pound lightly with your fist along the muscles of the outer thigh, which this exercise will help to strengthen (fig 3–14). If your leg becomes tired, try to imagine that someone else is lifting the leg for you. Breathe deeply into the abdomen, and try not to tense the abdomen, the lower back or any muscles not directly involved in the lifting. Then roll onto your right side and repeat with the left leg.

3–15   Standing, take a chair with a back low enough for you to swing your leg over its top. (If this is completely out of the question, you can swing your leg over the seat of the chair, or even over a couple of books on the floor – find the level which is comfortable for you.) Hold onto the back of another chair, a counter-top or whatever will give you enough support, and rotate your leg around the chair back, several times in each direction (fig 3–15). Now stop and tap your foot on the floor about ten times, while saying to yourself 'foot, foot, foot'

as you tap. Rotate your leg again, and visualize that your foot is leading the motion.

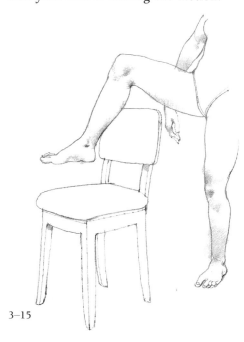

3–15

You may need to start out with only three or four rotations in each direction, but try to build up to fifteen or twenty. This movement will eventually strengthen your legs, but keep in mind that it is meant as a limbering exercise for the hips, and do not challenge yourself unduly by trying to swing your legs higher than you really can. This movement is especially good for increasing circulation to the entire pelvic area, and therefore has proved helpful in dealing with bladder infections, hemorrhoids and digestive problems, as well as muscle tightness.

As we have mentioned before, there is a strong connection between the hip joints and muscles and those of the spine, particularly the lower spine. The Spine chapter contains several sections with exercises especially designed to loosen the hip, which you are now ready to do. Please turn to the Spine chapter, to the sections titled Spinal Flexion, Sideways Stretches for the Lower Back and, of course, Loosening the Hips and Pelvis, and proceed with the exercises listed in these sections. We also recommend exercises 3–37 and 3–38 in this chapter.

Shoulders

The shoulder, like the hip, is a ball-and-socket joint, which means that potentially it has great range and freedom of movement. Potential aside, in most people the shoulder is the tightest area of the body. If you were to ask any group of people where they carry their greatest tension, a great many would say without hesitation, 'In my shoulders.' This tension is primarily a muscular tension, but its effect is to restrict the free movement of the joint. To create greater range of motion and banish shoulder tension, we need to work with two areas: the trapezius muscle of the shoulders and upper back, and the pectoral and intercostal muscles of the chest.

The shoulder is held in place by powerful, massive muscles – five layers of them in the back, three in the front. The outermost, and largest, muscle in the back is a roughly diamond-shaped muscle called the trapezius.

The trapezius muscle shows up throughout this book, and never as a friend. This is unfair, because the trapezius is a very important and helpful muscle. It helps to hold the head upright and to stabilize the scapula (shoulder blade) and clavicle (collarbone), and it participates in every movement of the shoulders. Obviously, to perform all of these functions, it has to be very strong. It is also one of the larger muscles, running from the spine to each shoulder and from the base of the skull to just above the lowest rib. Due to its size and strength, it can cause a lot of trouble.

People who work hard with the trapezius in the course of work or sports – lifting, carrying, digging, swinging a tennis racket or throwing a ball – may have trouble with this muscle if they strenuously repeat the same action in the same way over and over. Some fibers of the trapezius act to lift the shoulder blades, some to pull them down, and some to pull them backward. If one group of fibers goes into chronic contraction, it strains and inhibits the movement of the entire muscle. Moving so that you use all of the various groups of fibers – in other words, moving in a variety of ways – will help to prevent this problem.

Interestingly, it is people who do not use the trapezius vigorously who have the most trouble with it. Those whose jobs allow them little movement, who hold their shoulders and backs rigidly for hours at a time, are the ones who complain most of shoulder pain. This goes back to the point we made before: that strong muscles will rebel against disuse by going into spasm and staying there. Because we are not using them for the things they were originally used for – grabbing, reaching outward and upward, holding tight, carrying, swinging from branches – they store their unused energy in the form of muscle spasm.

The position of our shoulders and chest determines our posture and so both creates and reflects our body image. We use our posture to demonstrate how we see ourselves and how we relate to others. Maureen once watched two women having an argument, and their relative positions were crystal-clear from their postures. One was standing feet apart, fists on hips, shoulders flung back, chin and chest jutting aggressively forward – attacking. The other had her toes turned in, arms crossed on her chest, shoulders rounded forward and chin lowered – just as angry, but primarily concerned with defending herself. Many of us find ourselves in this position of needing to defend and protect ourselves from a world that seems to threaten us, and we reflect it in just that same posture, with the shoulders rounded forward and elevated and the chest caved in. Low self-esteem, a feeling of inferiority or the need constantly to defer to 'superiors' can also make us assume this cringing, 'humble' posture. Holding this position all the time can get to be an awful strain on the trapezius. Perhaps even worse, it cramps our chest so that we can never draw a really full breath. Shallow breathing is a sign of anxiety, and by itself helps to maintain anxiety.

Besides self-defense, our shoulders reflect our sense of responsibility. If our responsibilities seem too heavy, we often feel this sense of burden, of overload, squarely in the shoulders, which will unconsciously contract just as though they are carrying a real, physical load. The expression 'carrying the whole world on your shoulders', like so many body metaphors, describes a feeling based on tangible physical reality. If you feel that you have the world on your shoulders, your shoulders will begin to feel that way too.

The same muscles which provide mobility can also prevent it when they become contracted. Frozen from the back by the trapezius and rhomboids, the shoulders can be immobilized from the front by the pectoral and serratus muscles of the chest. These muscles contract for some of the same reasons that the shoulders do, partly because the forward-rounding of the shoulders depresses the chest cavity, keeping it from full expansion, and partly because we do not usually breathe enough to keep the chest fully mobile. A deep, full breath automatically raises and opens the chest, pushing the shoulders back where they belong – but how often do we take a full, nourishing breath? Many clients we have seen have found how little they really breathe and have been amazed – thinking that this trait is unique. In fact it is almost universal. Anxiety, concentration, pain – almost anything – can make a person forget to breathe. We read that Itzhak Perlman does not breathe, ever, while playing a long and complicated passage of Beethoven's violin concerto, because of his extreme concentration, so it is not just negative emotional states which make people forget their most basic function. (We would love to hear how this passage would sound if he did breathe while playing it.)

Chest tension is common in people who work with their hands at small-movement tasks – in other words, such work as writing, typing, or jewelry-making, as opposed to chopping wood. Tasks which bring the arms close to the body and hold them in one position for long times tend to depress and contract the chest cavity. There is also the problem that when we work with our hands we tend to exert much more effort than is necessary. We start this habit as children, struggling to gain the skills needed to write, and most of us never really get over it. Instead of using the smaller, deeper muscles in the arms and hands, which are better suited to such tasks, we tense our shoulders, upper arms and chest. In our massage classes, we train people to feel that they use just their hands to do massage, and in our movement classes we coach people through everyday activities such as writing, cutting vegetables and so on, showing them how much unnecessary effort they are making and how many unnecessary muscles they call upon to do their work. Letting go of the larger, stronger, external muscles and calling upon the more specialized inner muscles is an important part of improving your joint mobility.

Your shoulders love to move and hate to freeze. They will be happiest if you move them in as many ways as they can be moved — in, out, up, down, back, forward, clockwise and counterclockwise. When the shoulders relax, the entire body has a sense of lightness and release. Sometimes, however, working on the shoulders may be uncomfortable at first, as you become consciously aware of a deep layer of tension and restriction.

3–16   To feel whether your shoulders are tight, sit comfortably in a chair, with your back supported and your feet flat on the floor. Let your hands rest on your knees. If you prefer, you can sit on the floor, as long as your body is relaxed. This is very important, because your shoulders are very sensitive to tension anywhere in the body, and will usually respond to it by becoming more tense themselves.

Now slowly rotate just your left shoulder. Make this a slow, small-range movement, imagining that the edge of the shoulder — where the arm and the shoulder join, and not the shoulder blade — is leading the motion.

Rotate the shoulder ten times in one direction, then ten times in the other, breathing deeply and trying to keep the shoulder as relaxed as possible. Is it difficult to do this? Does your rotation feel smooth, or rough and jerky? Are you able to move the shoulder independently? Imagine that there is a string attached to your shoulder, like one of the strings on a marionette, and that someone else is pulling it. Tap with the fingertips of your right hand several times on the outer edge of your left shoulder, so that you can feel where the movement should be centered. Allow your shoulder blades to be moved almost passively.

Now place your right hand on your right shoulder and feel whether the muscles there are moving as you rotate your left shoulder (fig 3–16).

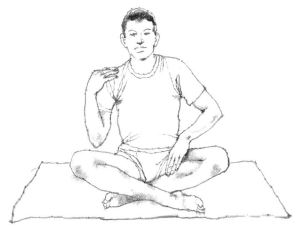

3–16

If they are, try to move the left shoulder in such a relaxed way that the right shoulder will not try to participate. Do this until you feel that the right-shoulder muscles are no longer moving. We recommend rotating the shoulder about fifty times in each direction. Rest and feel whether you notice a difference between the two shoulders; then repeat this exercise with your right shoulder.

This exercise may seem to make you feel more tense at first, as you discover how much tension you are carrying around in your shoulders. Inhale deeply to overcome the tension, and imagine that every muscle in your body is resting, except for those few which are moving the shoulder. Imagine the active muscles moving lightly, smoothly and easily. It may also help to tap on the chest, with a firm, quick tapping motion.

Office workers who take a five-minute break every hour or so to limber their shoulders will find themselves much less tired at the end of the workday. You do not need to move from your chair to take your shoulders through nearly all of their range of movement.

The following sequence of exercises is done with the arms hanging loosely at your sides.

3–17　Inhale deeply, then, as you exhale, bring the shoulders up as high as you can, reaching toward your ears with the outer edges of the shoulders (fig 3–17, right). Keep your shoulders elevated as you inhale for a slow count of five, then slowly lower them as you exhale.

Inhale, and exhale as you lower your shoulders as far as you can (fig 3–17, left). You should feel the muscles across the top of each shoulder and the muscles under your arms working to pull the shoulders down, but the arms should remain hanging at your sides. Keep the shoulders down while you inhale for a count of five, then exhale and let them come up again.

3–18　Breathe deeply in, and, while you exhale, bring both shoulders as far forward as you can without bringing them in toward your breastbone (fig 3–18, right). This motion will move your arms so that your palms face behind you; again, keep the arms as relaxed as possible. Inhale and hold, then exhale while you bring the shoulders as far backward as they will go without turning toward the shoulder blades (fig 3–18, left). Inhale and hold; exhale and relax. Repeat ten times or more.

3–18

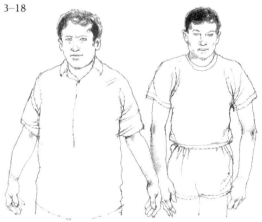

3–17

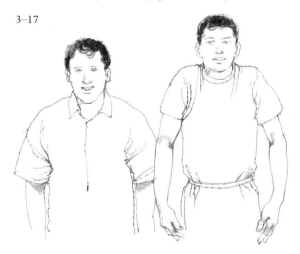

3–19　Repeat exercise 3–18, but this time allow your shoulders to round all the way in, turning toward the breastbone in front (fig 3–19, right) and toward the shoulder blades in back (fig 3–19, left). If your shoulders are normally rounded forward, hold this position twice as long in back as in front. Make sure that you are moving only your shoulders when

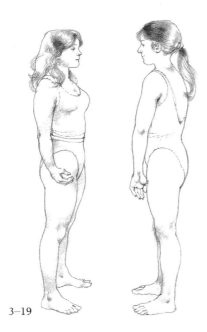

3–19

The next exercises will help you to tense and release tension in your shoulder muscles. Repeat each one five times, inhaling deeply before each movement and exhaling slowly as you do each one. Hold each position for a count of at least five.

3–20   Place your fingertips at the edge of each shoulder, and press your arms close to your sides, lowering your elbows as far as you can (fig 3–20, left). Then raise the arms, raising each elbow out to its own side and as high as you can (fig 3–20, right).

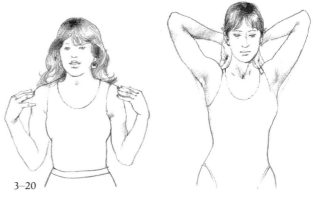

3–20

3–21   Bring the elbows forward, rounding out your upper back (fig 3–21, left). Bring the elbows back, toward your spine, pressing the shoulder blades together and rounding out your chest (fig 3–21, right).

3–21

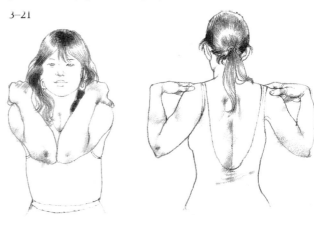

you do this; keep your neck straight, the top of your head level with the ceiling, and your back and abdomen relaxed. Repeat ten times or more.

Now rotate your shoulders again as you did for exercise 3–16, first one – about ten times in each direction, slowly – then the other, and then both together. A small rotation will mobilize the shoulder muscles just as effectively as a large one, and will be much more relaxing for them. Breathe deeply and feel the breath expanding your chest and increasing the distance between your shoulders. The looser your muscles, the more distance you can create between adjacent bones, and thus the less compression you will have in your joints. Pressure on a joint during movement is fine – when you move, you press on the joint and release it, press and release again, and this enables your cartilage to take in and expel lubricating synovial fluid. Tension without movement, on the other hand, decreases synovial-fluid circulation. Repeat ten times or more.

3–22 Move your fingertips so that they rest just below the base of your neck, and raise your elbows up toward the ceiling, as high as they will go (fig 3–22).

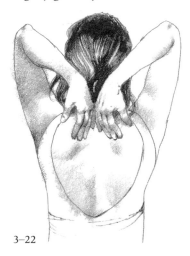

3–22

Notice how each of the above motions involves and activates a different set of muscles. It may be a good idea to finish this set by lowering your arms to your sides and rotating your shoulders twenty or thirty times to shake out any remaining tension.

3–23 Slowly raise both arms up and out to the side, then lower them. Each time you raise them, try, if possible, to elevate them a little higher above shoulder level than the time before.

3–24 Next, lift the arms to shoulder level and bring them forward, until your palms are touching (fig 3–24, left); hold, breathe and then extend your arms as far backward as you can, bringing the shoulder blades together. Imagine that you are trying to bring the backs of your hands to touch behind your back – or actually do so, if you can – and see whether you can get them to move a little further back each time you repeat this exercise. You may find

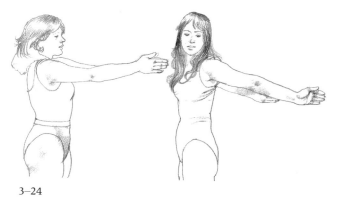

3–24

that if you look back at the stretched arm (fig 3–24, right) it will be easier for you to order it to stretch even further.

3–25 Holding the arms at shoulder level, rotate each arm about its axis as far as it will go about six times in each direction (i.e. a movement from palm-up to palm-down and back, but twist as far as the arm will go in either direction); now do the same while moving your arms in larger circles.

The shoulders and chest are dependent on each other in the same way as the lower back and the abdomen. When your body is working well, the two sets of muscles balance each other; when it is not, they can interfere with each other, each limiting the movement of the other. They often perform opposing functions; for example, the shoulder muscles pull the shoulder blades back, while the chest muscles pull them forward. For this reason, both must be equally strong and active.

In the Breathing and Circulation chapters, we have emphasized the need to expand our range of motion in both shoulders and chest, since you cannot really free the shoulders if the chest is still frozen – and vice versa. The shoulder joints, in particular, will not enjoy their full freedom of movement if either the chest or the shoulders is tight. Please turn now to the Breathing chapter, to the section entitled Stretching your Breathing Muscles, and practice the exercises listed there (1–7 to 1–14). Next, turn to the Circulation chapter's section entitled Creating Movement in the Chest and Shoulders and practice the exercises there (2–11 to 2–17).

Of course, the easiest way to move your shoulders is to have someone else do it for you. It may be that there is no other area in the body where passive movement is so helpful. This is because, as we have mentioned, the shoulder tends to work harder than it needs to, and to participate in movement where its help is not needed. This establishes an automatic nervous response in which your shoulder will contract a little every time you move any part of your body. You can change this habit – actually reprogramming your nerve response – by having the shoulder relax and let go and allow itself to be moved with no effort at all.

Massage is the best way to begin to loosen a shoulder. The person being massaged should either sit or lie on one side with a couple of pillows supporting the head. If the person has a neck or shoulder injury or problem, however, one of you should consult with a doctor about the massage techniques you use.

3–26 First squeeze, with both hands, the muscles that run along the top of the shoulders. Grasp them hard, pull upward on them and shake them, gently or vigorously as your partner prefers. Tap along the side of the neck and shoulder, all the way out to the shoulder's edge. Then, instead of tapping, palpate with all of your fingertips, in a rotating motion, up and down the neck and shoulder. On the neck area, you should not work hard enough to

cause pain, but on the shoulders people can often put up with a little pain, because the muscles there are tougher – in fact, the pain can sometimes feel like a needed release. Repeat the tapping and palpating massage on the other side. If your partner is sitting, push the head slightly down toward one shoulder while you work on the opposite side of the neck.

With your fingertips or thumbs, press deeply into the area surrounding the inner edge of the shoulder blade. Almost everyone has a knot of hard, tight muscle in this area, along with a buildup of connective tissue. This area can withstand a great deal of pressure, particularly if the connective tissue there is tough, and it may in fact need a lot of pressure in order to release its tension. If your partner can tolerate it, you can try pressing with your knuckles, or even your elbow, but start with very light pressure, increasing it only gradually, and reminding your partner to breathe deeply. His breathing will expand the upper back, creating an answering pressure against your massage, so that the muscles will be in a sense massaged from both sides at once. The deep breathing allows the person to feel the area better, as well.

3–27 Now take hold of the arm at the shoulder and wrist, and move it in rotation, making the circle as wide as you can, moving it ten or fifteen times in each direction. Take it in both hands and gently pull it straight out from the shoulder, shaking it vigorously. Pull it upward from the shoulder and shake again, then pull it down and backward and shake.

3–28 Put one palm in front of the shoulder and one behind it, and move it in rotation, stretching it as far forward and backward as it will go. Massage and tap with your fingertips on the upper chest area, and then rotate the shoulder again. If the person is lying on his side, with his back to you, press the shoulder forward toward the floor, then pull it back toward you to expand the chest. If he is sitting, place your palm behind one shoulder while you grasp the outer edge of the other, and turn him from side to side by simultaneously pushing one shoulder and pulling the other, alternately. Stand behind him, have him bend his elbows so that they point toward his back, then take hold of both elbows and pull them back toward you and upward, as far as it is comfortable for him. Still standing behind him, have him raise his arms above his head and bend them so that the elbows are pointing, as nearly as possible, toward the ceiling; take hold of both elbows and gently pull them back and downward, toward you. These stretches are good for the whole back.

You can do this helpful bodywork for the people you work with while they sit at their desks, and you can do it in your small therapy groups. It is a good idea to meet more often when you are working intensively on the shoulders, since this area needs more relaxing, more often than almost any other part of the body. Because of their sedentary lifestyle and their work, which often involves a lot of writing, typing and other work with the arms and hands, many people suffer with their shoulders; however, if your group prefers to concentrate on something else, do so by all means.

Knees and Ankles

These two joints are structured very differently. What they have in common is that both are weight-bearing joints, and both can be helped by many of the same exercises. The knee is the next-largest joint in the body, after the hip and shoulder, and one of the joints most frequently affected by both osteo- and rheumatoid arthritis. It is a very different structure from the ball-and-socket joints. Like the elbow, it is a hinge joint; it can bend and straighten (flex and extend), but its sideways and rotational movement is limited. There are several reasons for this. The knee is a major weight-bearing joint; when we take a step, the knee and ankle together momentarily take all of our body weight. Both are therefore designed for maximum strength, but the knee is less mobile. The knee has two joint capsules, an inner and an outer, and, rather than just being the joining-place of the thigh and calf bones, it has an extra bone, the patella or kneecap, which protects the joint in front and allows tendons to slide smoothly over the knee joint.

The knee is a complex structure, and an unusually rigid joint. In addition, most of us have a tendency to walk rigidly, which limits our range of motion. A synovial joint, as we have explained, needs freedom of movement to keep cartilage healthy. The knee's freedom of movement is limited to begin with. If any of the tissues that surround the knee is tense, mobility will decrease further. If there is weakness in a tendon or ligament, surrounding tissues will automatically tighten to keep the knee stable. Most of the exercises in this section are designed to strengthen and relax the tendons and muscles of the knee, to allow the joint its maximum freedom.

Most knee problems begin with the way a person walks. A stiff or unbalanced walk does as much damage as an injury; it just does it more gradually. Many people walk and stand with their toes habitually turned out or in rather than straight forward. In some people, this is structural, and can be partially or fully corrected. In many it develops as a result of tense or weak muscles in the back, pelvis, hips and legs – and therefore can be corrected fully. This type of gait can cause cartilage to wear out unevenly, putting much more stress on some areas of the joint than on others, and so may be the beginning of arthritis.

Even more common is a stiff-legged gait that keeps the knees locked, denying them even their natural range of movement. The two most common types of stiff-legged gait are shuffling, in which the person drags the legs, barely lifting them off the ground, and kicking the leg forward slightly with each step, but again without lifting it much off the ground or bending the knee. Shuffling sends the impact of each step – which should be absorbed by the foot and ankle – into the knee and hip joints, while kicking the leg forward sends most of it crashing into the patella. Nearly everyone we have seen with a knee problem walks with the latter type of gait, in both the injured knee and the uninjured knee. So the first thing we do is to retrain them in walking. For a complete description of this process, please turn to the Muscles chapter, the section on Learning to Walk.

3–29 The best way to begin work on your knees is to have them massaged. If you can get someone else to do this for you, by all means do so, but it should not be difficult to give yourself a very effective knee massage. You should sit in a comfortable chair or sofa, with your knees bent and your feet flat on the floor, or with the legs propped up in front of you, knees slightly bent and supported by pillows, or in any other position you feel comfortable in. Use a massage cream or oil so that you can rub firmly, but never roughly. Your knees will tell you how hard to rub – never hard enough to hurt. Massage with long firm strokes up from the shin, and up from the knee along the thigh. Interlace your fingers, rub the palms briskly together to warm them, and then rub with the whole hand in circles all around the knee area. Place your palms flat on the thigh, or to either side of the kneecap, and shake them, to ease the stress on the tendons and ligaments and soften any rigid connective tissue. Press with your thumbs and fingertips all around the kneecap, above and below, palpating and stretching the muscles (fig 3–29).

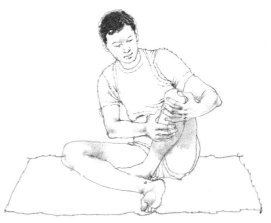

3–29

Tap with your fingertips all over and around the knee, including the back of the knee, and do this until the knee feels warmed and stimulated. This massage should be done before any kind of exercise session that works the knees, and is very helpful in preventing sports injuries. People with knee problems should massage their knees daily, for about fifteen minutes, for at least three weeks before going on to any more vigorous form of exercise for the knees. This is something you can do to make watching television less of a waste of time.

If you have arthritis or a knee injury, your knees may be too swollen or painful to tolerate much direct movement. In this case, you can start with exercises which move the knee indirectly, almost passively, without stress to the surrounding tissues. In the following exercises, the primary mover is the ankle, and so they are helpful for both ankles and knees. We suggest that you practice exercises 3–30 to 3–32 with one knee before changing to the other knee.

3–30 Sit in a comfortable chair, with your back supported and your feet flat on the floor in front of you. Hold one knee firmly with both hands and shake it from side to side, keeping the foot in place. Next, lift all but the heel of that same foot off the floor, so that the foot is completely flexed, and then lower the toes to the floor again. Try not to tense your thigh or anything else as you do this. Imagine that your toes are pulling the rest of the foot up with them, and that gravity pulls the toes down again. Repeat this several times, and notice how, although you are not 'moving' your knee, the muscles and ligaments around the knee are being moved, as is the patella. Even this slight motion is helpful to the synovial space and its cartilage. Continue this exercise, this time turning the ankle slightly so that you lower the toes first to the right then to the left, repeating this ten times. This kind of gentle sideways stretch is especially beneficial to the knee, which is most resistant to sideways motions.

3–31 Now, still keeping the heel on the floor, rotate the ankle in small circles, clockwise and counterclockwise. Concentrate on the movement of the toes, so that you will not tense your knee. Place your hands on your knee, and feel in front, in back and on either side as you move the foot, so that you can feel the movement within the knee.

3–32 Next elevate the same foot on a footstool or a cushioned chair, with a pillow or rolled towel under the thigh to keep the leg slightly bent. In this position, go through the same set of exercises as above: flex and extend the foot, point the toes to the right and to the left, and rotate the foot. This position will give you more range of motion, and you should be able to feel even more clearly the movement around the knee. When you have repeated each movement ten times in each direction, stop and rest the knee and see how it feels. Stand up and notice whether it feels different from the other knee. Even if you have been working on your weaker knee, it may feel warmer and more 'alive' than the knee that you have not moved.

Repeat all of the above three exercises with the second knee.

3–33 Sitting in your chair again, move both feet in small circles (one clockwise and one counterclockwise) without lifting them off the floor. As before, try not to tense your thighs or pelvis. If you do feel yourself tightening, notice where – thighs, hips, groin, calves, abdomen? Some people have a habitual tightness in one or more of these areas which is tied in with a knee problem. If this is the case for you, you may want to work on the tight areas concurrently with working on your knees. Breathe into the area to relax it, and imagine that your feet are doing all the work. At the same time, notice how much this small movement engages the knees, moving them in every direction they are capable of moving. This is the beauty of rotational movement. After about twenty rotations, reverse the direction of the circles.

3–34   Sitting on a chair, lift one foot a few inches off the floor and slowly rotate the calf, with the knee as the center of the circle. If it helps, you can hold your thigh with your hands (fig 3 34) or support it with a pillow, but if the knee is very painful it is best not to do this exercise. If it is only slightly painful, you can do several repetitions of the movement, then massage the area to take away any lingering discomfort.

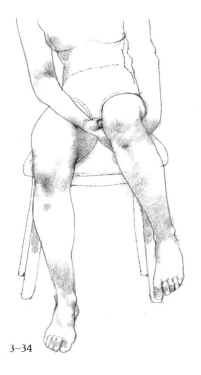

3–34

It is all right if you feel the muscles just above the knee tightening a little in this exercise, since it is meant to strengthen them as well as

to limber the knee. You will be able to see your increased strength as you gradually work up to fifteen rotations in each direction, but do not push yourself.

3–35   Lie on your back with both legs outstretched, and alternately bend and straighten one leg, keeping your foot on the floor. This exercise can also be done in a semi-reclining position, with the middle and upper back elevated and supported by pillows, the lower back and buttocks on the floor, making the movement less work for a weak back (see fig 2–30 in the Circulation chapter). The most important objective in this exercise is to avoid using your back or your abdomen to move your leg – do not let them work. If you feel them tensing, stop and relax them before continuing with the exercise. Knees get weak partly because many of us use the lower back to move our legs and hips, instead of making our leg muscles carry us. If you refuse to let your back or abdomen contract unnecessarily when bending the leg, this exercise will strengthen your lower thigh muscles as well as the knee ligaments. As soon as the leg begins to tire, stop and imagine that you are bending and straightening it effortlessly, as the foot leads the motion, and then try again.

You may find this exercise much easier with one leg than the other, but try to practice it equally with both. When you have done it with each leg, do it with both, bending one as you straighten the other. Then try it with the knees bent out to the sides. Your legs may feel wobbly and weak at first, and you may need to move them slowly, but this is fine, as long as they move for themselves.

Refer to exercise 2–25 in the Circulation chapter. This exercise encourages movement within the joint space of the knee rather than around it; you may be able to feel the bones moving slightly, with a small clicking sound. It is excellent for helping to disperse the fluid that can build up in an arthritic knee.

3–36   Lying on your back, with knees bent and feet flat, move the feet in circles on the floor, as you did while sitting (exercise 3–33). Breathe deeply to expand your lower back and abdomen and keep them from tightening, and imagine that the feet are leading the motion. You can make the circles as large or as small as is comfortable for you; the main concern is to let go of the back, abdomen and hips and increase the range of motion.

All types of passive movement are wonderful for the knees. Refer to the Massage chapter, exercise 7–26.

If you feel that your knees are strong enough, you can do most of the movements described there easily by yourself, but doing them with a partner is easier to begin with, and a great way to stretch without straining. The person being massaged needs to remember to let go as much as possible and let the other partner do the work. If a movement feels like too much of a stretch, do not tense to restrict it – just ask the massaging partner to stop doing it and do something more comfortable instead.

3–37   Last, here are some simple sitting stretches to get your knees more comfortable with sideways motions. Sit on the floor with your knees bent and pulled up toward your chest, feet flat on the floor, about three feet apart from one another. Your palms should also be flat on the floor, behind your hips, so that they support all your upper-body weight.

With your knees apart, lower both knees to the right until they touch the floor, or as far as you can stretch them comfortably (fig 3–37).

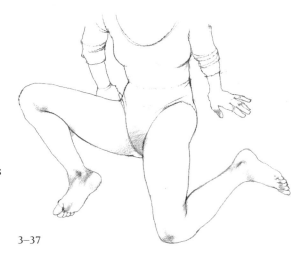

3–37

Bring them up, together, and lower them to the left. This is an exercise that we recommend for the hips and lower back, since it stretches the abductors of the hips – the muscles that move the leg sideways, away from the midline – but you can feel how it also gently stretches the ligaments on the inner and outer sides of the knee. Repeat the exercise at least ten times.

3–38   Sit in the same position as in exercise 3–37, and this time lower only one knee, in the direction of the opposite foot. Your left knee should bend toward the center line of your body, as if it were trying to touch your right foot. This is an exercise that should be done carefully and gradually. Do not force your knee down to the floor; let it take its own time stretching. Stroke the stretched knee with your open palm, rotating all around the knee area. Pound lightly with an open fist on the stretched hip. Repeat the exercise at least twenty times.

3–39 Lie down on the floor and bring your knees to your chest. Hug your thighs and kick with your legs one by one. Flex your foot as you straighten your leg; relax it as you bend the leg. Repeat this exercise at least twenty times.

Wrists

Even if your wrists have never given you a twinge, you should take care to work on this area. Most people tense their wrists whenever they work with their hands, tightening the muscles there to do the work which should be done by the fingers instead. The resulting tension can be felt all the way up to the shoulders. The wrists are prone to rheumatoid arthritis, tendinitis, and carpal-tunnel syndrome – probably because most people use their wrists with so much tension. The following exercises will show you how to relax your wrists, and how to use them without strain.

Practice exercise 2–20 from the Circulation chapter, either lying down or sitting with the forearms supported. Practice with only one hand, and then repeat the whole process with the other hand.

Practice exercise 2–21 from the Circulation chapter.

3–40 Tapping on muscles is one of our favorite bodywork techniques for releasing tension and bringing circulation quickly to an area. It is also one of the best ways to loosen your wrists, if you do it correctly. Try tapping on your chest or thighs as you lie on your back. Let your hands relax completely, with the fingers lightly curved as they normally are in repose. All of the motion should come from your wrist. Let it flop loosely, so that your fingers fall onto and bounce off the muscles you are tapping. The less you try to control the tapping, the looser your wrist will be, and the better the tapping will feel. If your fingers or wrists are rigid, the touch will feel harsh and prodding. It may help to imagine that you are gently shaking something from the ends of your fingertips.

3–41 Spread your fingers as far apart from each other as they will go, and hold them that way as you move your wrist in rotation (fig 3–41). You will be able to feel movement among the carpal bones – the cluster of small bones which compose the wrist – as you do this, as well as in the wrist joint itself.

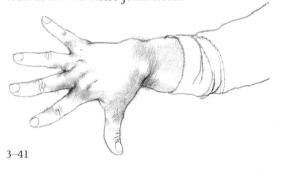

3–41

3–42 Passive movement of the wrist will relax your whole arm and chest. Ask your partner to hold your wrist and move it in rotating motion; to extend it as far as it will go comfortably by bending the hand backward, with the back of the hand toward the outside of the arm; and then to flex it by bending it forward, with the palm toward the inside of the arm. Your partner can hold your wrist, applying constant but gentle pressure on it, giving you a sense of lengthening. You can also do these types of passive movement by yourself.

Hands and Fingers

The fingers are one of the areas most frequently affected by various joint problems. Although most of us use our hands a great deal, we may not use them in a way which exercises the individual joints of each finger. Increasing flexibility and joint use in the hands is very easy. To begin your work on your hands, please turn to the Massage chapter, exercises 7–1 to 7–7 and 7–24. These exercises will show you how to take your fingers through their full range of movement, as well as increasing their circulation and muscle suppleness and strength.

More exercises for the hands and fingers can be found in the Musicians chapter.

If you are starting out with advanced stiffness or pain in your hands, you can make these exercises easier by doing them with your hand or hands immersed in a large bowl or basin of warm saltwater, which will help to drain swelling, improve your circulation and make any movement easier to do. Best of all would be to have someone else massage and passively move your hands in the ways we have suggested, then to do the exercises in warm water, and last to do them yourself as described. Remember that you are interested in achieving the fullest range of movement which is reasonably possible for you. If this range of movement is very small at first, do not be discouraged. Any movement at all, passive or active, is beneficial to your joints. Every small movement will eventually make larger movements possible.

CHAPTER 4

Spine
Balance frees you from pain

Eighty percent of the world's population suffers needlessly from back pain. Our purpose is to help change this reality. We strongly recommend this chapter to anyone who is reading this book, no matter what their special interest or problem may be. If you do not suffer from back pain, you can use the program offered here to prevent it. If you suffer from minor aches, this chapter will help you overcome them. If you do suffer from back pain, start with the chapter on Back Pain.

Hippocrates often found it useful to massage people's backs when he couldn't diagnose their problem. We share with him the concept that keeping the back healthy is very important for one's overall health: a good posture allows better breathing and circulation, more mobility and a general sense of well-being.

With the exception of victims of accidents and injuries, very few people should be suffering from back pain.

We are much more aware of the fronts of our bodies than of our backs. Some of the reasons for that are technical. For one, the nerve-endings in our backs are quite sparse. Second, there is less brain area in charge of the back than there is for one hand. In addition to those, there are the behavioral reasons. To mention just two: we respond to visual stimuli in front of us, and we move forward more frequently than backward. In order to balance the function of the body, we need to try first to balance its sensations. When you learn to sense your back, you bring it more circulation and more movement; you can reduce the stress on its various joints and support all of your body better.

Structure of the Spine

The skeletal spine consists of thirty-three bones called vertebrae, each separated from its neighbour by a flat, round cushion called a disk. The uppermost seven vertebrae support the neck and are called the cervical vertebrae. The next twelve support the middle and upper back and are attached to the twelve pairs of ribs; these are called the thoracic vertebrae. Next come the five lumbar vertebrae, at the lower back; then the five sacral vertebrae, which are fused into a single solid structure called the sacrum. The sacrum attaches to the hipbones on the sides. Last are the four small coccygeal vertebrae which comprise the coccyx, a vestige of the tails our ancestors had.

Each vertebra consists of a cylinder-shaped part, known as the vertebral body, and several projections, or processes, which stand out from the back and sides of it. Two of these projections meet behind the vertebral body, creating an opening, or foramen, between them. The foramina of the adjacent vertebrae create a tunnel, the vertebral canal, which serves the very important function of supporting and protecting the delicate spinal cord, a rope of nerves which, together with the brain, forms the central nervous system. Virtually all of the information about sensation and movement which passes between your body and your brain is carried through the spinal cord. From this central cord, nerve roots exit between the vertebral processes, branching again and again to reach nearly all parts of your body.

The disks consist of a semi-liquid, jelly-like center called the nucleus, which is held in place under strong pressure by a tough outer casing called the annulus. These disks cushion the vertebral bones and create space between them, enabling the spine to withstand pressure and absorb shock.

How Do You Create a Bad Back?

Almost any movement of the body will affect the back in one way or another. Movement which is performed sharply, strenuously, rigidly will have repercussions for the back, both in the spine itself and in the back muscles. Posture, too, influences the back more than it does any other part of the body, and chronic poor posture has an extremely degenerative effect on the condition of the spine.

There is no doubt that people have suffered from backache throughout recorded history. It does seem clear, however, that the current epidemic proportions of the problem are a more recent phenomenon. People who work at jobs involving heavy strenuous physical labor have always been the most obvious candidates for back troubles. It is interesting to notice, however, that, as fewer people work at jobs involving heavy labor and more people at sedentary jobs, the number of back-pain sufferers increases. All the evidence suggests that a sedentary job, and a sedentary lifestyle in general, will tend to make a person more vulnerable to spine problems – especially if he or she is also under a lot of emotional stress. While it is certainly true that a great many accidents are caused by strenuous movement of the back, it is also true that this usually happens when the injured person is habitually sedentary and has suddenly decided to become active, thereby pushing a weak back beyond its limits. A strong person in good condition, accustomed to using his or her back muscles in a balanced, coordinated way, will be less likely to be injured in such a situation. If the back is weak, tense and used incorrectly, you will very likely end up injuring it whether your work is active or sedentary.

We believe that movement is the key to a healthy spine – to creating it, to maintaining it and to restoring it when it has been injured. The vast majority of 'bad backs' will respond favorably to the right kind of movement. Movement is like a vitamin: if you have a deficiency, this will create obvious symptoms; but when it is restored to the body the symptoms will disappear. Unfortunately, most of us have to admit that our lives are deficient in movement.

Before technology took over so much of the manual labor in our lives, most people got plenty of exercise in the course of a day. Exercise was a fact of life, not an optional activity. Of course, people then had all kinds of problems resulting from the *way* they used their backs, but because they were active and engaged in a wide variety of movements they were able to keep many muscles strong and functional. Now, in order for many of us to get any exercise at all, we must plan our lives carefully in order to fit it in. Often we have to take a trip, and even bring special workout clothes, to get exercise. If we are lucky enough to find a physical activity we enjoy – walking, running, swimming, dancing, aerobics – and can do it on a regular basis, it becomes one of the great joys of our lives something that makes everything else easier because it imparts to the body such a sense of energy and well-being. For many people, however, even the thought of exercise is tiresome, and the performance of it is a tedious chore. To a body which has lost the habit and rhythm of movement, exercise comes to seem *unnatural*.

For this reason, we think it is very important to restore to people a sense of the pleasure of movement before teaching them specific exercises. Fans of running, swimming, aerobics or other forms of dance already know the sense of physical and emotional pleasure that these activities can give. Movement first of all increases circulation, aiding the blood in carrying nutrients to the cells and carrying toxic waste materials away from the cells; it increases the body's supply of oxygen, which further speeds circulation and refreshes the brain. It improves muscle elasticity – that is, the ability of the muscles to constantly change from contraction to relaxation – and prevents the buildup of hard connective tissue which can inhibit movement. It may also increase the body's production of endorphins. These

chemicals are produced in the brain and have an effect on the body similar to morphine, relieving pain and producing a feeling of mild euphoria.

With movement, as with most other things, how you do it is just as important as what you do. Movement alone is no guarantee of a healthy back. In fact, vigorous movement that is done without sensitivity to the body can sometimes do more harm than good – which is one reason why sports medicine has become such a profitable business. You must become aware of the condition of your back before you can use movement helpfully. If you have muscles which are extremely tight, you'll need to do exercises which will loosen them before using them vigorously. To avoid serious injury, weak muscles must be built up gradually, and the movements which relax a muscle may be very different from those which strengthen it. Most people have both tight and weak muscles in their backs, though the distribution of strain and weakness is different in each person. If you have tried some type of vigorous exercise and found that it didn't make you feel better, or actually seemed to make things worse, then you probably need to become more aware of your back and its particular needs. Self-Healing exercise is a very helpful – and often a very necessary – supplement to a program of more aerobic exercises. It will make any movement you do more effective.

It is also true that the pleasures of vigorous exercise are often not available to the back-pain sufferer, who may be starting from the basic position of flat on the afflicted back. Fortunately, the great majority of our Self-Healing exercises are done in this position. In Maureen's 'Relaxation through Movement' classes, usually over half of the participants have signed up in the hope of overcoming a back problem. Most of them will show up at the class at the end of a strenuous workday spent at a desk or in front of a computer, and the relief with which these people sink to the floor and roll onto their backs is obvious. Getting them up on their feet is a real chore, and Maureen usually does not even attempt it until after a good half-hour of gentle stretches and rotations to relax and limber every joint and muscle of the spine.

Movement is a way of extending your boundaries, of breaking through your limitations. This is as true for a physically active person as for one who is completely sedentary. The dancers and athletes in the class have as many problems with their backs and as much to learn about their bodies as the office workers. They may move more often and more vigorously, but often they are moving the same few overworked muscles in a mechanical and ultimately very stressful way. For these people, 'more movement' means movement of more of their muscles, increased lung capacity and better blood-flow. We can all move better than we do, no matter where we begin. You may be the world's fastest runner or strongest weight-lifter, but if you are moving without breathing deeply, or moving with stiff muscles, or moving in a way that places dangerous stresses on weak points, then you have as much to learn and as much room for improvement as anyone else. So whether you are starting from square one (the couch) or you are a champion marathon runner, if you want a healthy back you must bring increased movement to your whole body and increased awareness, sensitivity and even creativity to your movement.

If you are working seriously to improve your back, spend at least forty-five to fifty minutes working with it per day, and focus on eight to ten exercises in each session. Repeat each movement exercise at least thirty times, or else it will not be effective.

4–1 Standing We will start out on our feet, to get a true sense of how the back feels. First, you will want to take off your glasses, shoes, belt and anything else that might constrict your movement. Stand with your feet about hip-width apart and your weight distributed evenly on both feet, knees very slightly bent and arms hanging loosely at your sides. Your head should be neither tilted backward nor forward, but simply held straight so that the top of your head is parallel with the sky. Visualize your spine – including the neck – as being very long and very straight. Visualize your back as being very wide: your head goes up to the sky, and each shoulder goes to another part of the universe.

Breathe deeply and imagine that your back is soft and that each breath is expanding the different areas of your spine, especially if those areas feel 'sunken', as is often the case with the lower back. Let your breath fill you so that your shoulders separate, your chest and diaphragm expand, and your spine straightens.

If you think this seems like a lot of directions just for taking a stance, you are right – but there is a reason for it. Learning to stand can be the basis for developing good posture, by which of course we mean a posture which is good for the back. Notice what happens to you when you try to stand as we have suggested. Is it hard for you to keep your head straight? Do your arms feel uncomfortable just hanging there – wouldn't they really prefer to be doing something? Do your shoulders try to sneak back up into their usual position, somewhere around your ears? Stand first with your palms turned inward, then turn them outward – do the two positions feel quite different? How do you feel about standing on both feet; do you find yourself settling back onto one foot with the other hip and leg uselessly extended? Next time you go to a public place, look around at the people there and notice how they stand. You will find that almost none of them stand on both feet. It also becomes clear, if you take an analytic look at this common posture, how bad it is for the spine, completely distorting the vertebral alignment and distributing gravitational stresses in an unbalanced way. Most of us spend dozens of thousands of hours in this position. How could this not, ultimately, affect the spine?

If you feel comfortable with the stance we have described, that is wonderful. If not, then notice where your difficulties are and this will tell you – if you don't already know – where some of your major tensions are: the neck; the shoulders; the upper, middle or lower back; the sacrum or the hips. You will naturally want to concentrate on the areas that bother you the most, but keep in mind that you will need to work on the back as a whole in order to truly improve any one part.

Each part of your back supports the part above it. When your legs are strong and your hips flexible and balanced, your back will have good support. When your lower back is flexible and strong, your middle and upper back will be supported well. When your middle and upper back are strong and loose, your neck and head will not need to tense. If you suffer from neck pain, don't start searching for the cause in the neck itself – you will have to loosen your whole back before your neck is relieved. A weak lower back may create muscle stresses which result in shoulder pain. If you

are working on one area and your intuition tells you to move to another for a while, go ahead and try it. Tightness often results from a problem in another area of the body. A tight chest may result in mid-back pain. A tight back may result in wrist or finger problems. Keep searching for these connections in your body, because only through discovering the origins can you solve the local problem.

What this stance is aiming at is to get you as relaxed as you possibly can be and still stay upright. When you feel that you have relaxed as much as you can, you are ready to begin exercise 4–2, the spinal arch.

Return to this first exercise time and again, to see whether your back is more balanced. The more relaxed and mobile your back will be, the more your feet will put an even pressure on the floor.

4–2 Spinal Arch Stand with your feet about hip-width apart and your weight distributed evenly on both feet, your knees bent very slightly and your arms hanging loosely at your side. First form a mental image of your spine, then begin to *very slowly* bend forward, imagining that you are moving one vertebra at a time and making an arch of your spinal column. First the head will bend until the chin touches the chest, next the shoulders will curl forward, next the upper back, and so on as far down the spine as you can bend. You should make a special point of visualizing and trying to sense your middle and lower-back areas, which most people can barely feel, much less imagine moving independently. Each motion should bring the top of your head a little closer to the floor.

You may not be able to actually feel the individual movement of each vertebra at first; in fact, some of the vertebrae will undoubtedly feel completely rigid in your areas of greatest tension. You also may not be able to bend all the way over and touch the floor at first. It is important not to try to force this on your back. Bend as far as you can comfortably. When you start to feel a pull in the hamstring muscles in the backs of your thighs, bend more slowly – and remember to keep sensing the movement in your back. This movement will stretch both the back and the legs, but our main purpose here is to stretch out the back muscles and create space between the vertebrae. As you bend, visualize the spaces between the vertebrae and imagine them constantly widening.

Let your body hang loosely from the hips (make sure you are not holding your arms or your head rigidly) and sway gently from side to side (fig 4–2). This sway should have a slight up-and-down movement, like the elephant swing children do. This relieves pressure in the sacrum and loosens the hip and lower-back muscles.

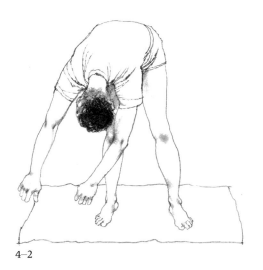

4–2

After about a minute of hanging loosely and swaying, you can start to uncurl your spine. To straighten up, you move in the opposite

sequence to the one you used to make your arch – that is, you begin at the base of the spine and *very slowly* straighten your spine, bringing the head up last. You will probably notice your back muscles tensing to try to help you pull yourself up. To avoid this, visualize your feet supporting you completely; bear down on them a little and mentally 'send' your weight down into your feet so that your spine can lift itself without effort. When you are standing upright, move your head in a rotating motion, stretch your arms up over your head and bend backward a little.

Now repeat the entire process from the beginning, several times. When you have done so, stand and again evaluate how you feel, just as you did in the beginning. Do you notice any changes in your stance, in your sense of being supported, in your posture? Most important, does your back feel longer, looser – in short, more expanded? If so, take note of what these changes are and how they feel. If not, it might be a good idea for you to begin with the exercises in the next section, which are done lying on the back. In this position you don't have to oppose gravity, and your back may appreciate that. You can also practice the sitting spinal arch, exercise 4–21, before you return to this exercise.

As you bend and straighten your spine, notice where your rigid areas are. Stop at that level, even if you have only moved your head halfway to your chest, and for a minute or so just move around that area, stretching to the left and right, rotating, or bending and straightening just that small area of the spine. Then keep moving, up or down. After several repetitions of this process – we recommend a minimum of six – you may find that you can bend much further than you could on the first try, and your spine may move more fluidly and easily. The movement has stretched and warmed your muscles, eased pressure on the vertebral joints, and stimulated a flow of synovial fluid in the spinal joints. Over time, the movement will also help to soften the disks and make them more flexible, as well as reducing pressure on the disks by increasing the space between them.

Vary this exercise by alternating between bending forward and bending toward each of your feet. This will stretch more of your back muscles. As you come up from the diagonal bend, continue the motion with your back by bending it backward and sideways with your arms stretched above your head, and then twist your torso to bend toward the other foot.

For the next two exercises, find a comfortable surface where you can stretch out flat on your back. Most beds will be too soft to allow you to do these movements properly, though some can be done on a very firm mattress. The best surface is a carpeted floor, though an exercise mat can be a good substitute – the larger the better, so that you'll have room to really move. It is a good idea to have a small, firm pillow or cushion handy to support the head. You may prefer to use it for all the exercises, or some of them, or not at all – experiment to see what works for you.

4–3   Lie on your back and begin to breathe deeply into your abdomen, chest and diaphragm in turn. As you concentrate on expanding the front of your body, feel the corresponding part of your back – the chest with the shoulders and upper back, the diaphragm with the middle back, and the abdomen with the lower back – and let that part of the back also relax and expand as you breathe. Feel where your back relaxes easily,

and feel where movement is restricted. Visualize your spine, and imagine it divided into not just three sections but nine, with the upper, middle and lower back each having an upper, middle and lower section. Stay with this visualization until you can really locate and sense your upper middle back, your middle upper back, your lower lower back, and so on.

Now imagine a line dividing the right half of your back from the left, right down the spine itself. Your back now has *eighteen* distinct sections. Visualize the lowest section of the left side of your back, and press just that area down toward the floor. Try not to use your abdominal muscles, your hips or other parts of the back to do this, but rather just the muscles in that small area. Breathe deeply throughout this exercise, since that will help you to relax the muscles you do not want to use. Go on to target each area of the back, and notice which areas seem to move easily and independently.

For some parts of your back, this exercise will consist more of a visualization than of genuine movement, but even this is good for the area in question. Visualizing an area automatically stimulates some of the nerves in that area, as well as the parts of the brain connected with those nerves, and eventually will make movement in that area easier. It is a good idea to do this exercise methodically at first, so that you make sure you have tried each separate area and felt its response, and then at random, to develop your ability to sense different parts of your spine at will.

4–4   Still on your back, bend your knees slightly and roll from side to side. As you roll to your right, press the back of your left palm on the floor to your right, and 'push off' with that palm as you roll to your left, imagining that your left shoulder is leading the motion (fig 4–4). Press the back of your right palm on the floor, and push yourself again to roll to your left. Rolling like this for five minutes, without tension, can be very effective in relaxing your back.

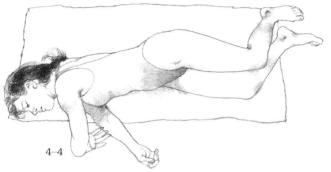

4–4

By now you are hopefully revived enough to get up off the floor. A word about getting up: if you get up the wrong way, it can put a real strain on your neck muscles. Getting up the wrong way means rising straight up from lying on your back, with your head leading the motion and unsupported. Since the neck muscles tend to be contracted in any case, this extra tightening is something you don't need. To avoid it, you can instead follow a simple and graceful procedure for rising. If you are lying on your abdomen or your back, first roll over onto your side – let's say the left side – so that your left arm is under you, your right hand palm down on the floor or bed, in front of your chest. Your chin should be near your chest. Without raising your head, push yourself slowly up, first with the right arm, then, as you lift your upper body, placing the left hand palm-down also and pushing up with both hands, until you are half-sitting sideways, with your legs stretched to the right of your hips and your weight mostly on the left hand. Do not tighten your abdominal muscles.

Now go onto your hands and knees, take your weight on your hands, and roll backward on your feet until you are squatting, knees apart, feet flat. From this position you can simultaneously straighten your legs and uncurl your spine upward as in the spinal arch (exercise 4–2), supporting your weight partially with your hands as long as you need to, with your head coming up last. Not only have you just gone from out flat to upright without so much as twitching a neck muscle, but anyone watching you will be sure that at one time you must have been a professional dancer.

If you simply want to move from lying down to sitting upright, follow the same procedure until you are sitting sideways. Now pull your legs into the cross-legged position, slowly allowing your head to come fully upright and your shoulders to fall back and downward, and don't take your weight off the left hand until the head is all the way up. You may find it easier at first to begin by lying on a bed rather than the floor. In this case, instead of sitting cross-legged, gently swing your legs over the side of the bed and to the floor before you straighten your neck to bring your head up.

Being even partially upright will immediately bring back to your spine some of the stresses of gravity, so be aware of any tightening that may follow standing or sitting up. Some muscle tone is necessary to keep you upright, of course, but check yourself for unnecessary tensions, such as in the abdomen, thighs, shoulders, arms or face. Try to release such tensions by breathing deeply and mentally 'sending' your breath into the area you wish to relax. Have the sense that your body is completely supported and upheld by the surface you are sitting or standing on. Let your shoulders drop and your hands rest naturally in your lap or on your knees if you are sitting, or allow them to hang loosely if you are standing.

Loosening the Hips and Pelvis — Relaxation of the Lower Back

The pelvis bears more weight and pressure than any other single structure in the body. This, in combination with a sedentary lifestyle, may cause the pelvic joints and muscles to grow rigid and 'frozen'. The following exercises will help to keep the hip joints limber, making it easier for you to walk, sit and stand, and providing a flexible base for movement of the back.

Hip Rotations

4–5 Stand with your weight distributed equally on both feet and the feet planted firmly, about hip-width apart. Notice whether you feel solid on your feet, whether the feet and legs feel relaxed, how much of the foot is actually touching the floor; then visualize that every part of your feet is bearing an equal portion of the weight of your torso, and that the torso is perfectly balanced on the legs and very light. Now rotate your entire lower body from the waist down, moving your hips in a circle (fig 4–5).

Your weight will shift naturally from one foot to the other as your pelvis circles. Don't tighten your abdomen or your buttocks as you move, and try not to let the upper body get involved in this motion, but concentrate on your pelvis, making a smooth, even circle with the hips. Rotate from twenty to forty times, both clockwise and counterclockwise.

4–6 When you have become comfortable with exercise 4–5, move your feet a few inches further apart and rotate the pelvis again, this time concentrating the motion on one hip at a time. Visualize the center of that hip's joint, and move the hip around that center (fig 4–6).

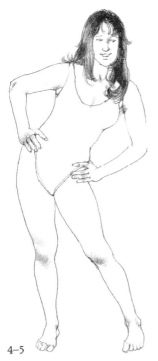

4–5

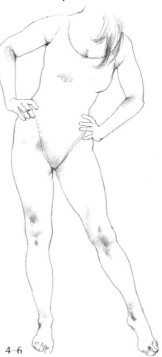

4–6

Your other hip will, of course, have to move as you do this, but it will be following a motion, rather than initiating one. Rotate the hip twenty times in each direction, and then switch to the other hip and do the same. Notice how your feet feel now. Is it easier and more comfortable to stand on them?

4–7 The next exercise is also done standing. If you have stairs, stand on the bottom step, facing the wall or the banisters; if not, then stand on a couple of large, thick books such as encyclopedia volumes, or on anything which will have you about six inches off the floor. With one hand, you may hold onto something – a chair back, counter-top etc. – for support. Stand on one foot, making sure that that foot is pointed forward and that your weight is evenly distributed on each part of the foot. You will be doing these movements with the unsupported leg.

First stretch the hip and leg muscles by pointing your toes toward the floor then flexing the foot so that the toes point back toward the shin. Now swing the leg, with the knee straight but not locked, back and forth from the hip. Let it swing easily about twenty times. Then lift it slightly out to its own side (i.e. the right foot out to the right) and move it in a rotating motion while holding it out, about six times clockwise and six times counterclockwise. Extend it behind you and do the same; then repeat with the leg lifted forward. If standing on books, swing the leg from the hip again, this time from left to right in front of you, and then from left to right behind you. Swing the leg across and in front of you (i.e. the right foot crossed to the left) and again move it in rotation, six times in each direction. Now repeat the entire series standing on the other leg.

4–8 Pelvic Lift   Lie on your back, knees bent, feet flat. Pressing your weight down onto your feet and your upper back and shoulders, lift your pelvis (fig 4–8) and move it in rotation, ten times in each direction. Rest for a minute or two, and then repeat; alternate resting and repeating four or five times.

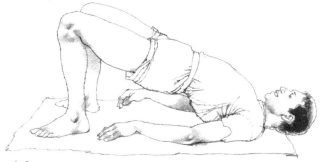

4–8

Besides loosening the pelvis, this movement is one of the best for strengthening the lower-back muscles. It will often relieve premenstrual pressure as well as menstrual cramping, constipation and gas. Pregnant women should consult with their medical advisers before practicing this exercise.

Spinal Flexion – Relaxation for the Lower Back

4–9   Lie on your back with your legs stretched out flat, and notice how much of your back is actually touching the floor. In the places where tension has contracted the muscles, there will be a space between your back and the floor. Now bend your knees and place your feet flat on the floor, about two feet apart. Notice whether this position flattens out the lower back, pressing it closer to the floor. This is the most comfortable position for many people, and the easiest on the spine. Take a couple of minutes to notice how each part of the back feels. Do you have pain in any area while the back is at rest? Does one shoulder or hip feel out of alignment with the other? Is there a sense of 'holding' even though you are not moving? Does either side feel different from the other? Do you find it easy to lie with the back of your head touching the floor, or does your head want to roll to one side (indicating that the neck muscles on that side are tighter than those on the other)?

With your knees bent and feet on the floor, roll slightly from side to side, and notice where you feel any restriction of your movement. Tilt your pelvis upward slightly and bring it down. Where does the movement pull; where does the back 'hold'? Remember all of these sensations, so that you can compare your feelings before and after doing the following movements.

Bring your bent knees together and pull them up to your chest, or as close to your chest as you comfortably can. Sometimes this simple movement by itself will relieve a mild backache or a sudden sharp pain. Remain in this position for a minute or two and visualize the muscles of the lower back being gently stretched, which is exactly what they are doing. When they contract through tension, they roll themselves up in one direction; when you flex your back as you are doing, you pull them in the opposite direction. It is important to remember not to do this movement strenuously; if it hurts, stop and do it more gently. There are many variations on spinal flexion. If your back is hurting, it is best to start with the easiest. Bend both knees but pull just one of them up to your chest, leaving the other foot on the floor. Holding the raised knee with both hands, move it in as large a rotation as

is comfortable. Be sure that your leg is not working during this motion — allow it to be passively moved by your hands. This allows the leg, hip and lower back to have the benefits of movement without any of the stress. Always remember to rotate both clockwise and counterclockwise, at least twenty times in each direction. After you have done this with one leg, lie with your legs outstretched and notice whether either leg feels different from the other, and what the differences are. Then repeat the motion with the other leg.

4–10 Next, try the same movement with one knee to the chest and the other leg outstretched. This is a greater stretch for the lower back and may not be comfortable if your back is really in bad shape. As your back grows stronger, though, you will probably prefer this larger stretch. Experiment with holding the knee with both hands and then with one hand. Holding it with one hand gives a wider range of movement, but again may not feel good at first.

4–11 Now pull both knees to the chest and rotate them, first together, holding them clasped to the chest, and then separately, holding one in each hand and moving one clockwise, the other counterclockwise. Last, hold your knees loosely and roll slowly from side to side (fig 4–11A). Repeat for about ten

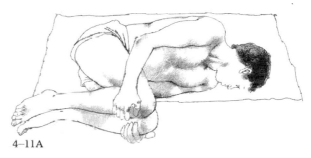
4–11A

rolls; then, as you roll onto your left side, extend both legs together straight out to the left so that they form a right angle to your torso (fig 4–11B). Repeat this motion to the right, and alternate several times.

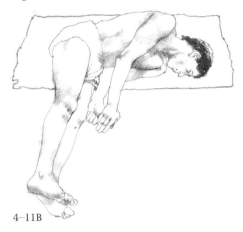

4–11B

Sideways Stretches for the Lower Back

These movements are especially important, because most of the movement we do in our normal activities involves a simple forward or backward, up or down type of motion rather than a sideways twisting, though our muscles are designed to perform all of these types of movement. Since we don't sufficiently use the muscles involved in sideways motion, they will tend to become stiff and so hamper the movement of our other muscles. Because these side muscles do not work, other muscles such as those which run parallel to the spine (the erector spinalis muscles) must work harder and so will tend to become rigid. Most of the back injuries which involve serious damage to the spine are caused by sudden sharp sideways motions for which the muscles were totally unprepared. The following exercises will give you a more complete range of movement, allowing you to keep all of your back muscles in working order.

Since you may be starting out with weak side muscles and rigid muscles through the midline of your back, you should remember, as always, to be sensitive to your back. Never try to move further to either side than is comfortable for you. You may find that you can move to the right easier than to the left, or vice versa. Don't try to force both sides to move equally. If you do these movements, you will strengthen your weaker side and relax your rigid side, and the motion will even itself out. Never strain to 'perform' any exercise – the tendency to strain is your problem to begin with. Your performance will automatically improve through conscious practice.

Start with exercise 2–28 of the Circulation chapter, which is the most basic and easy of the sideways stretches. It can often be done by people who find many other exercises too painful. Continue with exercise 2–29 of the Circulation chapter.

4–12   Still lying on your back with your knees bent, lift your right leg and rest it on the left, exactly as it would be if you were sitting in a chair with your legs crossed. Let the right leg relax and allow itself to be completely supported by the left, with the right foot hanging loosely. In this position, lower the knees to the right, making sure that the right leg stays relaxed, the left leg continues to work. Bring the knees upright again, then lower them to the left (fig 4–12).

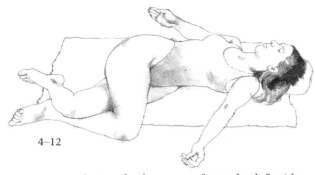

4–12

As you bring the knees up from the left side, notice that the right leg is now the supporting leg; it is under the left leg and must work to lift both knees. This exercise will strengthen the muscles of both thighs, as well as stretching the muscles of the lower back and hips. Its main value, however, is demonstrating the difference between a working and a resting muscle, so that you can learn how to relax muscles you don't need to use, working only those that should work. When you contract muscles that don't need to contract, you often create resistance or opposition to the movement you are trying to do, and end up unnecessarily doubling your effort.

4–13   Here are some more challenging stretches. Still lying on your back, place your feet about three feet apart, and lower your left knee toward your right foot, making sure the right knee stays upright (fig 4–13).

Ideally your knee should be able to touch

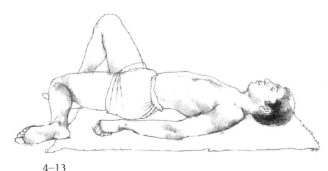

4–13

the floor, but if it won't go down that far just lower it until you feel a good stretch in the outer thigh muscles of the left leg. Pound lightly with a loose fist on the stretched hip and thigh muscles. Do the same thing with the right knee, then alternate thirty times.

4–14   If you are fairly flexible and have strong knees, try this exercise. Begin as in exercise 4–13, lowering the left knee toward the right foot, as close to the floor as it will go, then place the right foot on the bent left knee and keep it there while you take hold of the right knee and pull it down toward the left (fig 4–14). Don't pull to the degree that it hurts. Repeat this movement several times to each side.

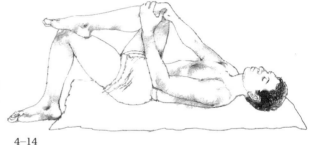

4–14

Now lie on your back with knees bent, and re-evaluate how your back feels. Are the tight places any closer to the floor than they were? Does either side feel different from the other? Is there any place that resists the stretches?

Exercises for the Abdomen and Lower Back

The muscles of the abdomen and the lower back are extremely interdependent: if one set weakens, the other suffers too. A distended abdomen (also known as potbelly) can be the sign of weak lower-back muscles which have allowed the abdomen to be pulled forward by its own weight. Very tense lower-back muscles may create corresponding rigidity in the lower abdomen, which often interferes with the digestive processes. This interdependence between abdomen and lower back is widely recognized, but has unfortunately given rise to some bizarre notions, such as tightening the abdomen to support the lower back, or strengthening the back so that a weak abdomen will not be injured.

It seems simpler and more reasonable to strengthen each part so that it can successfully and independently perform its own function; both that part and the rest of the body will then benefit automatically. The following exercises provide a very gentle stretch for the abdominal muscles, easy movement for the lower back, and stimulation to the digestive tract. The only restriction on doing these exercises is that some of them may be difficult for you if you have a very tight neck. It would be a good idea to try a few of the neck and shoulder exercises in this chapter first, to see whether your neck is stiff and, if so, to loosen it.

4–15 Lie on your abdomen on a firm surface, with your head turned to the side; do not use a pillow in this position, but do remember to turn your head to the opposite side every few minutes, in order to avoid stiffening your neck. Raise one leg (from the knee) and try to touch your buttock with your heel, pulling your ankle with your hand. If you cannot do this, it is partly because of tension in the thigh muscles and partly due to rigidity in the lower back. As the back relaxes, you will see that

you can bring the foot much closer to the buttock than at first. Now rotate the calf, making the circle of motion as large as possible. After about ten rotations in each direction, switch to the other leg.

Try to keep from tensing either your back or your abdomen as you do this exercise. If you feel yourself tensing, stop the rotation and instead alternately raise and lower both legs, as if trying to kick your buttocks (fig 4–15). This will shake out the leg and back tension so you can go on with the rotation. Visualize your toes as 'leading' the motion, or imagine someone else holding the foot and moving it for you. Remember to breathe deeply and relax your back; don't allow it to work during this exercise.

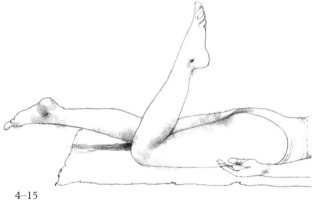

4–15

4–16 Remain lying on your abdomen. Now lift both legs simultaneously and move them both in rotation, first in the same direction – i.e. both clockwise or both counterclockwise – and then in opposing directions. Again, make these circles as large as possible. Next, with your knees touching and moving only from the waist down, move the two legs together as far to the left side as they will reach, and then as far to the right. This movement is more of a stretch and may be difficult at first, so lower the legs only as far as they will stretch comfortably. Repeat about six to eight times, then relieve any stress this motion creates by rotating both legs together, this time making a smaller circle.

Several yoga stretches are beneficial for this same general area, but they are a little more difficult than the preceding exercises and should not be done until you feel that your lower back is fairly relaxed. The first is called the Cobra, and is described in exercise 1–11 in the Breathing chapter.

4–17 To become the Bow – another yoga exercise – lie on your abdomen, lift your head, raise your feet and grasp an ankle in each hand (fig 4–17). Hold this pose for several breaths, pressing your abdomen toward the floor; then let go, stretch out, rest for a minute and then repeat several times.

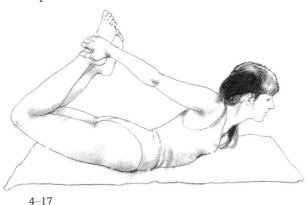

4–17

After doing the exercises in this section, again lie on your back with your knees bent, and see how your back feels. Breathe deeply and let your back sink into the floor while your chest and abdomen expand upward and outward. Do you feel any difference? Does your lower back feel as though it is closer to

the floor? What about your pelvis, and your shoulders? If you feel any discomfort after these exercises, pull one knee up to your chest, hold it there for a minute or two and then gently rotate it twenty to fifty times in each direction, and then repeat this with the other knee. This motion puts your back in a posture opposite to the posture used in the above exercises, and so balances the pull on your spinal bones and muscles. In principle, this balancing of motion (i.e. if you lean back you should lean forward; if you go right you should go left) is always good, but above all you must be sensitive to what your own body needs and wants.

Sitting Stretches and Rotations for the Lower Back

4–18 Sit cross-legged on the floor and begin to rotate your body from the pelvis up, as though it is a top spinning on a point in the exact center of your pelvis. Hold your spine straight but not rigid. By holding the spine straight all the way from the sacrum to the neck, you are limiting your range of motion and thus concentrating the movement in the lower pelvis and hips. Imagine that your head, rather than the back, is 'leading' the motion. After about twenty rotations in each direction, you can increase the range of the rotation, now allowing your lower spine to move freely and naturally. Your upper torso should remain completely relaxed, simply following the lead of the lower spine. When you are comfortable with this motion, continue the rotation and emphasize the movement of the lumbar (low back) area, deliberately making it concave as you lean forward (fig 4–18A) and convex as you curve backward (fig 4–18B).

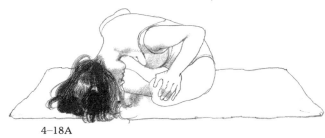

4–18A

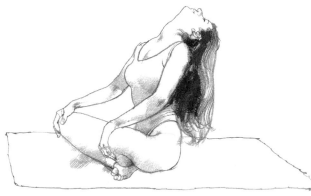

4–18B

4–19 It is in the lumbar and sacral areas that many of the most serious spine problems occur. Due to the pressures of walking and sitting, the vertebrae in these areas become compressed, which may cause damage to the disks or the nerve roots. In this exercise we will concentrate the movement in the lower back, starting just below the waist and working down to the coccyx.

Sit cross-legged with your hands holding onto your knees, and visualize your lower spine, starting with the first lumbar vertebra; then slowly begin to move the spine downward and outward, rolling backward onto the upper buttock area, creating a convex curve beginning at the waist and extending as far down as your spine will permit. Then roll your spine back to the position you started

with; repeat. Try not to tighten or push with your abdomen, but let the back muscles do all the work. Your back muscles may be very weak or rigid. This exercise will improve both of these conditions – in fact, it is one of the best and easiest ways of strengthening the lower-back muscles.

A variation of this movement is to try it sitting with knees bent and pulled up to the chest, arms around the knees and feet flat on the floor. You will find the movement even more limited in this position, so that when you return to the cross-legged position and repeat the exercise the movement will seem easy and expansive by contrast. At first we recommend doing this movement six times cross-legged, ten times with the knees pulled to the chest, and again six times cross-legged. Stop in the middle to visualize that you are doing the motion effortlessly, then return to the movement. When you have become comfortable with the exercise you can do it as often as you like, and preferably as often as possible.

4–20 If your lower back is strong and feeling flexible, continue with this exercise. Pull your knees up to your chest, cross your arms around your thighs, then roll backward until you are resting on your sacrum rather than your buttocks – or roll as far backward as you can without falling over – your feet off the floor. Then, in this position, rock yourself very slightly backward and forward. This movement will require you to tighten your abdominal muscles slightly, but try to keep this as slight as possible by breathing deeply into the abdomen and visualizing that your lower-back muscles are doing all the work to support you and to move you. As long as your lower back acts like one stiff unit, you may find that you have very little control over the rocking; any attempt to rock backward may find you rolling onto your middle and upper back.

Refer to the section on Learning to Walk in the Muscles chapter, and to the Nervous System chapter for exercises of walking and running backward, which are also beneficial for the lower back.

Exercises for the Middle and Upper Back

4–21 Now that you have limbered up your lower spine, make the spinal arch with your whole back while still sitting cross-legged. As in the standing spinal arch (exercise 4–2), the idea is to create an arch with the vertebrae, moving one vertebra at a time, working from the top down as you bring your head toward the floor and then from the bottom up. Bend your head first until your chin rests on your chest, then follow with the rest of your spine, curving slowly forward as far as you can comfortably reach. For some this will mean bending the chin to the chest; others will be able to touch their heads to the floor (fig 4–21).

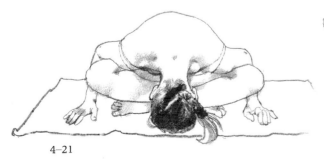

4–21

For most people, each repetition of this movement will enable them to bend slightly more. It may help to place your hands on the back of your neck and pull gently as you bend; this will give you a little more sense of elongation.

We recommend between six and ten repetitions of the sitting arch. Vary this exercise by alternating between curving forward and curving diagonally toward the knees, so that all of the back muscles – that is, those which run diagonally along the side as well as those which run vertically down the spine – may benefit from the stretch. Bend sideways and backward, tap on your chest to loosen its muscles, breathe deeply, and then bend forward to the opposite knee.

You can vary this exercise by changing your sitting position. If you can, do it kneeling, or sitting between your feet. If you are flexible enough, try doing it in a lotus position.

4–22 Lying on your back, bend your left leg and stretch the right leg out flat. Cross your bent left knee all the way over your body to the right side, turning your body slightly to the right (your left shoulder will come up slightly off the floor) until the inside of the left knee touches the floor to the right of you (fig 4–22A). Then, keeping the knee bent,

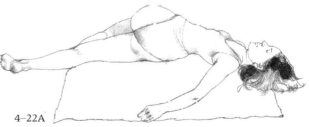

4–22A

move it back to the left until the outside of the left knee touches the floor to the left of you (fig 4–22B). Imagine that the knee leads the motion, as though someone else is holding

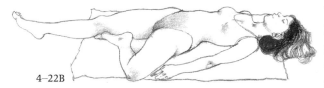

4–22B

and moving it for you. Repeat this five times, then reverse and do the same process with the right knee bent.

4–23 Lie with both legs out flat and your arms stretched out straight from the shoulders, and swing your right leg over your body to try to touch your left hand (fig 4–23). Your body from the waist up should stay on the floor; this is primarily a stretch for your back and hips, though it will stretch your shoulders as well. If you can actually touch your foot to your opposite hand, congratulations! You may at first be able only to reach in that general direction, but after alternating with the right and left feet about ten or fifteen times you may find yourself getting noticeably close to the hand you are aiming at.

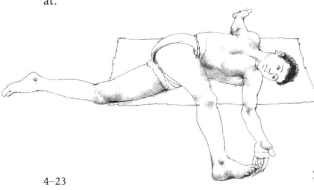

4–23

4–24 Three-way Twist Lie on your back, knees bent and feet flat, arms by your side. Very slowly, turn your head from side to side, so that your chin comes close to each shoulder in turn. Try to do this with no effort at all,

visualizing that someone else is gently rolling your head from side to side (if you can in fact get someone to do this for you at first, this is even better) and that your nose is 'leading' the motion; this will take pressure off the shoulder and neck muscles.

After about thirty slow rolls from side to side, combine this motion with alternately raising and lowering your arms. First raise your right arm and bring it back over your head until the back of the hand touches the floor; then, as you slowly return the right arm to your right side, bring the left arm up over your head. Continue this alternate raising and lowering of the arms while your head rolls from side to side, making sure that your head, with each turn, is turning *away* from the arm coming up; that is, when the right arm is coming up the head is turning to the left, and vice versa. This gives more of a stretch to your side neck flexor muscles.

This exercise has a third part, which will not only help you to move, stretch and relax your entire spine but will improve your coordination as well. Begin with your head turned to the right, your right arm at your side and your left arm up. Now lower your bent knees to the left, until the left knee is resting on the floor (fig 4–24).

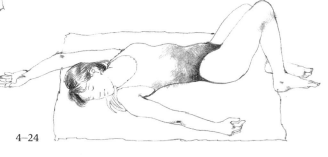

4–24

You will notice that both the knees and the arm are moving on the opposite side from that of the head movement. The purpose of this is to move your spine in as many directions simultaneously as possible – this is excellent for flexibility. Now turn your head to the left, put your left arm down, your right arm up, and lower your knees to the right – simultaneously. Do these alternating turns about ten or fifteen times; do them as slowly as you need to in order to do them correctly, and check yourself every so often to see if everything is in synch.

The windmill, exercise 1–10 from the Breathing chapter, is an excellent stretch for your upper back, neck, shoulders, arms and chest.

4–25 When you feel that your back and abdomen are strong enough, return to the Cobra exercise (1–11), and now try to lift your torso without using your arms at all. With your arms by your sides, use the power of the back muscles to lift the torso as a cobra would (fig 4–25). Hold this position for the length of two deep breaths, and then slowly lower yourself to the floor.

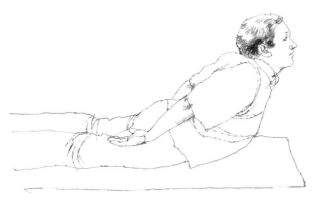

4–25

Practice exercise 1–13 from the Breathing chapter for the upper back, and exercise 2–15 from the Circulation chapter for the middle back.

Exercises for the Neck and Shoulders

These exercises can provide great relief for anyone suffering from stiffness in the neck and shoulders, whether it is a temporary or a chronic condition. They are excellent to do before falling asleep, to relax; or to get the blood flowing to the head upon waking. The change of posture stretches the neck muscles, allowing more circulation. These exercises will help prevent eyestrain and the effects of eyestrain by increasing circulation to the eyes, facial muscles and neck muscles which may tighten during intensive use of the eyes.

4–26 Head Rotation The most basic neck exercise is head rotation. First try it sitting up, with your back comfortably supported. Either sit on the floor with your back against the wall or, if this is uncomfortable, sit in a chair with a high back that you can lean your head against. Draw circles with the back of your head on the wall behind you. Visualize your neck as very long and completely flexible, and see the top of your head as parallel to the sky. Let your head begin to move slowly from side to side, stretching the neck as far to each side as is comfortable. Since your head is supported, allow your neck to completely relax as it stretches. Now begin to slowly move your head in rotation, as though it is moving around the perimeter of the circle you have imagined. The tendency of most people when first doing head rotations is to make huge sweeping circles with their heads, which only strains the neck muscles and does not ultimately relieve tension; so **keep the rotation small.**

You may notice that your head does not move in a smooth, even circle; tension in the neck muscles may make your rotation jerky and lopsided. If so, stop after twenty or so rotations in each direction, stretch your head toward each shoulder, and try to determine which side of the neck is the more tense. If it is the right, then stretch your head to the left, as if to rest it on your left shoulder, and in that position tap quickly and lightly with the fingertips of both hands up and down the length of your neck on the right. You should be tapping hard enough that your fingers will bounce off your neck. After about two minutes of this tapping, stretch your neck to each side again. Do the shoulders feel the same as they did? Now do the same thing to the left side of your neck, and then try the rotation again. You will probably find the motion much smoother and easier to do.

You may initially become dizzy during head rotations. This could be caused by a very tight neck, which is a problem you share with millions of people. To be on the safe side, however, you should consult a physician to find out whether your dizziness is caused by a condition that would contraindicate this exercise. Do only a few rotations in each direction, remembering to breathe deeply and continuously, and gradually increase the number each time you do this exercise. The dizziness will pass, probably in very little time. Palming – which means covering the closed eyes with the palms of the hands, breathing deeply, relaxing and visualizing blackness – can relieve dizziness almost immediately.

4–27   When you feel comfortable with head rotations sitting up, try them lying down on your back with your knees bent. Do not lift your head up from the floor while rotating; have a sense of the floor massaging the back of your skull. If this seems awkward at first, imagine that you are making a circle with your nose. What seems like a very limited motion is actually extremely effective in relieving neck tension. This exercise is excellent for headaches and fatigue, as it requires very little effort and has an immediately relaxing effect. Rotate your head about fifty times in both directions (clockwise and counterclockwise). You may want to alternate this exercise with 4–29.

We must unfortunately note here that some schools of bodywork are opposed to neck rotations, for reasons we have been unable to determine. All we can say is that we know of no evidence – certainly no documented evidence – that neck rotations are dangerous. Any movement can harm if done improperly, just as nearly any movement can be beneficial if done correctly.

4–28   Lace your fingers together so that they are supporting the back of your head. Relax your neck, and lift your head *with your hands* – don't let your neck do the work (fig 4–28).

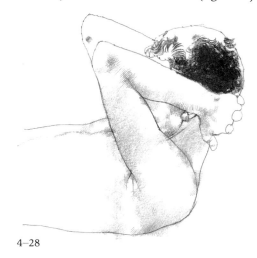

4–28

Keeping the neck completely loose, pull your head forward until your chin touches your chest. You may feel this stretch primarily in the neck and upper back, but notice that it stretches the lower back as well. Concentrate on the sensation in your lower back as you gently pull the head forward, and as you release the stretch. You may begin to have a sense of how all of the back muscles are connected, and how movement, or lack of it, in one part of the back affects other areas.

4–29 Lie on your back, stretch your arms behind your head, lace your fingers together, and rotate both arms together, making the circles as wide as possible without straining your neck or shoulders. Do this motion very slowly, so that at each point in the rotation you can feel where a pull is being exerted, and respond to that pull by visualizing the tight area loosening, lengthening and relaxing.

4–30 Shoulder Rotations Lying on your side with your head either supported by a thick pillow or on your palm, rotate your free shoulder twenty times in each direction, while your free palm rests on the floor in front of your chest (fig 4–30).

This position allows the force of gravity to stretch your shoulder as you bring the shoul-

der forward and backward. After rotating one shoulder in each direction, lie on your back and see whether you notice a difference between the two shoulders, and what the difference feels like; then repeat the exercise on the other side.

Refer to the chapter on the Joints for more exercises for the shoulders (exercises 3–16 to 3–28).

Exercises for the Whole Back

4–31 Return to exercise 4–5. After several rotations, remain in the same position and rotate just your upper body, from the waist up, keeping everything below the waist motionless (fig 4–31). Which of these motions feels easier to you? Return to the hip rotation, to feel the difference.

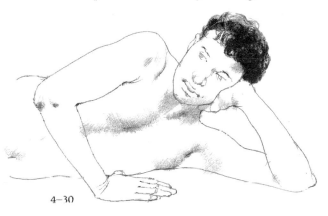

4–30

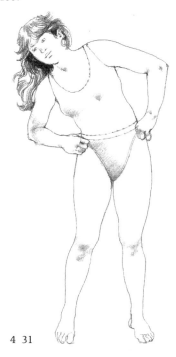

4 31

4–32   Return to exercise 4–17, and now try part two of the Bow: while grasping your ankles, use the power of your abdomen and the momentum of the movement to rock yourself back and forth, so that first your chest, then your abdomen and finally your knees will touch the floor. The first time you try this it may seem impossible, but, like any other movement, it will become easier with practice.

4–33   Return to exercise 4–3, and use your kinesthetic awareness to focus your attention on each part of your back. When you feel that you are able to truly sense each area of your spine, you can do the same exercise using a tennis ball under each targeted area in turn. Be careful to position the ball under muscles only, not under bones. This will increase the amount of pressure on the muscles and help them relax further, and of course will focus your attention on the area. Do this exercise only if your back is strong and flexible.

You may find that, when you get up from a chair, you tense many of your back muscles unnecessarily: it is the legs' role to get you up. One exercise with which you can practice getting up using your leg muscles is exercise 19–7 in the Back Pain chapter. Another one is this:

4–34   Sit on a chair with your feet apart, flat on the floor. Bend forward gradually, as in the sitting spinal arch (exercise 4–21), until your chest rests on your thighs (fig 4–34). Now straighten your legs as you get up from the chair – your back muscles will not try to help in this position. After your legs are straight, uncurl your back – vertebra by vertebra, again as in the spinal arch. To sit again,

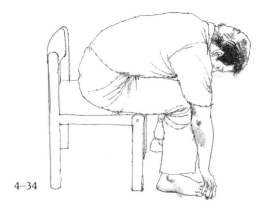

4–34

bend forward until your back is parallel to the floor, bend your knees to sit, and then straighten your back to sit up.

Back Bend

The back bend (exercise 4–37) may be dangerous for those whose backs are not strong, because it may lead to nerve pressure in such cases. Develop the ability to bend your back gradually. If it feels good, this will serve as a balancing exercise for the spinal arch. It will give you a good stretch for the abdominal and chest muscles, it will allow muscle fibers which are always partially contracted to contract fully and then relax, and it will ease their burden by activating muscle fibers that you don't normally contract. If you suffer from a slight lordosis, or swayback, this exercise may be especially beneficial for that reason.

The following two exercises will prepare you gradually for the back bend.

4–35   Stand on your knees, keeping them at least hip-width apart, and lean backward until your hands can hold your ankles (fig 4–35A). Return to an upright position using the muscles of your thighs.

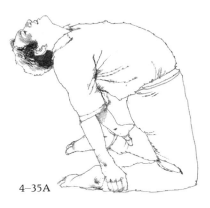

4–35A

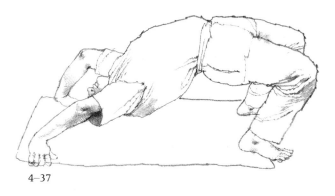

4–37

After practicing that several times, lean backward again, this time with an arched back, hold your ankles with your hands, and try to reach the floor with your head (fig 4–35B).

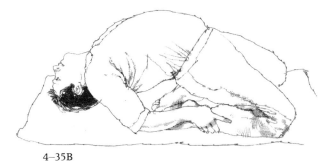

4–35B

4–36 Stand with your back to a wall, about two feet away from the wall. Lift your arms, bend backward and bring your palms to the wall. Now start climbing down with your palms on the wall. Gradually move your feet further away from the wall. To get up again, climb with your palms up on the wall.

4–37 Back Bend Lie on your back, your knees bent and your feet flat on the floor. Put your palms next to your ears, with your fingers pointed toward your shoulders, and lift yourself onto your palms and feet (fig 4–37). The more you practice this exercise, the more curved your back can be in a full back bend.

Feel the stretch in your chest and breathe deeply. Return to the floor gradually and carefully.

Stretching with the Help of a Friend

4–38 If your back is strong, you can give a friend a very relaxing stretch. All you will need is a little bit of balancing and the help of gravity. Stand back to back with your friend, and bend your knees so that your upper back is against your friend's concave middle–lower back. Pull your friend's arms above your shoulders (fig 4–38A). Use the muscles of your

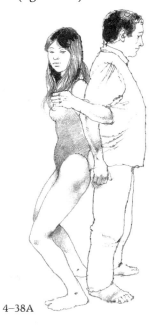

4–38A

thighs to lift your friend off the ground as you bend forward to prevent the gravitational weight from working against you (fig 4–38B).

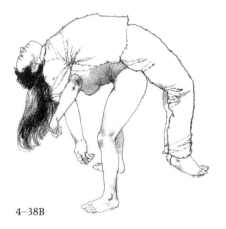

4–38B

As your friend lies stretched on your back, feet off the floor, you can bounce him a little by bending and straightening your legs slightly. Your friend's own weight will give his back a stretch. This exercise will be effective only if your friend feels safe, as otherwise he will tense up.

Other Back-Relaxers

There are several exercises in the Muscles chapter which are excellent for limbering and relaxing the back muscles: both exercises 5–39 and 5–40 are good additions to your back regimen.

If your back is strong, practice exercise 6–22 from the Nervous System chapter.

Finish your back session by lying, once again, flat on your back, knees bent, feet flat. Without lifting any part of your torso off the floor, slowly press your lower back down against the floor, then release it. Repeat this three or four times, remembering to breathe deeply and to keep your abdomen relaxed. Now press your middle back against the floor, hold for two or three deep breaths, and release. Do the same with the upper back, the shoulders and the neck. Now simply lie still and feel each part of your back. Do you feel that any part of your spine is looser, less constricted, more in contact with the floor, larger, lighter or simply more 'there'? If so, you are beginning to build a healthy back.

CHAPTER 5

Muscles
The key to understanding and changing your body

For a human being, movement is life. Even when you appear to be completely motionless, there is a ceaseless flow of movement within your body. Your heart pumps, your blood flows, your digestive organs move food through your system, your lungs and diaphragm expand and contract with each breath, nerves relay messages to and from the brain at amazing speeds, and hormones travel through your bloodstream to regulate all of these functions. Most of your body's cells are producing some kind of motion most of the time. This motion is essential to our existence.

Most of this movement is automatic and involuntary, and much of it is carried out by the part of our muscular system known as involuntary muscle. The circulatory and respiratory systems and digestive organs contain a tissue called smooth muscle tissue, while the heart is in a muscular class all by itself, composed of tissue called simply cardiac muscle. Because the movements these muscles make appear to be automatically performed by our bodies, it may seem that they are beyond our control, but this is not really true.

We possess another set of muscles, called the skeletal or voluntary muscles, composed of more than 600 moving parts, whose move-

ment we can direct. These muscles are called skeletal because almost all of them attach to bones, making it possible to move our limbs and head and spine. They are composed of long, thin fibers arranged in parallel bundles. These fibers contract and relax to create, or to allow, movement. The smooth muscles and these skeletal muscles are different from each other in both appearance and type of function; what they have in common is that both control movement. While it may seem that our skeletal muscles are responsible only for controlling our outward motions – the motions which we perform voluntarily – the truth is that our outer movement has a very strong influence on our inner, or involuntary, movement as well. In our opinion, external movement is our single most effective healing tool, precisely because it facilitates all of our essential inner movement.

This is why exercise is good for you. The benefit of exercise is not just to keep the muscles themselves in shape, though this by itself is extremely important, since about 40 percent of our total body weight consists of muscle tissue. The benefits of movement extend to every body function, and to functions of the mind as well. Why is walking better than driving? You will get where you are going either way. For your schedule, driving may be better. For your body, walking is better — for many reasons:

- because it moves your joints, causing them to circulate the synovial fluid which keeps them from deteriorating;
- because it increases your circulation, strengthening your heart and blood vessels;
- because it increases your respiration, strengthening the action of your lungs and increasing your body's supply of oxygen, which it needs for every action it performs;
- because it strengthens the muscles themselves, increasing their tone and coordination.

Walking may also aid digestion, nerve functioning and even brain function. Many of the great thinkers and writers were also enthusiastic walkers, and many have commented how this exercise seems to clear and quiet the mind and spirit.

Self-Healing is primarily a movement method. The health of your muscles is so vitally important. Of course, it is essential to your well-being to have a body that is flexible, supple, relaxed, free of pain and capable of doing whatever you ask of it. That by itself would be reason enough to give your muscles a lot of attention. But when we realize that muscle movement plays a vital part in the body's inner rhythms as well, our understanding of the muscles expands. We begin to see how truly interconnected all parts of the body really are.

The skeletal, or striated, muscles have a wide middle part, called the belly of the muscle, which tapers at each end. The two ends are attached by tendons to two different bones, and usually one of these bones moves more

than the other when the muscle contracts. (There are several exceptions to this rule, such as in some muscles of the face.) In general, the place where the muscle is joined to the less mobile of the two bones is called that muscle's 'origin', and the place where the muscle attaches to the more mobile bone is called its 'insertion'. This is only a very general rule, since some muscles actually have several origins or insertions. Muscles are connected to each other by fascia, or connective tissue, a kind of tissue which is found in every part of the body, which holds each part in its place and connects each part to its neighboring parts. In his book *Job's Body* (Station Hill Press, Berrytown, NY, 1987), Deane Juhan says of connective tissue, 'if all other tissues were extracted, the connective framework alone would preserve the three-dimensional human form in all its details.' We will discuss connective tissue in more detail later.

Movement usually involves the coordinated action of several muscles. One muscle will be the primary moving agent, while other muscles must relax to allow the desired movement to occur; and still others must contract to maintain the body's balance and stability during the movement. To perform the body's desired movements effectively, the muscles must be able to contract and to relax, with equal ease, whenever we need them to. Difficulties begin when either contracting or relaxing becomes difficult or impossible for a muscle. What we will be working to achieve is a balance between tone — a necessary degree of contraction — and relaxation. We want our muscles to be loose and supple but not weak; strong and well-toned without being overly or unnecessarily contracted.

People have come to use the word 'tension' as though it is synonymous with 'stress', but this is not accurate. Muscular tension is often increased by emotional or physical stress, and that excess is not desirable. Some tension, however, is needed in all muscles to maintain normal resting tone which allows for posture, the positioning of bones and any movement we attempt. The tension we want to eliminate is unnecessary tension – the contraction of muscles that ought to be relaxing. Everyone suffers from some degree of unnecessary tension.

Excess muscle tension comes mainly from two sources. It may develop when we overuse a muscle until it becomes chronically contracted and cannot relax. This may come about as a result of hard labor; it may just as easily come about as a result of holding one position for too long, or of unconsciously tightening a muscle due to emotional stress. Muscle strain may also result from attempting to use a weak, seldom-used muscle as though it were a strong one. (This is how 'weekend athletes' damage themselves.) We all have a tendency to rely heavily upon our stronger muscles, overusing them until strain results, and to neglect to use the weaker ones, which in time only weakens them further. If we are not mindful of how we move, we end up using only relatively few of our muscles to perform every action we do. We thus create patterns of movement in which everything we do makes the situation worse. To promote better muscle function, we must: (1) keep all of our muscles in regular use, by practicing motions that bring them into play, (2) use only those muscles which are appropriate for a particular action, and (3) relax when the action is completed!

The most destructive type of muscular tension is that which is created simply by holding the body rigidly, without moving it. As we have said, muscles may become over-contracted as a result of hard exercise, but when they are moving they at least have the benefit of the increased circulation and respiration that movement brings about. When muscles contract without performing any actual movement, they are 'working' very hard but not reaping any of the benefits of work. They are burning up oxygen without helping the body to bring any more in; they are using up the chemicals which allow them to work, without helping the body to reproduce those chemicals. This type of tension can make you feel completely exhausted – not the rather pleasant exhaustion that follows a day's hard exercise, but a depleted, sick feeling of fatigue.

This type of motionless muscle contraction may be brought on by sitting, standing or even lying in the same position for too long a time, or by having to hold or carry something, or by having repeated the same motion, through tension, so often that the muscles 'freeze' into the position required for that motion. Walking on concrete in hard, non-flexible shoes causes your feet and legs and hips to repeat, under stress, exactly the same motion over and over in a way that can 'freeze' your muscles and weaken muscles which are not in use (in this case, the peroneals, which move the feet sideways). The uneven impact on the joints and muscles is harmful for both. The situation is similar with constant repetitions of any type of movement. An assembly-line worker, a musician or a typist may develop muscle cramps in the hands, wrists or shoulders from repeating the same gestures thousands of times while in a state of physical tension. But all can prevent those problems by changing the positions in which they stand or sit, by working only those muscles that need to work (you do not really need to tense your shoulders and neck in order to type) and by exercising their hands, arms and backs in patterns which relax the hard-working muscles and activate the ones which are never, or seldom, in use.

Muscular problems do not develop because of movement, nor because of many repetitions of movement, but because of tension which either prevents movement or keeps it from being beneficial. Very often this tension is the result of an unconscious holding of parts of the body for hours at a time, often caused by emotional stress of some kind, or by intense mental concentration which may cause you to forget you have a body. Our muscles carry a double burden: besides performing our every action, they also reflect our emotional and mental states. Emotional stress may be held in the muscles, in the form of contraction and spasm, long after the original emotional upset occurred. A severe enough emotional trauma may still be reflected in the body's muscles for *years* afterward.

Anatomy books, in denoting the functions of the various muscles, include for the facial muscles the task of expressing our emotions. Actually, though the face is the primary communicator of emotions, the whole body can reflect and express them. Anyone who has had or given a massage has seen how some emotions seem to be locked into the muscles themselves and how those feelings can sometimes be released when the muscle contraction is relieved through touch. Certain emotions seem to be more closely related with specific parts of the body, such as anger and frustration with the jaws, grief with the chest, anxiety with the abdomen, exhaustion and depression with the neck and shoulders, and so on. Bodywork therapists refer to these holding patterns as 'body armor', particularly in reference to tension in the chest. **Our number-one killer, cardiovascular disease, with its accompany-ing symptoms of high blood pressure and congested blood vessels, is, we believe, directly related to excess tension in the chest muscles. Strokes, we have found, are closely related to excess tension in the neck muscles. Excess muscle contraction in the back may trigger neurological problems such as multiple sclerosis. Relaxing muscle tension is, therefore, not just important – it could be a lifesaver.**

It is important to understand just what happens when a muscle remains contracted when it ought to relax. On the most surface level, a tight muscle impedes the motion of other related muscles. As we have seen, when a particular muscle needs to move, certain other muscles must relax to allow that movement. If they cannot let go of their contraction, the movement is distorted or becomes completely impossible. Movement of the tight muscle itself is of course made much more difficult: if it cannot effectively relax in order to contract again, it must simply remain more or less static. On a deeper level, chronic muscle contraction interferes with the efficient functioning of both the nervous and the circulatory systems. A tight muscle puts extreme pressure on capillary walls, often crushing them completely. That places a greater strain on the remaining larger blood vessels, which are narrowed and hardened as a result of the pressure. Nerve impulses, which must be passed from one nerve to another until they reach the brain, are impeded if the muscles through which they run are knotted. This can easily be seen in the fact that very tight areas often become numb, regaining their full feeling only when the tension is released.

We cannot always distinguish whether stress has its roots in emotional tension or in physical tension. Patterns of tension tend to be cyclical rather than linear. What is clear is that one type of tension, if unrelieved, will almost always lead to the other as well. If your body is tense or in pain, the discomfort will eventually make you feel emotionally upset as well. Also, the mind associates certain body states with particular emotions, so that being in that physical state may actually help to create the emotion associated with it. For example, a slumped posture can actually make a person feel depressed, or shallow breathing induce a sense of anxiety. Muscle cramps may be a reminder of feelings of anger or agitation.

Conversely, if you are undergoing emotional stress, your body is almost certain to reflect it immediately. This is so obvious as to need no proof. What is medically known about the body's response to emotions could fill endless volumes, and we are continually learning still more. You do not have to know physiology to see that when people are angry their faces flush, when they are afraid they tremble, and when they are anxious it can be read from their expression and posture. Look a little deeper, and you will also find contraction of muscles, constriction of the blood vessels, changes in blood chemistry and heart rate, changes in the structure of the stomach lining and profound changes in nerve activity — all produced instantaneously by strong emotions. There simply is no way we can have an emotion without our bodies' reflecting it in some visible, tangible and biochemically unmistakable manner.

For this reason, among many others, the analogy of the body as a machine does not hold up: the functioning of machines is not influenced by their emotions. Machines are affected only by physical factors, whereas we are affected by innumerable influences. Because of this, we must learn to truly know

ourselves, and be sensitive to our changing needs. When our bodies do not perform as we want them to, we should try to find out what the problem is and solve it if possible, rather than doing what most people do — trying to force the body, by any means possible, to do what the will requires. The body's needs are as legitimate as those of the mind, and your body will always find some way of convincing you to respect its needs, even if total collapse is the only thing which will work.

Choosing the right exercise at the right time is part of being sensitive to your body. Many ironic comments have been made (mostly by professional couch potatoes) about how people have literally killed themselves trying to be healthy, dying of heart attacks during jogging and tennis. What must be considered is that these people were nearly always living high-stress lifestyles. Stress or jogging alone would probably not have killed them, but the combination of contracted chest muscles, constricted blood vessels, and a heart overworked by high blood pressure and the exertion of trying to force blood into narrowed arteries — in other words, a stress-wracked body trying to respond to unusually heavy physical demands — can be deadly. It is criminal, if you consider suicide a crime, to behave as though you are simply the owner and operator of a body which must do whatever you ask of it. Whether we like it or not, we are one with our bodies. If we try to act otherwise, asking the unreasonable or impossible of the body, it will certainly remind us of this fact.

Excess muscular tension is not restricted to the skeletal muscles: it can occur in the smooth-muscle tissue as well, manifesting as spasms of the stomach and duodenum (the first part of the small intestines, where most of the digestive process takes place); spastic-colon syndrome; closure of the pyloric sphincter, which controls the passage of ingested food from the stomach to the duodenum; and so on. A spasm is an involuntary and often prolonged contraction of a muscle. In fact, many digestive disorders can be traced to contraction – and hence lack of movement – in the digestive tract. When semidigested food is trapped somewhere in the gastrointestinal tract, it can cause acidity, toxicity, ulcers, diverticulitis, colitis – problems ranging from hiccups to colon cancer (one of the most common forms of cancer in junk-food-loving, sedentary America) and including constipation, diarrhea, gas pain, bad skin, bad breath and obesity.

We have never met anyone who did not have tight neck muscles at least occasionally, or anyone who did not sigh with relief when the neck and shoulders were massaged. When these muscles, normally rigid with strain, are relaxed either through massage or through exercise, people experience feelings of renewed energy, lightness and freedom, and even of clearer thinking, as circulation to the head is increased. Tension in the neck is a 'normal' problem, but it is still a problem. We believe that release from normal, everyday tensions is as vital as food to the body, and ought to be a part of our everyday maintenance.

Extraordinary muscular tension is another matter. Whether it is caused by overwork, destructive use of the body or emotional trauma, it can alter the body's structure – perhaps even permanently. One task of the muscles is to hold the bones in their proper places; thus, if a contracted muscle on one side of the body exerts a strong pull on weaker muscles on the other side of the body, the body's entire alignment can be distorted, causing one shoulder or hip to be held higher,

one leg to seem longer, and creating every imaginable distortion in the position of the vertebrae.

Muscle tension can distort the body in innumerable ways, causing pain and perpetuating emotional difficulties. The jaws, for example, are moved by powerful muscles. They are involved in the expression of anger, and always have been. We may not actually gnash our teeth any more, but we certainly grind them, compressing our jaw muscles as we do so. This can lead to TMJ – temporomandibular joint syndrome – a painful contraction that extends from the jaw to the temple; to neuralgia and migraine; to permanent changes in the location and structure of the jaw and teeth. It may be even more dangerous if the jaw tightness is powerful enough to affect the neck muscles as well. It is interesting that this jaw tightness seems to be caused by repressed, rather than expressed, anger – it is almost as though the jaw muscles are forcibly contracting to keep the mouth closed. Perhaps the original idea was to keep oneself from biting one's adversary; now it seems to be aimed at holding in angry words. In any case, it is very typical that a repressed emotion will create muscular tension, and that this tension will then play a part in perpetuating that emotion.

Tension in neck muscles can move the head forward, causing the shoulders also to round forward, compressing the chest, restricting breathing, tightening the pelvis and lumbar region, and making for a heavy, stiff-legged walk. Apart from posture and gait distortions, the worst effect of tight neck muscles is to constrict the large blood vessels of the neck. The blood vessels run between the muscles, and when the strong muscles tighten around them the effect is similar to what happens when you step on a hose through which water is pouring: the water does not get where it is supposed to go, or it does so only in a thin trickle, while pressure is increased around the compressed area and at the water's source. Thus neck tension can deprive the brain and the facial muscles of their full circulation, while increasing pressure in the blood vessels in the neck itself. You may not necessarily be hurting when your muscle tension is extreme, for the strongest level of tension, which is also the most dangerous, causes numbness. If you suffer pain, you are probably doing better: at least you are aware that you need to do something about it.

Arms become tense partly as a result of chest and shoulder tension and partly as a natural result of the fact that we use them for everything we do. Nearly all of us earn our living with our hands, one way or another, whether it is hauling wood or operating a computer. Not only do they get tired from so much use, but they also feel any tension which may be associated with the task they are performing. Any sense of being overwhelmed, any sense of effort or strain – emotional or physical – goes directly into the muscles of the arms. Very few people know how to use their arms without tension, making only as much physical effort as the task actually requires. This habitual tension produces carpal-tunnel syndrome, an acute ache in the hands, wrists, and forearms; tendinitis; stiffness in the trapezius, the large, diamond-shaped muscle that spans the shoulders and upper back; fatigue from working much harder than is really necessary; tightness in chest muscles; and circulation problems which may lead to high blood pressure and heart trouble. A poorly trained bodyworker will suffer pain and stiffness in the shoulders, arms and hands, as well as general

exhaustion, after only two or three clients. A basic part of the training of Self-Healing practitioners is learning how to avoid this overexertion, and we can truthfully claim that any of us could work a full day without any problems in the hands, shoulders or back. The simple secret lies in avoiding unnecessary effort.

Perhaps this particular tension has its roots in early childhood, especially in learning to write. We all tense our hands when we write, as well as tightening our shoulders, stiffening our necks, pressing harder than necessary on the pen, compressing our jaws and foreheads, and breathing shallowly. If you have ever watched small children writing, you can see this in its most exaggerated form, but most of us never quite outgrow it. As a writer, Maureen has often experienced how profoundly unnatural it is to have to channel communication – normally an oral activity – through her arms and hands, and maybe this is part of why writing is often so difficult.

Many people use their hands automatically and unconsciously to express anxiety – wringing the hands, tapping the fingers, twisting the hair, tearing up paper, and doodling. This is a sure sign of tension in the shoulders, neck and jaw. Because of contracted muscles in these areas, the hands feel restless and their nervousness is expressed through these nervous movements. This kind of severe neck and shoulder tension is, in our opinion, part of a pattern which may contribute to a stroke. The constriction of muscles around the large blood vessels of the neck which we described earlier can lead eventually to the momentary cutting-off of blood to the brain which is the cause of a stroke. There are three contributors to a stroke: (1) a poor diet; (2) an innate tendency for atherosclerosis, a condition resulting in thickening and/or hardening of the arterial walls; and, in our opinion, (3) extreme muscle contraction in the neck. In many cases, one would not get a stroke without number 3.

It should be clear by now that the issue of muscle relaxation is vital to a healthy body. There are a number of ways to achieve it, but many of these have undesirable side effects. We have found gentle, undemanding movement to be the most effective means of relaxing the muscles, and we recommend that our clients make this part of their daily maintenance. Some clients (especially those whose problems were caused in the first place by a total lack of exercise) ask indignantly, 'Am I going to have to do these exercises for the rest of my life?' Well – if you envision a completely stress-free life, then the answer is 'No.' The rest of us need something to counteract the physical effects of daily stresses. We all have our individual ways of coping. This way has many advantages: no drugs, no alcohol, no need to spend money or buy special clothes or even leave the house. The only side effects are increased well-being, energy, flexibility, strength and overall relaxation; the only investments are your time and attention. You give time and energy to many different things in life – is it not worthwhile to give them to your health and well-being?

As with so many other of the exercises in this book, you will be doing things consciously that you have, up until now, done unconsciously, adding the element of kinesthetic awareness to movements that may have been mechanical. What you do may not be as important as how you do it.

When working to improve the quality of your movement, there are three aspects to focus on.

The first of these is *isolation*, or learning to use the right muscle, or muscle group, for a particular action. If you tense your neck when trying to lift something, you not only exhaust your neck muscles doing something they are not equipped to do, you also use different arm muscles from those which would have been used had the neck been loose. This means that you are writing off many important muscles. When you tighten up many more muscles than you need for a specific action, your nervous system will be working very monotonously. This is destructive for the nervous system and for the muscles which need the neurological stimulation. You may end up with poor coordination, very contracted muscles, damaged joints, limited blood flow and lack of grace. What isolation means, therefore, is working one muscle or muscle group while resting the others.

The second aspect is learning how to use muscle contraction, effort and resistance to strengthen your muscles in a balanced and helpful way. There are plenty of books, videos and instructors around who will tell you that it is good to strengthen your muscles, and tell you how to do it. Some of our clients came to us – with back strain, muscle sprains, joint damage, torn tendons, tendinitis, and other exercise-related injuries – as a result of knowing only this kind of muscle work. If you strengthen only some sets of muscles and neglect their opponents, if you strengthen your muscles without relaxing them, you can cause yourself much physical harm.

The third aspect is to develop a sense of elongation through movement. This includes visualizing that the muscles are long as well as physically stretching them in a balanced way. Overstretching, just like overtensing, is unhealthy and weakening for the muscles.

When you strive for flexibility but do not contract after stretching, or when you stretch some muscles and leave their opponents stiff, you may suffer postural and structural damages – torn muscles, tendons and even ligaments – and these are slow to heal.

When we teach exercises, we design the program to reflect the principles above. A person is introduced to movement in stages. The first stage is readying the body for movement, through relaxation and kinesthetic awareness. When you are relaxed and sensitive to your body, your exercises will be much more effective, since you will be better able to sense which muscles you are using, which movements are genuinely helpful, where change is taking place, and so on. For this stage we use massage, passive movement, visualization and very gentle exercises whose main purpose is to increase your body awareness.

The second stage of exercise is movement done without the resistance of gravity, or with very little resistance. This includes movement done in water, where gravity's pull is reduced, and some exercises which are done lying on the back, which require very little resistance. Even this kind of gentle exercise activates the muscles enough to improve their circulation, their elasticity and, to some extent, their strength.

The third stage is non-vigorous movement which yet requires some resistance to gravity. An example of this might be sitting cross-legged and slowly curling the spine forward so as to lower the head toward the floor.

The fourth stage, of course, is vigorous exercise which encourages muscle contraction and builds muscle size and strength.

In the following exercises, we will deal with all of these aspects of movement. The main purpose of these exercises, however, is to make you aware of your own movement: how it feels now; how it can feel when you try to do it in different ways; how your body responds to different types of movement; where your strengths and weaknesses, tensions and flexibility, lie. All of the exercises in this book involve using your muscles; the exercises in this chapter are about getting to know those muscles.

The Lower Body

5–1   Let's start with your feet, since they support your entire body and never really get the attention they deserve.

Stand up, barefoot, and find your natural stance – the one you automatically fall into when you need to stand for any length of time. Chances are that your stance is unbalanced, with all or most of your weight supported on one foot, the hip on that side thrown out to the side, the spine curved sideways in that direction, and the other leg more or less dangling. This stance often evolves because the muscles are stronger on one side of your body than the other, and these strong muscles will pull your whole body toward their own side. Most people have a tendency to walk and stand more heavily on one foot than on the other, and this can affect posture, spine alignment and the amount of stress placed on the leg joints.

Now stand with your feet hip-width apart and try to distribute your weight evenly on both feet. Feel how your feet meet the floor. Is your weight on the balls of the feet, or the heels, or the toes? Is it more on the outside or the inside of the foot? Try to balance yourself on each foot in turn by lifting the other foot and holding it suspended for a minute. Where do you place your weight on the supporting foot? Do you feel a difference between the two feet in terms of how well they support you? Usually one foot will feel considerably stronger. Now lift one foot, hold it up for a few seconds, and then let it fall so that it strikes the floor with some impact; do not stop it, just let it relax so that it drops to the floor. Which part of the foot hits the floor first, or with the greatest force? This is probably the part of the foot you lean on the most heavily when standing or walking. Repeat the foot-drop ten or fifteen times, and see whether you can drop it so that all parts of the foot hit the floor evenly and at the same time. Do this exercise with the other foot, then do it so that you move each foot alternately. Does one foot come down more heavily or more stiffly than the other? By now it should be obvious which is your stronger foot, if it wasn't already.

5–2 Foot Massage Sit in a comfortable chair, or on the floor with your back supported by a wall, and take hold of one foot. If you noticed, while standing alternately on each foot, that one of your feet supported you better, take hold of the other one now. This foot is probably the weaker and tenser of the two. You will now learn how to give yourself the most effective foot massage you will ever receive.

With the lower part of one leg, just above the ankle, resting on the other thigh (knee bent), hold your ankle with one hand, your toes with the other hand, and slowly rotate the foot. Let your leg muscles relax, as all the work is done by your hands. Stretch the foot as far in each direction as you can comfortably, pulling slightly on the toes. Then let go of the

ankle and rotate the foot by itself. (Whenever you make a rotating motion, be sure to circle in both directions, clockwise and counter-clockwise, for an equal number of turns.) Tap with your fingertips around the ankle and up the shin, and feel how this brings circulation into the foot.

Give your toes a lot of attention. Take hold of all of them and move them together in rotation, and then rotate each one individually. First hold the toe and rotate it passively, then let go and see if you can get it to rotate on its own – or even to wiggle individually (fig 5–2A).

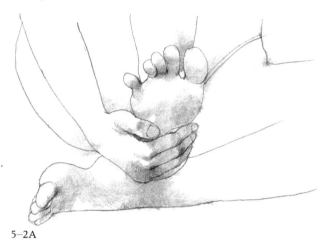

5–2A

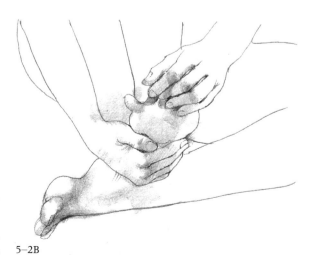

5–2B

You may need to hold onto all the other toes in order to help one move by itself (fig 5–2B). At first you may find that only the big toe can move by itself, but if you are patient you may get each toe to perform. We are accustomed to using the foot as though it is just one big, undifferentiated block, but in fact the foot is much like the hand in structure, with a similar number and arrangement of joints and bones. It is capable of great sensitivity, agility and flexibility, as some people with disabled hands have proved.

Taking each toe separately, press down on the toe with one finger while simultaneously pressing upward with the toe against the finger, so that the toe resists the finger's pressure. Reverse this by placing the finger underneath the toe and pressing up while the toe resists by pressing down. Do this sideways: press on your toe to one side, while trying to resist that pressure with the toe. Then press with your finger to the other side, and resist again with the toe. Now try to rotate your toe again without the help of your hands. Does it rotate any better than before? Stop and imagine that you are rotating the toe, and then rotate it again.

If you run into initial difficulties, remember that there are people who can draw, play music, drive, type and feed themselves with their toes – and they probably started off feeling just as limited as you do. With visualization and practice, you will be able to access your mobility, and along the way you will bring circulation to your feet as well.

Massage the arches of your feet with your thumbs, gently at first, then with gradually increasing pressure. The muscles of the arch are often very tight if the foot has remained for too long in one cramped position; often shoes are shaped so that they force the foot into an unnatural shape or angle. Massage along your instep with long strokes of the thumbs, from the toes toward the heel (always massage toward the heart). The tibialis anterior muscle runs all the way down the calf, into the instep of the foot; by massaging the instep, you are relaxing the leg muscles from your knees almost to your toes.

Continue to massage every part of the foot. See whether you can distinguish each muscle from the surrounding muscles as you massage it. Can you feel where the muscles overlap and intersect? Can you feel how a particularly tight muscle can cause tightness in the surrounding muscles? With your fingertips, try to trace the tibialis anterior through the instep and up the shin; then try to follow the flexor digitorum longus muscles, which run from the sole of the foot into the back of the calf. Stroke, pinch, and palpate the calf muscles; they will love it.

How does the foot feel now? Is its color different from the other foot? Stand up and feel how the two feet support you; has the stiff foot now become the relaxed foot? Now, of course, you will have to give the other foot the same treatment and see how they measure up to each other.

Exercises in the Bathtub

Exercising in the water is excellent for anyone whose muscles have been weakened by disease or lack of use, since it tones and strengthens the muscles without tiring them. Although you may be using exactly the same muscles as you would use out of the water, the sense of effort is much less, since your muscles will not feel as much of the resistance created by the pull of gravity. We have all been told that you can only strengthen muscles through hard

work ('no pain, no gain') , but it ain't necessarily so. Practice these exercises for ten days,
twenty minutes per day, before continuing
with more vigorous exercises.

You will need to fill your bathtub to practice
in deep water, so expect to splash. If you do
not have access to a bathtub, you can hopefully
practice the exercises for the pool or seashore,
described later.

5–3 Sit in the bathtub with your knees
slightly bent and your toes touching the
bathtub wall. By bending and flexing your
foot, bring your heels to the wall and away
from it. Repeat this movement at least twenty
times – do it 100 times if you can.

This is an extremely relaxing motion. On a
stressful business trip, for example, if you can
only find time to relax in the bathtub, alternate
between this exercise and exercise 5–4 –
spending more time with this one.

5–4 To get a sense of truly effortless movement, recline against the back of the tub with
your legs outstretched, and slowly bend and
straighten each leg in turn; then bend one as
you straighten the other. Your feet should slide
on the floor of the bathtub. Imagine that the
feet are leading the motion. Repeat this thirty
to forty times. Now bend forward, stretching
your arms toward your feet, and, as you sit up
slowly, rake your calves and your hamstrings
with your fingers.

5–5 Bend one knee, hold it with your hands
and bring it to your chest, and then throw
your leg back to the water. Now do the same
with your other leg. Repeat fifteen to twenty
times with each leg.

5–6 Bring both knees to your chest and let
yourself slide into the water (if your ears are
not sensitive and if you can avoid bumping
your head). Throw both legs into the water,
and, as they hit the tub wall, push yourself up
with your feet. Repeat this five or six times.
Return to exercise 5–4 and repeat it 100 times.

5–7 If possible, position yourself in the
bathtub on your abdomen, holding on with
your arms to a bar or to the side of the bath
so as not to slide in. Now bend your leg and
rotate it in deep water – only your foot should
be out in the air. Repeat with the other leg.

Exercises in a Pool

You do not need to know how to swim in
order to enjoy, and benefit from, moving with
very little gravitational resistance in a pool.
We shall describe a few of the endless possibilities for movement – experiment for yourself.

5–8 Stand with the edge of the pool at your
side, in water which is at least up to your
waist. Hold the side wall of the pool and,
facing along the side wall, let one of your legs
move freely, as if it is weightless. Have a sense
of lightness and ease of motion. Now bend
and flex your foot several times. Move your
straight leg in large circles, feeling a stretch
in your hip at all angles. Remember to circle
both clockwise and counterclockwise. Now lift
one knee forward, and, as you move it slowly
sideways and backward, bend it and kick with
your lower leg again and again – forward,
sideways and backward as high as you can.

5–9 Stand with your back to the wall, and bring your knees one by one to your chest. Pull each knee to the chest for an extra stretch, and then let your leg drop.

5–10 Hold the side wall of the pool with both hands, and climb up the wall with your feet until they are about two to three feet below your hands. Then try to straighten your legs – that may give you quite a stretch. In that position, keep 'marching' with your heels only – keeping your toes and the balls of your feet at their place on the wall.

Spend about two more months with the following exercises for the legs.

5–11 Lie down, preferably on a carpeted floor, but a blanket or a mat on the floor will do. Lie stretched out flat, with your toes pointing up to the ceiling. Slowly point and flex one foot at a time. When the foot points, the toes should be lowered toward the floor; when it flexes, the toes come backward, toward the shin. Feel which muscles are involved in pointing, and which in flexing. Now try to do this exercise in as relaxed a way as you can. Imagine that there are strings attached to your toes which someone else pulls to move your feet. Make as little effort with the rest of your body as possible, while still pointing and flexing the foot as fully as possible. Which muscles does this move in your legs, hips, back?

5–12 Gravity is the most readily available form of resistance. To strengthen the same muscles as in exercise 5–11, you can resist their motion using your own body's weight. Stand up, lift yourself up so that you are standing on your tiptoes, then rock your feet backward until only your heels are on the floor. You will probably need to hold something to keep your balance, but be sure that you are just balancing, rather than holding yourself up – all of your weight should be on your feet. Repeat this rocking motion thirty times, and try to stretch your feet a little more each time.

5–13 Lie on your back again with your legs stretched out flat, and rotate one ankle. As it rotates, notice which other leg muscles are involved in this motion. You may be tightening muscles all the way up your leg as you turn the ankle; try not to do this. Imagine that your toes are leading the motion and the rest of the foot is passively following, and allow as many as possible of your leg muscles to relax. Rotate the ankle at least fifty times in each direction, then rest while you imagine that you are still moving your foot. Visualize your ankle rotating effortlessly and smoothly, with no help from the other leg muscles. Now rotate the same foot again, and see whether you notice any difference in the way it moves. Stop and notice how that ankle feels in relation to the other one – looser? warmer? lighter? – before you go on to repeat this exercise with the other ankle.

5–14 Sit on a chair, and rest your left calf on your right thigh. Rotate your left ankle several times in both directions. Now hold the toes of your left foot with your right hand, and, as you rotate the foot, resist its motion with your hand. Do this very slowly, and be careful not to put painful pressure on the ankle. Repeat with the other leg.

5–15 Stand up, and, keeping both feet flat on the floor, shift your weight in a circular motion: lean heavily on your heels, and then on the left sides of your feet; slowly move your weight onto your toes, and then to the right sides of your feet. Rotate in this manner twenty times.

By relaxing the feet and increasing their blood supply, you have already provided a stronger base for the working of the leg muscles. Most popular exercises for the legs are designed for only two purposes: to slim them or to increase the muscle strength. What we are trying to do, however, is to help the legs to move in a way that improves not only their own functioning but also the way they function in relation to the rest of the body.

5–16 On the floor again, roll over onto your abdomen, with your head turned to one side. Bend one leg at the knee, and rotate the calf of that leg, both clockwise and counterclockwise (fig 5–16A). Imagine that the foot leads the motion, that the calf is weightless, the knee moves fluidly and without effort, and the thighs, hips and back are completely at rest. The more muscles you can relax, the more it will become clear which muscles are really meant to be used in this motion and how much effort is actually required for the motion – not very much.

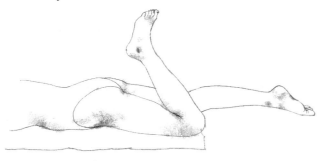

5–16A

After you have repeated this exercise with each leg, raise both calves and let the right rest on the left, while rotating the left calf (fig 5–16B). The purpose here is to let the right leg be completely passive, allowing the left to do all the work. Does the right leg allow itself to be carried? Reverse this motion, resting the left leg on the right, and see whether it is easier or more difficult on this side to allow the leg to relax. Does one leg seem to be stronger than the other? Is one leg stronger and the other leg more relaxed? Or is one leg both stronger *and* more relaxed?

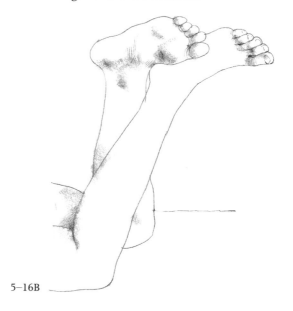

5–16B

5–17 Lying on your back, lift one leg, grasp the thigh of that leg above the knee with both hands, with the foot hanging loosely, and shake the thigh muscles vigorously. Move your hands up to mid-thigh and shake the leg again. As your hands move up your leg, be aware of the different muscles you are touching, and of their sensations. Feel where they are tight and where they are loose, where they resist the motion and where they allow it. Stretch both legs out flat and notice whether you can feel a difference in sensation between them. Now stand up and see whether there is a difference in how your legs support you. Do you stand more solidly and firmly on one than on the other? Is there a difference in the way each leg joins the pelvis and hip? Does one thigh or calf seem to be working harder than the other to bear your weight? Repeat the exercise with the other leg.

5–18 Lie on your side, bring the upper knee to your chest, then take hold of the ankle, draw the foot back as close to the buttock as possible, and then pull the knee backward behind you, as far as you can (fig 5–18). Repeat this movement five or six times, then get up and sit in a chair and notice how the two sides of the pelvis feel. The side you moved may feel looser, larger, lighter, warmer, more alive. This is an exercise which dancers or athletes will do standing up, but it loosens the pelvis and the front of the thigh just as effectively done lying down, and is far less rigorous. (If you are strong and in good shape, you may prefer to do this exercise standing up and holding a table for balance.) Now lie down again and repeat the exercise on the other side.

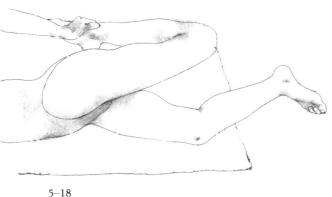

5–18

5–19 Lying on your back with both knees bent, slowly straighten your right leg until it lies flat on the floor. Then slowly bend the right knee, drawing your right heel toward your right hip, while at the same time allowing the left leg to straighten until it is flat on the floor. Now bend the left leg while you straighten the right. Your feet should always be touching the floor, and every movement should be done slowly and fluidly. Place your hands on your abdomen and feel how the muscles there tighten as your legs bend and straighten; feel also how the muscles in your thighs and hips are working.

Now try to imagine that your feet alone are performing this motion, as though someone else is holding and moving them, or as if they are strong enough to move without the assistance of your entire lower body. Breathe into your abdomen and let go of the tension there. Relax your hips and thighs and put all of your attention into your feet. See how much unnecessary muscle tension you can eliminate while doing this motion. Also notice which muscles are working the hardest. We do not expect you to be able to isolate the exact muscles and cite them by their Latin names, but do try to get a sense of where they are – on the inside of the thigh? the upper part of the hips? the outside of the thighs? Everyone's body works differently from everyone else's; what we want is for you to get a sense of how *your* body works.

5–20 You can create resistance without using weights for strength training. Sit with your back to a wall, knees to your chest and feet flat on the floor. Try to straighten one leg while creating resistance to the movement by holding first the shin (fig 5–20A), then the back of the thigh (fig 5–20B), with both hands.

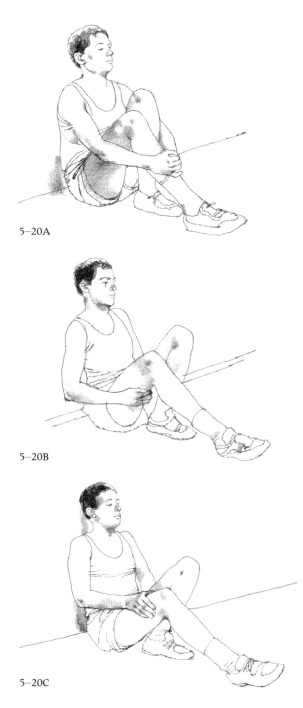

5–20A

5–20B

5–20C

Your leg has to work against the pressure of your hands. When the leg has succeeded in straightening itself, try to bend it again while pushing with both hands against the front of

the thigh (fig 5–20C). (Do not resist the leg's motion so hard that you strain your shoulders, just hard enough to make the thigh muscles work.) Repeat this exercise many times.

5–21 Next, stand facing a wall. Hold a chair or counter-top, if you need to, to balance yourself, place the sole of one foot flat against the wall, and slowly lean forward so that the knee bends toward the chest. This movement automatically creates resistance: when the body leans forward, the foot and ankle resist the motion; when the leg straightens, the pelvis resists. This exercise stretches the entire back of the leg and the groin area of the supporting leg, and passively works the hamstrings and the muscles of the shin area. To relax from this exercise, bend your upper body toward your lifted leg, to stretch the muscles that have worked.

5–22 To loosen tight muscles in the hips and outer thighs, lie on your side with a pillow under your head, roll forward until your upper knee is resting comfortably on the floor, and begin to lightly strike the tight muscles with a loose fist. Do not pound with the fist itself, but rather let the motion come from the wrist. Your hand should bounce lightly off the muscle after it strikes. (You can also purchase bongers, which have a rubber ball attached to a flexible handle and are designed for this purpose, and these may give you a much longer reach.) Move up and down the leg from the knee up to the hip and behind to the buttocks. Most people are surprised to find how much tension they carry in the buttock muscles, but it really is not strange, since these muscles do so much of the work of supporting us when we stand or walk.

5–23 The next exercise may be something of a challenge for the thigh muscles, but if you have warmed and loosened your muscles with the preceding exercises you will find it much easier to do. Sit with the buttocks between the feet, the inner thigh and calf resting on the floor and the feet pointing out to each side. From this position, raise yourself up onto your knees, using the power of the thigh muscles alone to do this. As before, try not to allow the back and abdominal muscles to do the work for you; even the buttock muscles, which do participate in this movement, should be as relaxed as possible. Make your thighs work. Lower yourself slowly to the left, so that you end up sitting on your left heel, and notice where you feel a stretch in this position. Raise yourself up again, remembering to use only the thighs, and lower yourself onto your right heel (fig 5–23). Continue this pattern – lowering yourself first between your thighs, then to the left, between the thighs, to the right, and again between, as slowly as possible – four or five times. Then stand, feet apart, weight evenly balanced on both feet, and see whether you feel any difference in your stance from how it felt

in the beginning. Strengthening your legs will give your whole body a much more solid foundation to rest on and to move from.

5–24 Lie on your back, knees bent, feet flat on the floor. Move your legs so that the feet are tracing large circles on the floor, with one moving clockwise and the other counter-clockwise (this may sound complicated, but you will find that they move this way naturally). Again, imagine that the feet are leading the motion, and relax your abdomen and lower back. Focus your attention on the muscles of the legs. Now let one leg rest while the other circles, making the circle as large as possible, then move both legs simultaneously again. Do not forget to change directions: the leg which circled clockwise should also circle counterclockwise, and vice versa.

5–25 Do exercise 3–10 in the Joints chapter. Now massage your inner thighs from the groin to the knees, and focus on the areas where you felt the most resistance.

You can relax the outer thigh muscles by placing a tennis ball under the thigh and then pressing the thigh down against the ball (fig

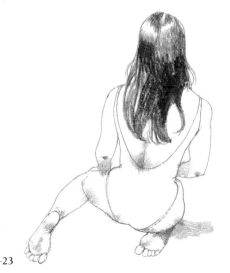

5–23

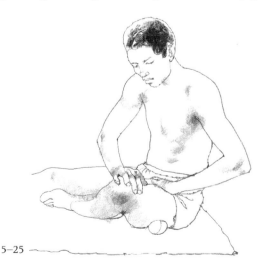

5–25

5–25). Move the ball from one point to another, all along the underside of the thigh.

Last, press down on the knees while at the same time resisting the motion with your thighs. Make your thigh muscles work; do not let your back or abdominal muscles do it for them. Press as hard as you can and resist the pressure as firmly as you can. Now press without resistance. Do your thighs allow more movement than they did at first?

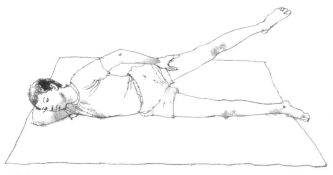

5–27

5–26   To stretch the muscles of both the inner and the outer thighs, as well as the hips and lower back, practice exercises 3–37 and 3–38 from the Joints chapter. Always remember to breathe deeply, so that your abdomen will constantly expand and release, and keep your abdomen and lower back from trying to participate in the movement.

Now, for a more challenging stretch, slowly lower both knees, simultaneously, toward the midline – that is, toward each other. Do not push this stretch too far; you should be able to feel quite a stretch in the hips and thighs, but do not force your knees to the floor.

Repeat exercises 3–37 and 3–38 at least thirty times with each leg, and then do the same with resistance: as you bring your knee up, press against it with your hand.

5–27   Lie on one side with both legs straight, and lift the upper leg. Imagine that your leg is weightless, and that your foot is pulled up with a string. Now bring the leg down, and repeat the motion.

After lifting and lowering each leg seven times, do the same with resistance: lift the leg while you press down on the thigh with the palm of your hand (fig 5–27). Press as hard as you can to resist the upward movement of the leg, so that the thigh muscles will have to

work hard. Make sure that they, and not the back, hips or abdomen, are working.

When you have raised the leg as high as you can, bring it forward so it is perpendicular to your body, and lower it slowly while pressing upward on the thigh with your hand. The effects of this exercise are similar to those achieved with Nautilus machines; the difference is that you can automatically vary the amount of resistance and so avoid straining the working muscle.

5–28   Now sit cross-legged, in the position known in yoga as the half-lotus, with the left foot resting on the right thigh. Do you feel any strain or tension in this position, and, if so, where? When you reverse the position, with the right foot resting on the left thigh, do you feel any pain or tension, and is it in the same places as on the other side? For a few minutes, lie or sit comfortably and massage the areas that hurt or strain in this position. You can stroke with your fingertips, rub vigorously with your palms, and tap percussively with a loose wrist and relaxed fingers. Try placing your palms flat on the tight area and shaking them so that they vibrate the muscles under them. If you have pain or tension around the ankle, squeeze and stroke the foot and calf close to the ankle; if around the knees, tap on them and rub them. Return to the half-lotus and see whether it is more comfortable now.

Holding the half-lotus position and grasping your knees, rotate your whole upper body from the pelvis up, making the rotation as large as you can. Do this motion both clockwise and counterclockwise, first with the right foot uppermost, then with the left. Does this help to make the position more comfortable to hold?

If you are fairly flexible, try these same exercises in the full-lotus position, with each foot resting on the opposite thigh. At least attempt to sit in this position for a minute or two, if only to see where your muscle tensions are, but do not stay in this position for longer than that if it is uncomfortable for you. This exercise activates muscles that you do not use regularly.

Learning to Walk

When a baby learns to walk, it has essentially taught itself a complicated series of movements and gravitational shifts. Many muscles must be used to pull off this extraordinary balancing-act. This is such a terrific achievement that it is a shame that the process of learning to walk usually stops right there, after the child has figured out how to get from place to place on two feet while balancing to stay upright. It would be nice if we could also show the child how to walk well, placing equal weight on each foot, lifting the feet high enough to allow full movement of the foot's muscles and bones, bending the front knee while straightening the back knee, and all without tightening the hips, knees and ankles. Unfortunately, most children learn their style of walking by observing their parents, and so harmful movement patterns are unconsciously perpetuated.

The way you walk may of course be altered along the way by many other factors, but the adaptations you make will almost always be completely unconscious. It is a very unusual thing for a person to decide to walk in a particular way, except perhaps as part of an act or impersonation. A style of walking may be common not only to a family but to an entire cultural group. Early white settlers noticed that Native Americans walked with their toes pointed inward. Maya Angelou, in her book *I Know why the Caged Bird Sings*, remembers that her black community suspected that white people were not completely human because (among other things) they walked 'on their heels, like horses, instead of on the balls of their feet like people'.

5–29 When you have done something the same way for long enough – and since infancy is a very long time – it becomes very hard to change the way you do it. One way to involve muscles that are usually not part of our walking pattern is to walk (barefoot, if possible) on an uneven surface. When you step in sand or on grass, when you climb up a hill or descend from it, each step calls for a slightly different positioning of the foot, and hence of the leg, hip and back. If you can, walk several miles a day on a soft surface for two months.

Many of us, when we walk, strain our hips, lower back and abdomen, moving the legs from this region instead of by the power of the leg muscles themselves. The more you keep your attention and awareness on the feet and legs, and the less you use your lower back and hips, the more efficiently you will walk. What is efficient movement? It is movement which enhances body function rather than detracting from it. Walking is a motion

109

designed to be performed by the legs. If you use principally your leg muscles for walking, you will strengthen them and increase their capacity for walking. If you walk using principally the power of your back and hips, which were not designed for that purpose, you will simultaneously exhaust them and weaken your legs.

The pelvis is one of the three major stress-bearing areas of our bodies, along with the knees and the neck. Because of the limited movement we have in our daily life, it becomes stiff. The way most people walk is one reason for this stiffness. When we walk with rigid feet, tense ankles and locked knees, all the shock of the impact of every step is conducted directly into the pelvic joints, instead of being evenly distributed and absorbed along the way by the other joints. This kind of walk contributes directly to arthritis of the hips and knees, and also to the fragility of the pelvis so often found in older people. Ideally, the impact should be taken by the foot first, then by the ankle, then by the knee, and last and least of all by the hip. This can happen only if the feet and knees are strong, relaxed and flexible. All the work you have been doing on your feet, legs, hips and pelvis will be the first step toward a stronger pelvis, and will naturally improve the activities your legs do the most: standing and walking. You will find that standing will bring less strain and fatigue, and walking will be easier and more beneficial to the body as a whole.

With time, stiff, uneven walking can lead not only to damage in the ankles, knees and hips, but also to back problems such as sciatica and to extreme hardening of connective tissue, which often develops in the inner or outer thigh muscles.

5–30 Being aware of how you habitually walk is the next step. The best way to observe your own walk is to walk with shoes – since you normally do wear them when you are out walking – on a hard floor, so that you can hear yourself walk. Walk around the floor in your usual way, at your usual pace, and pay attention to how your walk feels, looks and sounds. Does one of your feet make more noise than the other when it hits the floor? Do you drag either or both of your feet? Do you tend to kick them out ahead of you? Are your knees or your ankles locked in place? Do you tiptoe, or slam down on your heels, or walk on the outsides of the feet only? (You should have some clue about this from your previous work on your feet.) Now walk so that you heavily exaggerate whatever peculiarities you have discovered in your walk, and see how this feels, in the legs, in the hips and in the back. To a lesser degree, this is what your walk is doing to your body with every step you take.

In our movement classes, we often ask one student to walk across the room and have the rest of the class imitate the walk, to demonstrate how individual a walk can be and to give each student the sense of how different patterns of tension affect the body.

So, when you begin to correct the way you walk, do not be surprised if it feels completely unnatural at first. You may feel as though the movements you are making look bizarre and exaggerated, but if you watch yourself in the mirror as you walk you will see that this is not the case.

5–31 There are three very simple things to remember in stress-reduced walking. The first is to bend your knees when you step (fig 5–31). It may seem strange even to have to mention this, but it is amazing how many

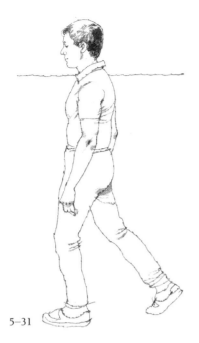

5-31

people walk with completely locked knees, either dragging their feet so that they barely leave the floor or actually kicking the foot out in front with every step. You can correct this by imagining with every step that you are stepping over some small obstacle, like a stick. This will give you enough lift to bend the knee sufficiently, but not enough to look as though you are marching – though at first it may feel that way.

The second thing to remember is to put each foot down with equal impact. Almost everyone walks more heavily on one foot than on the other, as any shoe-repairer can tell you. Listening to your walk will help you to correct this. Practice walking so that each foot makes the same sound when it hits the floor.

The third key is to put the foot down with the heel first, and then roll the foot until the weight is transferred to the ball of the foot and the toes. The weight should be distributed evenly on each part of the foot in its turn. This is much easier and more natural if you are

bending your knees. Many people have a tendency to walk heavily on their heels, a tendency which becomes even more pronounced when they walk quickly. Others land heavily on the balls of the feet, which can create a swayback and weaken the lumbar area.

The muscles of the thighs, hips and buttocks are extremely strong – some of the strongest in the body – and are therefore capable of developing extraordinary tension. If you find you have a lot of difficulty in changing the way you walk, it may be due to habitual tightness in these areas. Sometimes a muscle tension may be so deep and so persistent that any movement that the muscle tries to perform will only make the tension worse. This is where bodywork and massage techniques can be most helpful.

The Abdomen and Back

The back muscles, particularly those of the lower back, also help to support our upright posture – a difficult task, for which they need to be supple and strong. But, with most people, the lower-back muscles tend to be both tense and weak: tense because we tend to limit their range of mobility, and weak because this tension restricts the circulation and limits even further the easy movement which naturally strengthens muscles.

Many people believe that they must strengthen their abdominal muscles to support the lower back. This idea is on the right track, but it misses the point. It is true that a weak abdomen will put additional strain on the lower back, which has as much stress as it can cope with even under optimal conditions. However, it is as wrong to speak in terms of

111

asking the abdomen to support the lower back as to want the lower back to support the abdomen: both sets of muscles have their own specific functions, and both must be strengthened so that they can function efficiently and as independently as possible. Moreover, this principle applies to every muscle in the body.

Strengthening and relaxing the abdomen does take some strain off the lower-back muscles. It also aids digestion, especially in the intestines, and may make a potbelly smaller if it was caused by slack muscles. Breathing also improves when the abdomen is relaxed enough to expand fully with a deep breath.

The lower abdomen has less connective tissue holding it than does the upper abdomen – only one strong sheet instead of two, which is one reason why it tends to herniate. The lower abdomen will benefit much from releasing the tension in it, because of the improved circulation it will get. All the releasing exercises for the lower back are good for hernia, as is exercise 5–4 in this chapter.

The first three abdominal exercises should be done in your bathtub. Do these water exercises every day for two weeks, and then go on to the exercises that follow.

5–32 In water deep enough to cover all of your body, slowly bend both knees and bring them up to your chest. Hold them there for a few seconds, then slowly straighten them. Do this five or six times.

5–33 Bring the knees to the chest, hold them there with a hand on each knee, and move them both together in rotating motion, pressing the thighs against the abdomen as you do so. Rotate them about ten times in each direction. Then massage the abdomen under water with your palms, pressing as deeply as is comfortable.

5–34 Because you are in the bathtub anyway, you may as well try the next exercise. You may find that it helps your digestion and internal organs.

Sit in the bathtub, inhale and blow out your cheeks. Do not exhale as you slide and sink into the water – your head included. Slowly release the air through your mouth until you feel you have emptied your lungs. Sit up again, breathe normally, and repeat the exercise five more times.

The following exercises are done outside the water.

Lie on the floor on your back. Bend and straighten your knees alternately, quickly, 100 times. Keep your hands on your abdomen and try not to use the muscles of your abdomen for this motion. This exercise is good for the lower abdomen, including a herniated lower abdomen.

Bring your knees to your chest, hold your knees with your hands and move your knees in circles in opposite directions. Relax your abdomen, thighs and back. Let your knees be moved passively by your hands. Now hug your knees and rotate them together.

Now you are ready for more vigorous exercises.

5–35 Lying on your back, place your feet flat on the floor and lift up one hip at a time, as far as you can, until you feel the muscles on that side of the abdomen gently stretching (fig 5–35). This is a good exercise to relieve constipation and gas pain.

Return to exercises 5–32 to 5–35 when you relax from the following, more vigorous, exercises.

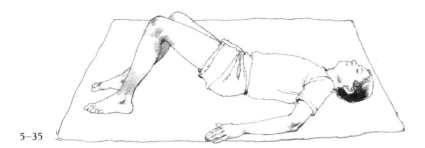

5–35

5–36 Lie on your back, bend your knees and bring them to your chest, and straighten your legs upward, perpendicular to your body. Now lower your legs slowly toward the floor. Keep your feet flexed – this will help your back not to tense during this exercise. After doing this several times with both legs, do it with each leg separately.

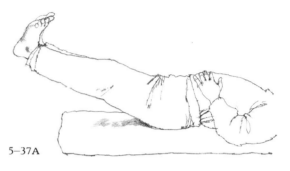

5–37A

5–37 Lie on your back, with your legs stretched. Begin by breathing deeply 'into' the abdomen and fully expanding it with your breath, at least five times. Now lift both legs a few inches off the floor, feet together (fig 5–37A), and rotate them six times each way. Move the feet hip-width apart (fig 5–37B), and repeat the rotation.

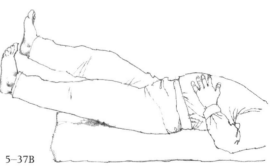

5–37B

In all of these exercises, you must remember to keep your feet flexed and to not allow the abdominal muscles to strain. It is helpful to massage the abdomen as you move the legs, and to imagine that it is the feet which are pulling the legs up with them, rather than the abdomen straining to hold the legs up. Now hold the feet hip-width apart, but with one foot higher off the floor than the other (fig 5–37C) and repeat the rotation. Do the same with the other foot held higher.

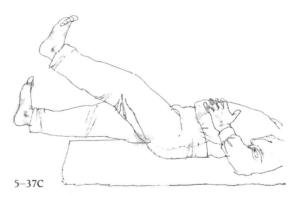

5–37C

5–38 Lying on your side, with your head supported by a firm pillow, or by your arm, do the same series of leg-lifts described in the previous exercise (fig 5–38A, 5–38B and 5–38C). Keep one upper arm in front of you for balance, but do not use it to help in the movement. Imagine that the feet are lifting the legs, and breathe deeply as you move.

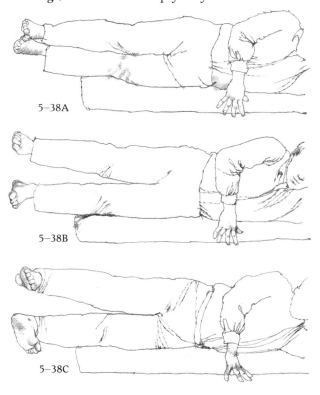

5–38A

5–38B

5–38C

The Torso

To relax and strengthen the back muscles, nothing can compare with massage. The back, being the center of the body, ends up – rightly or wrongly – being involved with nearly every movement we perform. Like the hips and legs, it can become so tense that any movement we attempt may just increase the tension. To put it quite simply, the back muscles are over-worked and there is nothing they appreciate

more than to lie perfectly still and let someone else's hands ease their tension and restore their circulation.

For many areas of the body, self-massage is perfectly adequate, but this becomes difficult with the back. Refer to exercise 7–17 in the Massage chapter for some ideas, which would be an excellent preparation for back exercises if you can't get a massage from someone else. (The sooner we all learn to expect massage as one of our daily requirements and inalienable rights, the happier and healthier we will be!)

5–39 The next exercise will help you to find out where your back tensions are. We caution those who have a serious back problem or are worried about their backs to get their doctor's approval before doing this exercise, since it can be somewhat rigorous for the spine.

First, get a broomstick or a thick dowel, place it on the floor, and lie down on top of it so that it lies directly under your spine. Breathe deeply and try to relax your back muscles. To anyone lying on top of a broom-stick for the first time, that last direction will seem pretty ridiculous – how can you relax when it hurts so much? – but the surprising truth is that the pressure of the broomstick does not have to hurt: it hurts only in those spots where the muscles are tense, and it will stop hurting if you can relax the muscles. That is why this exercise, though it seems like a form of torture, is so effective – you have such a good incentive to relax! So try for a time to bear the pain. Visualize your back muscles lengthening, flattening and softening, breathe deeply, and imagine that your breath flows into the painful areas. Tell yourself: I am breathing deeply; my back is relaxing, growing longer and wider and flatter; my spinal muscles are as soft as butter, melting over this broomstick; my vertebrae are softly cushioned and separated by large spaces. You may like to dictate this or something like it onto a tape to listen to while you do this exercise.

It may take several sessions of trying before your back becomes comfortable with the broomstick. If it is impossible at first to lie with your whole spine on the broomstick, place it so that only part of your spine lies on it, and introduce your back to it bit by it.

As you lie on the broomstick, you can do the following exercises.

Place your hands under your head and lift it, bringing your chin to your chest, making sure not to strain your neck (fig 5–39A). Many people feel less or no pain in this position. Lower the head and lift it again, three or four times.

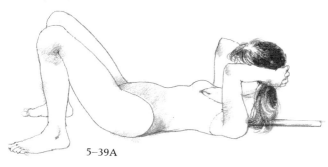

5–39A

With your head resting on the broomstick, bring one knee up to your chest, breathe deeply, lower the leg, and bring the other knee to your chest (fig 5–39B).

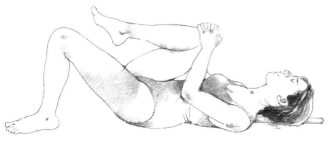

5–39B

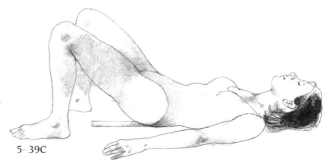

5–39C

Place both feet flat on the floor, tilt the pelvis up to stretch the lower back, and breathe deeply (fig 5–39C). Lower your pelvis to the broomstick.

Then concentrate on your head. Sense each side of your face separately, and visualize each side relaxing separately. Imagine each eye in turn as large, liquid and soft. Follow the sensation of each eye inward, to the deep inner parts of the brain, and imagine that your brain, too, is a muscle that softens and relaxes. Mentally relax your skull, and the skin covering it, even to the roots of your hair. Let your forehead relax. Sense your jaw, and the relative tightness and heaviness of it and of your tongue and teeth. You may also find it relaxing to palm your eyes (see exercise 8–5 in the Vision chapter).

When you roll off the broomstick, lie on your back for a few minutes, pull one knee up to your chest, hold it with both hands, and rotate it, clockwise and counterclockwise, forty or fifty times. Then do the same with the other knee. This will erase any after-effects of the pressure on your spine.

Now notice how your back feels. If you have an area that stays sore after you get up off the broomstick, or an area that was particularly troublesome when you were lying on the broomstick, make that your target area.

For more back exercises, turn to the Spine chapter, which is devoted entirely to exercises for the spinal muscles. You may like to begin with the exercises for your specific target area; we suggest, however, that you try all of the back movements in the chapter, so as to completely relax the entire back and keep it in balance. You should also massage your back, with the help of the instructions in the Massage chapter, or arrange for a member of your Self-Healing group to exchange massages with you.

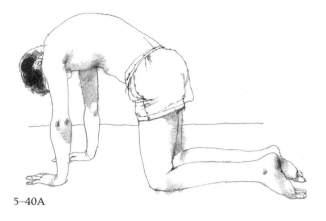

5–40A

5–40 The following series of movements is designed both to isolate – that is, to use specific muscles for specific purposes – and to coordinate different parts of the spine. These movements are done on hands and knees, as shown. The first is known as the Cow–Cat in yoga. For the first part, the Cow, slowly bring your head up and backward; then, imagining that you move one vertebra at a time (beginning with the neck vertebrae and working down to the coccyx), let your spine curve into a concave shape, with your abdomen at the lowest point and your head and rear somewhat elevated. Then, again imagining that you move one vertebra at a time, beginning at the coccyx and slowly working up to the head, arch your back into a convex shape, like the back of an angry cat (fig 5–40A). Your middle back will then be at the highest point and your head and rear lowered and somewhat tucked in. Alternate these two movements several times, taking at least a full minute to go from the Cow to the Cat position. Try to focus your movement in the back muscles themselves, without too much tensing of the shoulders or abdomen. Notice how far your awareness extends – can you actually sense the movement of the vertebrae all the way down the spine, or are there areas where you simply cannot

feel it? You may like to do this motion in front of a mirror, as seeing the motion may help you to feel it more, and to locate your sensation in the area which is actually moving. This exercise helps to re-create the natural spaces between vertebrae, balances the distribution of pressure on the intervertebral disks, and improves circulation and so makes movement easier throughout the spine.

There are so many ways to move the spine while on all fours that it is difficult to list them all.

To relieve tension in the lower back, rotate your buttocks, keeping the arms and legs as stationary as possible. You can then vary this motion by allowing your thighs to rock forward and backward in a rotating motion as you rotate the hips, which will make the range of the rotation larger and work the thigh muscles.

Next, rotate your entire torso, so that the weight shifts forward onto your hands and back onto your knees as you rotate.

Now keep your pelvis as stationary as you can and rotate the chest and upper back. Do this first with the weight remaining equally distributed on both hands at all times, so that the rotation involves more of an up-and-down motion; then rotate so that your weight shifts

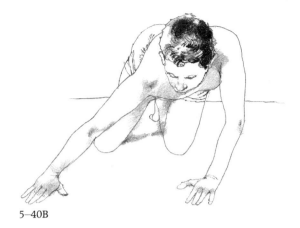

5–40B

from one hand to the other, giving more of a side-to-side motion (fig 5–40B).

Now keep your entire torso stationary and your weight on both hands, and rotate your shoulders – first together and in the same direction, and then alternately, so that one shoulder will be up while the other is down.

Last, lower your head to the ground with your back arched so that the top of your skull touches the floor and takes some of your weight (fig 5–40C), and rotate your whole torso so that the pressure moves around the top of your head in a circular motion.

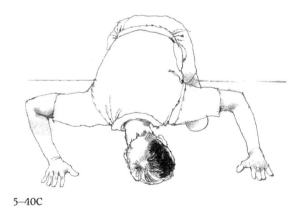

5–40C

Of all the exercises in this book, these are the hardest to describe. If you have a hard time understanding these directions, just get on

your hands and knees and start moving in whatever way feels best to you, then begin to experiment with different types of movement. Use these suggestions as a starting-point, and go on to see how many different ways you can find to move your spine. Any and all of these movements will benefit the spinal muscles.

5–41 Swimming is a wonderful opportunity to isolate your torso from the rest of your body. As you swim, imagine that your toes are pushing you and your fingers are leading you, and that no effort needs to be made by the feet, calves, thighs, back, arms or shoulders.

5–42 Breathing deeply provides the best way to become aware of the anterior (frontal) torso muscles. Lie on your back with your knees bent, or, if it is comfortable for you, with your knees bent out to the sides and the soles of the feet together, so that the legs make a diamond shape. This position opens up the groin and pelvis and slightly stretches the abdominal muscles. Try both positions and see which is better for you; if both feel good, notice in what ways the two positions feel different.

Place your hands flat on your abdomen and inhale slowly and deeply, allowing your breath to swell your abdomen, then move the hands up to the diaphragm and let your breath expand it, and last move your hands to your chest and feel how your breath lifts it. Begin to expel the breath slowly, feeling first how the chest deflates, then the diaphragm and last the abdomen.

Now breathe normally for several breaths.

The Neck

Your neck has a sixteen-hour-per-day job holding up your head, which is a fairly heavy load. Your neck muscles may be among the tightest in your entire body. The side neck muscles may be so hard to the touch that they could be mistaken for bone. This book is full of exercises to relax these and other neck muscles; you can find them in the chapters on Breathing (1–10, 1–24), Circulation (2–18), the Joints (3–26), the Spine (4–2, 4–21, 4–26, 4–27, 4–28), the Nervous System, Massage, Vision, and Back Pain. The following exercise is just to give you a sense of your own neck muscles.

5–43 Sit comfortably, and rotate your head slowly (fig 5–43A). You will notice immediately whether the motion feels like a smooth roll or a series of little jerky movements. You may also notice creaks, crackles or crunches as the head circles; these are nothing to worry about, but they do indicate stiffness in the neck. Now move your head up and back, extending your throat, then down and forward, until the chin touches the chest. Notice any tightness or pain in the throat or the back of

the neck. Tilt your head to the left and then raise your chin up as far as possible, stretching the side muscles on the right, then repeat the same motion to the other side.

You can test the flexibility and strength of your neck by using resistance. Most people find they have more strength than flexibility, but the neck needs both. Place your hands under your chin to raise the head, and then palm-down on the top of your head to lower it. Try to lower your chin to your chest while at the same time pushing upward on it with your fingers. Then try to raise your head while you push down on it with your palm. Which is stronger, your hands or your neck?

Holding your head with both hands, try to move your head up and down, and in circles, with no resistance from the neck at all (fig 5–43B). Will your neck relax enough to allow your head to be passively moved, or does it insist on participating?

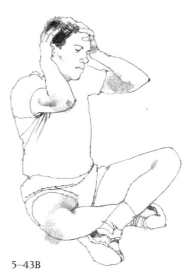

5–43B

Try this same exercise with someone else holding and moving your head (fig 5–43C). Can you relax for someone else better than you can for yourself? If you have a hard time

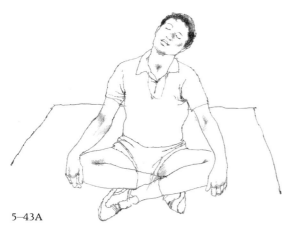

5–43A

5–45   Standing or sitting on a chair, move your whole arm in large circles (fig 5–45). Imagine that your arm is light and long, and that your fingers are leading the motion. Tap your fingers on a hard surface 100 times, and then move your arms in circles again.

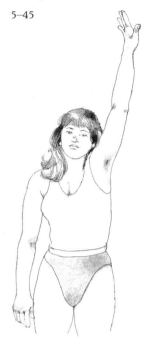

5–45

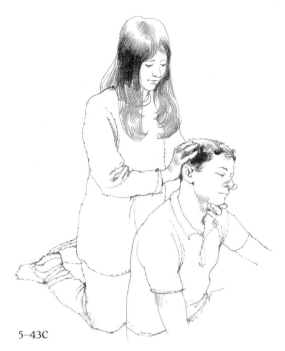

5–43C

relaxing your neck, practice the neck exercises that we have referred to for some time, then come back to these and try again.

Arms

5–44   This exercise is done in a pool. Stand in water up to your chest, and let your arms float, loosely, with your palms resting on the water. Rotate your torso slowly from side to side, and let your arms follow the rotation. Feel how light your arms can be when they move, how they are separate entities from your torso – as if tied to it with strings. Try to memorize the feeling. Now hold your left forearm with your right hand and move your left arm back and forth several times on the water. Don't let your left arm participate – it is the same loose, passive, floating entity that it was before. Now do the same with your other hand.

Do the same exercise holding weights in your hands. Start with light weights, and increase them gradually as you get stronger.

5 46   Sit on a chair or couch and support your elbow with an armrest, a desk or pillows. With your hand hanging loosely from your wrist, move your forearms in large circles. Imagine that your fingertips are leading the motion, and that the muscles of your arms are not doing any work.

Now move your forearms while holding weights in your hands. Gradually, as your arms strengthen, increase the weight.

Return to exercise 1–13 in the Breathing chapter. Practice it for five days, increasing the number of stretches up to 100. Only then continue with the following exercises.

5–47 Push-aways   Stand facing a wall, stretch your arms in front of you, and lean your palms on the wall (fig 5–47A). Slowly bend your elbows as you transfer more of your weight to your arms, and then straighten them, pushing yourself (slowly) from the wall. Inhale while bending your arms, exhale as you push yourself away. After repeating this five times, rotate your hands inward, so that your fingers are pointing downward, and again bend and straighten your elbows five times.

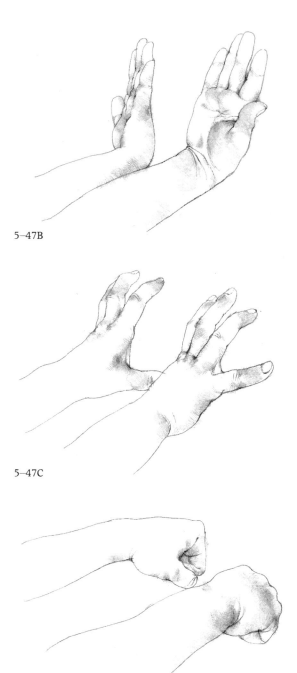

5–47B

5–47C

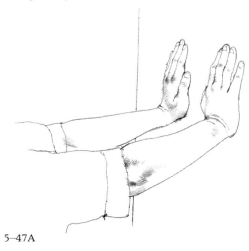

5–47A

Do the same with the backs of your palms against the wall (fig 5–47B), with your fingers rather than your palms against the wall (fig 5–47C), and with your knuckles (fig 5–47D).

5–48 Pull-ups   Hanging from a bar and pulling your whole body's weight up is definitely a vigorous and strengthening exercise.

5–47D

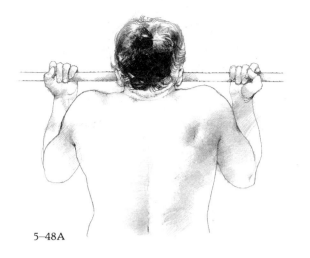

5–48A

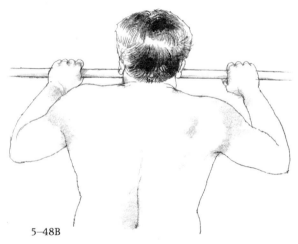

5–48B

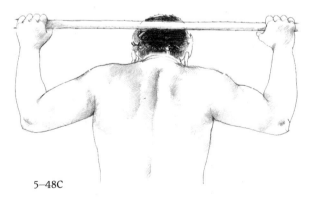

5–48C

What you want to avoid is using the same muscles again and again. You can vary how you hold the bar – with either your fingers or the backs of your palms facing you (fig 5–48A and 5–48B). You can also vary the angle at which you raise your body – try bringing your head and shoulders to the other side of the bar, rather than keeping them at the same side as the rest of your body (fig 5–48C).

The Face

Last of all, let's become aware of the muscles of the face. These muscles are strong and extremely mobile, designed for the task of expressing and communicating our feelings, from the strongest to the most subtle. Often our emotions will leave their mark on the face long after the feeling has passed, in the form of muscular tension held in the jaw, around the mouth, the eyes, the forehead and so on. Moving and massaging the facial muscles often brings a sense of emotional release, as we erase the after-effects of difficult emotions.

5–49 Look at the diagram of the face muscles on page 122. Then look in the mirror, and touch each individual muscle and, as you touch it, experiment with different motions which will move that particular muscle. See how many different directions the muscle will move in, and how many different types of motion will cause it to move. Maureen used this exercise to learn to move each eyebrow separately and to wiggle her nose, so if you have ambitions in this direction you will find this exercise helpful.

121

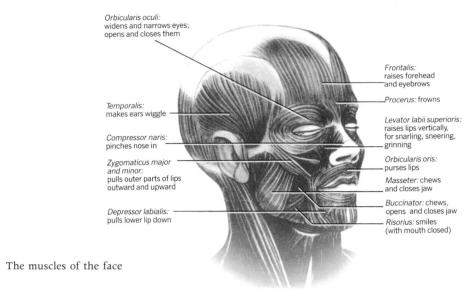

Orbicularis oculi:
widens and narrows eyes;
opens and closes them

Frontalis:
raises forehead
and eyebrows

Procerus: frowns

Temporalis:
makes ears wiggle

Levator labii superioris:
raises lips vertically,
for snarling, sneering,
grinning

Compressor naris:
pinches nose in

Orbicularis oris:
purses lips

Zygomaticus major
and minor:
pulls outer parts of lips
outward and upward

Masseter: chews
and closes jaw

Buccinator: chews,
opens and closes jaw

Depressor labialis:
pulls lower lip down

Risorius: smiles
(with mouth closed)

The muscles of the face

5–50 The muscles of the jaw are especially powerful, and can become very tight during times of intense concentration or strong emotion – particularly anger. Open your mouth and stretch your jaws as wide as possible – slowly – noticing whether there is any sense of restriction in the movement, and, if so, where. Do this several times, trying to stretch the jaws a little wider each time, then let your jaws hang slack while you massage them with your fingertips. Is there any tenderness or pain? This is an area where you can massage deeply. Start just below the ear and move down and inward toward the chin, both above and below the jawbone. Then tap firmly with the fingertips; let your wrist be completely loose so that the hand moves freely, rather than jabbing with the fingertips themselves.

Move the jaw again, opening the mouth wide (will it stretch wider than before?); moving the jaw to the left, right, forward (toward the mirror) and backward (toward your throat); and moving the jaw in a complete circle. Now close your mouth and repeat all of these motions, concentrating on your chin

rather than on the jaw itself. Then open your mouth and stretch your jaws wide again, and let yourself yawn several times, as fully as you can. Sometimes even the thought of yawning is enough to bring on a huge, satisfying yawn. Feel how the yawn relaxes the jaw, throat, forehead and eyes.

For blinking exercises refer to the Vision chapter, and for rotations of the eyes refer to exercises 8–2, 24–12 and 24–13.

Using Weights

We would like to refer you again to the section on isolation toward the beginning of this chapter.

Many people who work with weights to build up their bodies unconsciously recruit muscles not needed in the movement and, as a result, strain and damage those accessory areas, for example, the abdomen and the knees. Your most important goal should be to undo this habit.

The second concept which may need some adjusting to is 'no pain, no strain and lots of gain'. If you are in your twenties or thirties, make a serious decision now. You can either develop the strongest body you could possibly have *now*, meaning 'for the next five years', but have a tendency to suffer injuries in your forties, or you can have a body that is agile and strong and builds up strength throughout many years. It can be stronger in your forties and fifties than in your early thirties, and remain fit and capable in your seventies.

By isolating your muscles and working them separately, you will allow your nervous system to work more efficiently and to support your muscles. Practically this means a few things:

- First of all, work with weights light enough that you can use them without strain. For example, use forty pounds rather than fifty, or sixty rather than seventy, and you will not recruit as many accessory muscles as you would have with a heavier weight.
- Second, use your joints to their full range of motion. At each angle you will be using a different combination of muscles or muscle fibers. Moving a joint slowly and smoothly will allow each of its muscles to strengthen.
- Third, work on muscles which are usually not activated much. For example, lifting your arms or legs sideways (abduction) and bringing them back (adduction) will develop the side muscles which do not participate much in most daily activities.

There are several other principles for healthy use of weights.

The muscles of your upper arms or your thighs may be very strong, and can enjoy working with very heavy weights, but your wrists or ankles, which also take part in the lifting, may not be strong enough to do so

without damage. Work on strengthening your wrists with lighter weights before challenging the arm muscles. Use weights that you can rotate your wrist with. Work on strengthening your shin muscles (which flex your feet) before using their help to strengthen the thighs. The shin muscles need much more work than the gastrocnemius muscles of the calves, which in most people are overdeveloped anyway.

Use your breathing to help you with your exercise. Exhale when you make the effort, inhale when you relax. For example, when you build up your shoulder muscles by lifting a weight with a straight arm, inhale before lifting the arm, and exhale slowly as you lift your arm slowly up. When you build up your biceps by bending your elbow while holding a weight, exhale as you bend your elbow. To build up the triceps, the opponents of your biceps, you would need to lift the weights as you straighten your elbows. Again, exhale as you make the effort.

Use visualization. After lifting the weights several times, stop and visualize that you are lifting them without effort, that your movement is smooth and easy. Now lift the weights again.

There is nothing like a healthy challenge for the muscles. There is, on the other hand, nothing as destructive as an overkill strain on your body.

By now, you should have some sense of the difference between appropriate and inappropriate muscle contraction. Your muscles love to be used in the ways for which they are designed. By activating as many of them as possible, as well as resting them when they need it, you can keep them working well and happily, to the benefit of your entire body.

CHAPTER 6

Nervous System
Reprogram your control system

Your nerves are your body's communication system, information bank and messenger service. Everything that happens within your body does so because of information carried to and from the brain by your nerves. Everything you feel, everything you know, everything you do is made possible by the cooperation between your nervous system and the rest of your body.

Different nerves serve different, specialized functions, but all nerves have important features in common. For example, like some other specialized body tissues, nerve cells, or neurons, do not divide to reproduce themselves. Neurons respond to electrical or chemical stimuli, and conduct electricity themselves. They all have projections, with which they are connected in a network, allowing each neuron to receive the electric information it needs from other neurons or from sensory organs, and to send information to other nerves or to muscles or glands. Nerve impulses – the charges which carry information that ultimately directs every activity of body and mind – are received by projections called dendrites, are interpreted in the cell body, and are sent on through the cell's axon toward the next target.

The workings of your nervous system could be compared to the working of electronic circuitry, though no man-made system comes anywhere close to its intricacy. When a neuron is stimulated by an electrical charge, it undergoes chemical changes which create a small electrical impulse and cause the excited neuron to expel chemicals from its axon into the dendrites or the cell bodies of neighboring neurons. Outside the brain, neurons usually do not actually touch each other; their contact is through this chemical spill, which empties into the tiny space that separates the neurons. This contact between neurons is called a synapse. The expelled chemicals, called neurotransmitters, cause changes similar to those which happened in the first neuron to happen in the neighboring neurons, and in this way the original electrical charge is carried from the first neuron along a pathway which may include many other neurons. These electrical charges, or impulses, will carry sensory information about the external or internal environment of the body to the brain, and will carry commands for various types of movement back from the brain to all other parts of the body.

Since the nervous system is so complex, and since it extends into every part of the body, it is easier to understand it if we study it in sections or divisions. The first division usually made is between the central and the peripheral parts of the nervous system. This is mostly a geographical, or anatomical, division rather than a functional one, since for the most part the peripheral and central parts work together as a unit – an extremely complex and astonishingly well-coordinated unit, but a unit nonetheless.

The central nervous system consists of the brain and the spinal cord, a dense rope of nerves, which are bundles of neurons, that runs the length of the spine and is enclosed and protected by the vertebral column. The vast majority of our nerve fibers are contained within the central nervous system. Nerves that lie outside the brain and spinal cord are collectively called the peripheral nervous system. The peripheral nervous system connects to the central by means of pairs of nerves. There are twelve pairs of cranial nerves, ten of which connect the brain to various parts of the head, face and throat, while the others – the vagus and spinal accessory nerves – connect the brain to points in the torso. From the spinal cord, between the vertebrae, exit the thirty-one pairs of spinal nerves, branching again and again to connect with other nerves and ultimately to reach every part of the body – every organ, muscle, joint; every inch of the body's surface.

Within the peripheral nervous system there are again a number of major divisions. To begin with, there are neurons which carry information to the brain from organs, blood vessels, skin and sense organs. These neurons, and the pathways that they travel through the body, are called afferent, from the Latin for 'carrying toward', since they carry information toward the brain, which is always considered as the central point of the nervous system.

They are also called sensory neurons, since all the information they carry is gathered through our physical senses. Four of these – sight, hearing, smell and taste – are called the specialized senses. The organs responsible for these senses are all located in the head and nowhere else. The sense of touch, on the other hand, can be found in any part of the body. Different types of nerve receptors are designed to respond to different categories of touch-sense, such as pressure, temperature, and texture, but every part of your body is supplied with each type of receptor. Some areas, such as the lips, hands and genitals, are much more richly supplied with nerve receptors than is the rest of the body.

Then there are completely different sets of neurons which carry commands from the brain to the rest of the body. These are called efferent, or 'carrying away from', since they lead away from the brain. These respond to orders from the brain, usually with motor impulses intended to move some specific part of the body in some specific way.

Again within the peripheral nervous system, there are neurons which control voluntary actions, such as most kinds of muscle movement. If you are bitten by a mosquito, the afferent nerves in this system – also known as sensory nerves – will carry information from the bitten place to your brain about the location and the intensity of the itch. Having received this information, the brain will activate the efferent nerves – which are called motor nerves, because they prompt a motion – which are needed to move your hand to the proper area and scratch it until your sensory nerves inform your brain that the itch is gone. These nerves involved in movement of the skeletal muscles are called somatic nerves. You may not always be aware of this kind of activity, but it is not automatic: you have the ability to choose, in this case, whether to scratch or not to scratch.

Then there are nerves – known as the autonomic nervous system – which control involuntary, unconscious functions, mostly of smooth muscle tissue, such as digestion, circulation and respiration. These too have afferent and efferent pathways; the difference is that their activities usually go on without our being conscious of them. For example, if the pressure within a certain blood vessel has grown too high, the nerves that service that blood vessel will tell the brain, which will then activate self-regulating functions in the autonomic nervous system which will bring the pressure down.

And for the final division – one which will be very important to us in our use of therapeutic relaxation – there are the two divisions of the autonomic nervous system. These two divisions are called the sympathetic and the parasympathetic. It might be more helpful to think of the sympathetic as the 'arousing' part of the autonomic system, and the parasympathetic as the 'calming' part. The sympathetic mainly controls our emergency-related response, while the parasympathetic controls relaxation and digestion. These two systems perform often opposing functions, and by so doing they balance each other. For example, the autonomic system, as a whole, controls the rate of your heartbeat. The job of the sympathetic nervous system is to speed up the heart rate when this becomes necessary, while the job of the parasympathetic is to slow it down. The sympathetic nervous system contracts the bladder sphincter, the parasympathetic nervous system relaxes it; and so on.

The sympathetic nervous system is perhaps the most direct link between your emotional mind and your body, translating emotional states almost instantaneously into physical changes in your body. Why call emotions 'feelings' if not because we very physically feel them? The sympathetic nervous system responds especially to anger and fear and anxiety. Much of our chronic or recurring physical tension has its roots in the activity, or rather in the overactivity, of the sympathetic nervous system. Since this physical tension has such a widespread destructive effect throughout the body, it is crucial that we understand its source, and learn to defuse it.

You may be interested to know that the source of emotional reaction is linked both with the older, more primitive parts of our brain, which we share with other animals, and with the very highest centers. When these highly developed parts of the brain have made the decision that we have something to be angry or scared about, nerve impulses travel very rapidly and eventually cause the release of stimulating hormones at various organs or, in a dire emergency, into the bloodstream. This can have a very disturbing effect on your body.

In a life which is not dominated by anxiety, it is the parasympathetic system which is the more active, taking care of digestion, elimination and so on, to feed, cleanse and regulate the body. When anxiety becomes too frequent or too prolonged a visitor, the sympathetic nervous system takes over, and, instead of balancing the actions of the parasympathetic nervous system, it inhibits them. One of the major functions of the parasympathetic nervous system is enabling you to relax. You may not be aware of what really happens when you cannot relax.

What happens to your body when you are

subjected to severe stress? And why? Many of the changes seem designed to give us the power to fight an enemy or to flee an aggressor, which is why the response is named the 'fight-or-flight' response. It involves all parts of the nervous system, as well as the endocrine system. The role of the autonomic nervous system in this is usually to increase the activity of the sympathetic nervous system. Your heart rate will speed up, your lungs move more rapidly. Your digestion will be inhibited, from the salivary glands (this is why anxiety produces a dry mouth) to the entire twenty-five feet of the intestines, seemingly on the assumption that the body has more urgent business at the moment than pushing food along. All the sphincter muscles, which act as gates between different parts of the digestive system, will close. The liver will release large quantities of stored sugar into your blood-stream; the skeletal muscles will have more glucose available and will increase their con-traction. This is what makes the terrified person able to run so fast or the infuriated one to hit so hard.

Fear will cause blood to drain from some surface areas and some organs, and will auto-matically draw the body into a defensive half-crouch known as the startle reflex: shoulders and head thrust forward, abdomen drawn tightly in, knees bent, hands tensed. It will also cause the eyes to move furiously in a manner designed to produce a broad general picture – useful perhaps for spotting potential dangers, but without clear and precise details. Fear will also, interestingly, ensure that the frightening experience is vividly, immediately, imprinted on the memory cortex, in a way that anger will not necessarily do. For purposes of simple survival, it is very useful to remember which things are dangerous, so that we can

recognize them if they come around again to threaten us. The problem is that the mind tends to be very associative, and will dredge up our fear memories and the mind/body state that accompanies them if we are reminded even of something similar to the thing that scared us. We end up being unnecessarily uneasy much of the time.

So here you are, heart pumping wildly, epinephrine and sugar swirling through your blood, the blood itself flowing so rapidly that it actually forms eddies and whirlpools and overheats, with overlapping streams of blood creating friction and becoming sticky within the blood vessels, making it harder for the heart to pump it along. Your lungs are bringing in vast amounts of air which you cannot keep in your lungs long enough to utilize, so that most of their work is wasted. A large pro-portion of your muscles are contracted and will not relax again until either they are force-fully used or the epinephrine has left your bloodstream. Your stomach cannot digest its contents, nor your intestines get rid of theirs, until the sympathetic nervous system lets go of its grip.

At this point, you are lucky if you indeed have somewhere to run, or someone to punch, because your body is primed for it – is, in fact, demanding it. The problem for the vast majority of people reading this book is that they do not have access to these forms of physical release. Most of our present-day anxieties are caused by less tangible things than the life-threatening predators that the sympathetic nervous system was probably designed to protect us from. Financial worries, job pressures, fears about our performance in career, study or relationships, upsetting situ-ations which are difficult to change – these are the adversaries most of us face. These are the things that activate the sympathetic nervous system in exactly the same way that falling into a crocodile-infested river would do. Swimming like hell to get away from the crocodiles would use up the epinephrine and the blood sugar, work the contracted muscles in the arms and legs so as to force them, eventually, to relax, make use of the accelerated heart and lung activity – in short, provided you did manage to escape the crocodiles, your body would naturally balance itself, letting the sympathetic nervous system shut down and the parasympathetic nervous system do its work of getting things back to normal. Without full relaxation the nerves would not be able to return to functioning at their normal capacity, and our nerve response would in time be dulled. Without full relaxation one could not survive in the jungle.

When our problem is not crocodiles, when our problem is, say, a mean and overly demanding boss who merely reminds us of a crocodile, then what happens is that we are stuck with all the effects of sympathetic-nervous-system arousal, unable to 'work it off' as the body intended us to do. Our blood remains flooded with sugar and arousing hormones, which leave us with a tense, shaky, overstimulated feeling. Our muscles remain contracted. Our hearts and blood vessels continue to work much too hard, for a long time after the initial arousal. We remain on sympathetic-nervous-system alert, and the signal to the parasympathetic nervous system to resume its functions is delayed. This is where mental anxiety is transformed into chronic physical tension, the two of them combining to produce stress.

You can probably get a sense of which health disorders are clearly stress-related. First and most deadly on the list is cardiovascular

disease – heart attack and high blood pressure, caused by exactly the conditions present in sympathetic-nervous-system arousal, and the number one cause of premature death in the West. Next, digestive problems of every description, from ulcers to colon cancer – among the most common of the fatal cancers – caused by frequent shutdowns of the digestive system. The colon shuts down in times of extreme tension, but often we respond to this tension by eating, further increasing the colon's burden. Unnecessary tension in the back muscles leads to back pain. These are only a few of the disorders that result from overexcitement – without climax and release – of the sympathetic nervous system. Arguably, stress reduction could add many years to your life.

Most of us do not spend our lives under siege from a full-scale sympathetic-nervous-system attack. We would not survive very long that way. What most of us do suffer from is a disturbance in the balance between the workings of the sympathetic nervous system and the parasympathetic nervous system, with the sympathetic nervous system dominating. Many of us have created lives which encourage this, with noise, challenges, pressures and stimulation being far more common than quiet, rest and contemplation – when in fact, for our health, we need both stimulation and rest. We have become sensation-junkies, stimulation addicts, who associate wracked and over-worked nerves with being fully alive. Or, to put it more politely, we crave excitement. What we need to understand is the cost to our bodies of too much excitement.

To restore a healthy balance between the two branches of the autonomic nervous system, two things are necessary. First, when the sympathetic nervous system has been aroused, it has to be allowed to come to a climax – that is, we need to let the body do what the sympathetic nervous system has programmed it to do: work hard, let off steam and then relax. The degree to which we need to do this depends on the degree to which the sympathetic nervous system has been excited. If you find yourself at the point where you are shaking with rage or terror, jittery with anxiety, or just so tense that you cannot let go, then your sympathetic nervous system has been powerfully activated and requires a powerful release. The best thing to do would be to run, walk very fast, hit a punching bag, pound a pillow or take a lot of expendable, breakable objects into the basement and throw them at the wall as hard as you can – while you are still upset. It will help you calm down a lot faster. Some psychotherapists give their patients pieces of hose and have them beat chairs, pillows or other objects, in the hope of giving them exactly this sort of release, and if the patient is in fact under the sway of the sympathetic nervous system this will indeed help.

Overstimulation of the sympathetic nervous system does not always produce such a strong reaction, however. Usually symptoms are milder: constipation, diarrhea, insomnia, or just a general sense of stress might let you know that your autonomic nervous system is not yet back in balance. It is very important to pay attention to these signals, not to suppress them, because they are the only clues you may have that a serious problem is developing. Just as vigorous – even violent – physical exertion helps after a strong sympathetic-nervous-system alert, so milder exercise helps you recover from general stress. It will use up your increased blood sugar and

flush the excess epinephrine out of your blood. It will deepen your breathing and regulate your circulation. It will help your digestive system to resume its regular functioning. In short, it will convince the sympathetic nervous system that it has done its work and can now rest.

It may seem a little strange to think of consciously influencing the function of a system designed for automatic functioning, but in fact the idea is not new at all. Yogis have taken it a step further, into consciously controlling the autonomic nervous system they have proved to the satisfaction of scientific observers that it is indeed possible to slow or speed up the pulse, raise or lower the blood pressure and body temperature, and lower the rate of respiration – all of the autonomic functions we have mentioned. All of these can be influenced by conscious control. You do not even need the rigorous training of a yogi; what you need to do is to understand how your autonomic nervous system works, and to become more aware of how it is affecting you.

The second technique necessary to balance the autonomic nervous system is to learn to imitate – and thereby encourage – the action of the parasympathetic nervous system. To do this, you have to seek out things which calm and relax you. By now it should be quite obvious why you cannot usually relax just by telling yourself to, when exactly the opposite order has been spread throughout your body. It is not just your mind that is tensing you; it is nerves and muscles and organs. These can all be persuaded to relax, but you must address them directly, both mentally and physically. There are a number of ways to do this, and we can all find the way which best suits our needs and likes.

Calling on the Parasympathetic Nervous System

Probably the best and easiest way to begin is with breathing. The sympathetic nervous system speeds up breathing, the para-sympathetic nervous system slows it down; your entire body will take its cue from your rate of respiration. By consciously slowing and deepening your breathing, you direct your entire autonomic nervous system into the calming mode.

Working with thousands of people, we have found again and again that very few people breathe as deeply as they should. When people begin to learn to relax, the first thing they usually discover is how little, how seldom and how shallowly they breathe, and how easy it is to forget to breathe when they are con-centrating on something else. When they try to breathe deeply, they do it with the same sense of strain they bring to other physical activities. Forcibly dragging a huge gulp of air into your lungs is not going to deepen your breathing – your lungs will just expel it almost as fast as you bring it in.

To breathe deeply, fully, you need to inhale slowly, to keep inhaling slowly until your lungs cannot hold any more breath, and to exhale even more slowly, exhaling until your lungs are virtually emptied. Your lungs have millions of tiny air pockets, called alveoli. The average breath brings in 500 ml of air, about one-ninth of the maximum possible inspir-ation. A shallow breath such as this fills only the upper alveoli. Inhaling slowly will allow all of them to expand to their full capacity, taking in the maximum quantity of oxygen. This is important because it is in the lower

alveoli that the greatest exchange of oxygen and carbon dioxide takes place.

All your body's cells depend on oxygen to provide 'fuel' for their activities. Your cells are constantly using oxygen, which they take from the blood. As they do this, the level of oxygen in the blood drops and the level of carbon dioxide increases. Oxygen-depleted blood goes to the lungs, where it exchanges its surplus carbon dioxide for a new supply of oxygen. The carbon dioxide is then expelled from your lungs when you exhale. As with so many other processes, your body's interest lies in maintaining a balanced state, in this case between oxygen and carbon-dioxide levels. This is why exhaling is just as important as inhaling. You need to virtually empty your lungs of their carbon dioxide, to make room for fresh oxygen.

Whether or not you suffer from neurological problems, if you can manage to follow this chapter we suggest that you spend six months working with it. If you do find some parts difficult, defer them until they become easier for you, and consult your support group and, if possible, a Self-Healing practitioner.

6–1   The following exercise will help you to breathe more fully. First assume a completely relaxed position, either sitting or lying down, with your head and back supported and your limbs at rest. Close your eyes, and empty your lungs by exhaling through your nose until you feel the lungs are completely empty. You may feel your diaphragm area (just under the ribcage) drawing inward and upward as you do this. Then *slowly* begin to inhale, through your nose *only*. Let the oxygen enter the lungs gradually, taking the time needed for each part of the lung to fill itself. Try to feel this happening. Visualize your lungs as you do this, and picture the alveoli swelling like tiny balloons. Your ribcage will expand outward and your diaphragm will press downward as your lungs swell. Let yourself continue to slowly inhale for a count of ten.

When you feel that your lungs have reached their fullest capacity, do not exhale; hold the breath in for a count of thirty. Then *slowly* exhale, and keep exhaling until your lungs are as empty as they were at the beginning of this exercise. Do not inhale. Stay without breathing for as long as you can, and then again slowly inhale. Do this whole process three times.

If you began this exercise with a rapid pulse rate, you may now discover that your pulse has slowed. This is partly because your body automatically associates slow breathing with a slower heartbeat. It is also because oxygen-poor blood forces the heart to work harder, while oxygen-enriched blood makes the heart's job easier.

You have also stretched and strengthened the tissues of your heart, lungs and blood vessels, as well as the muscles of your chest, abdomen and ribs. Anxiety causes these muscles to be held rigid; breathing lets them expand, contract and relax. All of these areas are responsive to sympathetic-nervous-system arousal.

6–2   To make the breathing exercise even more effective, do it as follows. Inhale slowly and fully, and, while holding the air in your lungs, simultaneously push the chest out and draw the abdomen in, then push the abdomen out and pull the chest in. Alternate this way — chest in, abdomen out; chest out, abdomen in — five or six times, then slowly and fully exhale. Before inhaling, repeat the same movements

with your abdomen and chest, again five or six times. Repeat this entire process three times. Then relax and breathe normally, and take stock of how your body feels. You may notice more sense of relaxation in your muscles, particularly those of the back and shoulders.

We strongly recommend that you turn now to the Breathing chapter, which contains further exercises to deepen your breathing and increase your awareness of what breathing does to your body. There simply is no more effective aid to relaxing your body and calming your mind.

6–3 Massage   The following massage instructions are written for the massage therapist. If you are the one being worked on, please give this to your practitioner to read, since massage designed for the nervous system is a little different from other techniques.

A good massage will do everything the parasympathetic system is supposed to do; and if it is good enough it will even do this over the strenuous objections of the sympathetic nervous system. It is hard to think of many things which will transform a body so completely. For this purpose, however, keep in mind that a slow and gentle massage is the most effective. Rough or overvigorous massage is not appropriate on a body that is already suffering from overstimulation.

The best way to begin a massage which is specifically for the purpose of calming and relaxing someone is by working on the back, along the spine but not on it, at the roots of the peripheral nervous system. Relaxing the muscles of the spine will send messages of relaxation throughout the back, arms and legs. Releasing the upper-back muscles makes movement of the chest freer and easier;

releasing the lower-back muscles does the same for the abdomen, so that both respiration and digestion are enhanced. If the spinal cord carries the sensation of relaxation to the brain, this can be communicated to every part of the body. Remember, the brain responds to sensory information with motor commands. When the senses – in this case, the sense of touch – carry pleasurable and soothing feelings to the brain, it will tend to allow muscles to relax, the better to enjoy those feelings.

Do not try to begin this kind of massage with deep pressure, since the tension in this case is not just in specific muscles but throughout the body. A light tapping and shaking motion is much more effective. Activation of the fight-or-flight mechanism tenses muscles for immediate and vigorous movement, contracting muscle fibers and connective tissue, while simultaneously releasing epinephrine and stored sugar into the bloodstream. Unless these tissues are allowed to loosen, the irritating substances in the blood remain in the tissues. Tapping and shaking creates a movement in the tissues which satisfies the muscles' craving for movement and flushes out the arousing substances, so that relaxation and normal function can return. Deep pressure may simply create a resistance that causes the muscles to tighten further; it should not be used until you feel that the process of relaxation has begun.

When you tap, let your wrists flop loosely, rather than prodding with the fingertips. When you shake, place all your fingertips on the area, press down very gently, and shake the area without lifting your hand off it. You can begin either at the top of the spine or at the bottom – ask which feels best – and work your way along the entire length of it. Then you can tap, shake and gently knead the muscles of the shoulders, under and around the shoulder blades and down along the back to the buttocks. The buttocks tighten strongly during anxiety, in response to the closing of the anal sphincter, and so should be massaged along with the back to release anxiety.

Massage of the scalp also aids in deep relaxation. It is not known whether massaging the head directly affects the cranial nerves. The visual cortex of the brain underlies the lower part of the back of the head. It seems that, when the eyes are strained, the muscles which cover this part of the skull become tense. Whether the reason is neurological or postural, massage of the back of the neck and of the head has a calming effect and can improve vision.

Some sympathetic nerves have their endings in the scalp, where they cause the hair to stand on end during fear or excitement. Massage of the scalp is extremely pleasant after the hair follicles have been stimulated in this way; it seems to bring the stimulation to a climax and allow it to pass. For whatever reason, scalp massage feels wonderful and is one of the quickest ways to relax a jittery person. Here, tapping is in most cases less pleasant and effective; the muscles are thinner and do not absorb the percussion very well. Shaking is good, and so is a gentle, palpating 'pinch' – the type of motion you use when you wash your hair. Taking thick handfuls of hair and very gently pulling it is a good technique as long as it does not hurt.

After extensive massage of the spine and the cranium, your client should be showing definite signs of relaxation. His posture should be looser – even in a person who is lying down, the difference will be obvious. The muscles under your fingers will feel softer and probably warmer. His breathing should be noticeably deeper and slower. Often you will hear gurgling or rumblings from the abdomen, indicating that his digestive processes have resumed. The massage is creating a condition wherein the relaxing messages of the parasympathetic nervous system can be heard by the body.

Breathing exercises may be helpful now. Have him lie on his back, and lead him through the breathing exercise described above, or other exercises from the Breathing chapter. You can make these exercises more effective by massaging the chest, the upper arms and the upper pectoral area where the arms and chest connect; by tapping lightly along and around the sternum and clavicle (breastbone and collarbone); and by pressing lightly with both palms on the chest or abdomen. Please refer to the Massage chapter for a more detailed description of massage techniques.

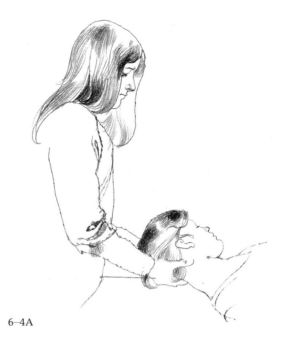

6–4A

6–4 The next most useful bodywork technique is *passive movement*. This will not work early in the massage session, because the person's muscles are still under orders to contract and to work, and it will be very difficult for her to allow you to move them. The arms, especially, will resist relaxation. Picture a sleepy child being carried by a parent, limp as a rag doll. This is the effect you want to achieve now.

With your client still lying on her back, slide your palms under her skull to completely support it, and lift it up about three or four inches. Turn the head slowly from side to side (fig 6–4A). You do not have to move the neck at all; just turn the palms of your hands so that the head rests first on one, then on the other. Some people find it very hard to allow this movement, as the neck muscles are so used to tensing that they cannot relax. If you find your client's neck tight and difficult to move,

first ask her to let you move it, then show her that you can easily support the weight of her head and will not turn the head sharply or painfully. Often this will be enough to get a person to let go. If not, try to get her to focus on breathing exercises, which will both relax and distract her.

After turning the head from side to side until the neck seems looser, you can raise the head from below and bring the chin toward the chest. With the neck bent in this way, again move the head from side to side several times, lower the head toward the table, then raise it again and repeat the motion. Be sure at all times that you are completely supporting the head; think of a newborn infant, whose neck must be supported at all times, and treat your client as if her neck were equally limber. This will give her the same sense of looseness.

Next, move the legs. Most people find it easier to allow passive movement of their legs than of their arms, perhaps because the legs

133

are heavier and require more effort to raise or move them. Refer to the Massage chapter, exercise 7–26, for passive movements of the leg. In addition to those, you can hold the legs at the ankle, lift them slightly, and shake them vigorously. If you can get another person to participate, you can have one of you stand on each side of the client, lift the leg, and toss it back and forth to each other (fig 6–4B). This is not only delightful to do or to have done to you, it is also extremely relaxing, since it requires that the person being moved totally lets go of the limb. This has a powerful releasing effect on the lower pelvis.

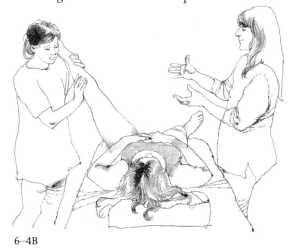

6–4B

Last of all, move the arms. You may find it easiest at first to have the person lie on her side, with a pillow under her head. In this position, you can place one palm on either side of the shoulder and gently rotate it, making sure that she does not hold the arm stiffly while you do this. Then lift the arm and rotate it from the shoulder, making the rotation as large as comfortably possible. Have her lie on her back and stretch the arm in as many directions as you can – sideways, upward, or sideways and upward simultaneously. Hold the arm by the wrist and simultaneously shake

and stretch it. Lift it straight up, as though she were pointing forward, hold it by the wrist, and shake it, letting the whole arm sway as if blown by the wind. When she is relaxed enough to let you do this, the autonomic nervous system has begun to balance itself.

Naturally, these instructions are not just for therapists and massage practitioners. If you feel that you could use this treatment yourself, show this chapter to your favorite massage partner and suggest that he get to work (and be available for him the next time he gets stressed out). Giving a massage is much more pleasant than witnessing an anxiety attack. We strongly recommend that you either see a massage therapist or trade massages with someone in your Self-Healing support group, preferably twice a week for a month, before continuing with the other exercises in this chapter.

Letting Go Internally

We have already mentioned that the digestive system shuts down completely during sympathetic-nervous-system arousal. During most of our lives, food is being continually processed through the alimentary canal, which includes the mouth, esophagus, stomach, intestines and rectum. This requires frequent movement of the smooth muscles in these organs. When food is not processed normally, we suffer in two ways: we fail to receive the nutrients from our food, and we retain toxic matter that would normally be eliminated. Why are high-fiber foods recommended in fighting cancer? Simply because they encourage the passage of these toxic materials out of the body as quickly as possible. But when the sympathetic nervous system has ordered shutdown of the digestive system, tightening the smooth muscles and closing the sphincters to hold everything frozen in place, even high-fiber food will not help.

The sphincters are, for the most part, ring-shaped muscles which surround the openings of portions of the digestive tract and act as valves, opening and closing in response to pressure and to commands from the autonomic nervous system. The first one in the alimentary canal is at the top of the esophagus; it opens during swallowing to allow food to enter the esophagus. The next is between the esophagus and the stomach (the lower esophageal sphincter). The next is the pyloric valve, between the stomach and the small intestine, followed by the ileocecal valve between the small intestine and the large intestine. Last are the anal sphincters, voluntary and involuntary, at the end of the rectum. (The bladder, though not part of the alimentary canal, also terminates in a sphincter muscle which keeps urine from entering the urethra. This sphincter is also controlled by the autonomic nervous system.)

When the sympathetic nervous system is on full alert, all of these sphincters will contract tightly to make sure there is no passage of food within the system. Movement of food stimulates various digestive secretions and processes, and the body that is geared for fight or flight wants to delay these processes, saving its energy for what it considers more urgent matters. This leaves the digestive system in a sort of state of suspended animation. Digestion will return to normal when the body relaxes — when the sympathetic nervous system switches off and the parasympathetic switches on. If this switch is not fully made — if the body remains in a state of semi-tension — then digestion is chronically hampered.

Exercising and releasing tension in the sphincter muscles is one more way to signal the parasympathetic nervous system that it can now proceed with its calming, normalizing activity. We are indebted to Paula Gerber, in Israel, for developing the sphincter-release exercises which we use in our work with the nervous system. These sphincter exercises are designed to create first maximum tension, and then — as a result of this tension — maximum release in the sphincters. These exercises, by the way, have been consistently effective for patients who have multiple sclerosis, a nerve disease whose symptoms may include loss of bladder control.

6–5   We begin with an exercise that may be familiar by now – the spinal arch. Stand with your feet hip-width apart and your arms hanging loosely at your sides, and begin very slowly to bend forward, curving your back as you bend. Imagine that you curl forward one vertebra at a time. First lower your chin to your chest, then continue the forward movement with the head as you let the shoulders, the upper back and the middle back, follow. Let your arms drop forward loosely and hang in front of you, following the motion of your body. Bend as far forward as it is comfortable for you, and hang there for a few seconds. Visualize the change that this posture creates in your spine: imagine the spaces between the vertebrae enlarging, and visualize the convex curve of the usually concave lower back. Let the muscles which hold the spine erect relax and expand; they do not have to work in this position, but they may continue to tighten (since they are used to doing so) unless you consciously direct them to relax.

Now inhale a long full breath through your nose, hold it in, and then exhale slowly and fully, through your nose again. Inhale again, exhale fully, and, without inhaling again, contract your anal area as tightly as you can and hold the contraction for fifteen seconds. Let go of the contraction, inhale, exhale fully, and, without inhaling, contract your bladder sphincters, as if keeping yourself from urinating, for fifteen seconds. Let go of the bladder contraction, inhale, do not exhale, puff your cheeks, and alternate between releasing them and puffing them for ten seconds altogether. Keep inhaling as you work with your cheeks. Now exhale, do not inhale, and contract your anal muscles again. Do you feel you have better control over them? Breathe normally. You may find that you now automatically breathe much more deeply, almost as if the letting go of the contraction created a vacuum that sucked air into your lungs.

See if you can bend any further. Now straighten up slowly, uncurling your spine as gradually as you curled it, imagining that you move each vertebra separately in turn.

Repeat the whole process five times. This is a good exercise to do daily.

This exercise can also be done by women with the muscles of the vagina. Sexual and sexually related emotional tension or trauma cause many women to unconsciously tighten the vaginal muscles, and this contraction may often be so powerful that it affects the bladder and the anus as well. Releasing vaginal tension will help release the entire pelvic floor, and will help to condition the uterus by encouraging it to relax as well.

As you do the exercise, be aware of the muscles that surround the sphincter you are working on. Unconscious tightening of the anus, bladder or vagina can tighten muscles in the buttocks, thighs, abdomen and lower back, which can be relieved by release of the sphincter contraction. We are all subject, to some degree, to this unconscious tightening, since we very frequently have to delay defecation until such time as it is polite or convenient. The same applies to urinating and to passing intestinal gas. When the need to do these things arises and we, for whatever reason, do not relieve the need, the sphincters — and their surrounding muscles — tighten automatically and stay in a partial paralysis until we let out whatever needs to come out. This exercise allows the sphincters to tighten completely and then to release completely. Earlier we mentioned how vigorous, even violent, exercise can work off stress by allowing a climax of tension, and thus shut off the sympathetic-nervous-system signals. This exercise is of the same order.

This exercise, by the way, is good for the peripheral nervous system not only because of the sphincter release but because the stretching of the spine relieves pressure on the spinal nerves. As we mentioned, peripheral nerves branch off from the spinal cord between each pair of vertebrae. If the bones are too close to each other, they press on these nerve roots. When this happens, the nerves are less able to conduct messages to and from the brain, and so nerve functioning is decreased — with one exception. The pressure on the nerve can be extremely painful, and *that* message has no trouble reaching the brain at all.

6–6 Lie down on your back with your knees bent and your feet flat on the floor, hip-width apart or wider; this position will give you more awareness of your pelvic sensations. Can you tell whether you are holding tension in your pelvic area, and can you tell where that tension is centered? Before you begin the next exercise, go back to exercise 6–1 and repeat it several times, noticing whether it helps the pelvis to relax. It would also be a good idea to empty your bladder before going on with this exercise.

Now close your eyes and contract the muscles around them as hard as you can; hold each thumb against the four fingertips and squeeze them together as tightly as you can; squeeze your lips tightly together (fig 6–6). Now, holding all of these areas contracted, inhale through your nose and exhale sharply, with a forceful 'ch! ch!' sound, through your mouth; tighten the bladder for a count of fifteen, and release it. Relax your eyes, hands and mouth before you inhale again. Breathe normally for several breaths.

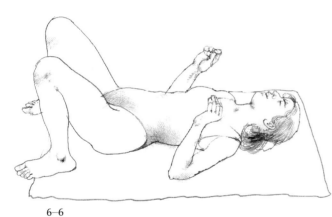

6–6

Next, repeat the whole process as above, but this time, instead of tightening the bladder as if to keep from urinating, press down on it as though you are trying to expel urine. This gives you a completely different kind of release: instead of increasing the retentive contraction to a climax, it opposes it, exerting pressure in the opposite direction. Imagine how tiring it would be to keep your hand balled into a tight fist for hours at a time, and what a relief it would be to finally stretch the fingers in the opposite direction, or to shake the hand loosely. This is similar to what you are doing to your bladder sphincter.

This exercise should also be done with the anal sphincter, first tightening it as though to prevent defecation, then pushing as though to eliminate (if you have ever suffered from constipation, you will be very familiar with this kind of pushing). Try to use the abdominal, buttock and lower-back muscles as little as possible, concentrating the effort on the anus itself. Women can go through the same process with the vaginal area.

Another exercise which more indirectly releases pelvic tension is the pelvic lift, exercise 4–8 in the Spine chapter. By the way, this movement, if done about 1,000 times, can produce contractions so intense that it is used to bring on a delayed period or to relieve constipation. It is not recommended for the early weeks of pregnancy. To balance this exercise, lie on your back with your knees pulled up to your chest, hold one knee in each hand, and move the knees in rotating motion.

The upper sphincters – of the esophagus, stomach and small intestine – can best be tightened and released through breathing exercises. Please refer to exercise 1–14 in the Breathing chapter.

Kinesthetic Awareness

Much of this chapter may seem to you like a review of the previous chapters. By now, almost none of the concepts we are discussing are completely new to you; we are simply presenting them in greater depth, with more emphasis on how and why they work, now that you have already experienced the fact that they do work. Kinesthetic awareness is your feeling-sense of your body. We have involved it in every exercise we have done so far, asking you not just to do something but also to pay attention to how it feels to do that thing – not just whether it feels bad or good, easy or difficult, but the particular sensation in the specific part of the body which is moved.

This awareness of your sensations is important because it helps you to do exercises more effectively. It is even more important, however, because it helps to keep your brain and nervous system alive and functioning. When you pay attention to a specific part of your body, you stimulate the nerves which connect that part to your brain – and thus you also stimulate the brain.

Paying attention to what you feel, to what each part of your body feels, will strengthen your kinesthetic awareness. One of the best ways to increase your capacity to do this is to move in ways that are unusual for you. Repetitive movement leads to diminishing sensation, not only because your conscious mind loses interest but because you are creating an imbalance in nervous system function. Overloads on some motor pathways and underloads on others can lead to numbness and motor exhaustion.

The opposite of sensation is numbness. Numbness can develop in, for example, the student or office worker who feels compelled to remain, fixed at a desk, immobile, for long periods of time. Many such people may feel that they have no alternatives, and had better suppress their growing stiffness and discomfort. Consequently, they shut out these feelings which are replaced by numbness.

People make themselves numb for a combination of physical and mental reasons, including, as in this case, perceived necessity, as well as lack of correct use, repetitive movement, and a failure to imagine new ways to move. Moving in new ways will take the load off these nerves and allow other nerves to function.

This may be part of why dancing is so enjoyable. When we dance, we use all kinds of movements that do not occur in everyday activities. We highly recommend dancing, yoga and many other types of activity that get you to move in new ways. A more basic suggestion, however, is simply to do movements that bend or stretch you sideways. People tend to move mostly either back and forward, or up and down, rather than sideways. This is why most back and knee injuries tend to happen as a result of a sharp sideways motion. Our muscles do not, as a rule, get enough sideways stretch, and so tend not to be prepared for it.

For an introduction to sideways movements, we refer you to the Spine chapter. Begin with the spinal arch, exercise 4–2, and continue with the section Sideways Stretches for the Lower Back.

The Central Nervous System

When we work on the central nervous system, we are doing nothing less than re-creating the way we feel and function, from its very source. To work on the central nervous system is to re-create feeling and function at their source. To change your walk, for example, work not just with the legs but with the nerves that supply the leg and with all parts of the brain involved in its movement. You are probably aware of the possibilities of learning new things, such as riding a bicycle or juggling three oranges, but you may not be aware of how much relearning you can do of activities you have done all your life.

One small example will suffice to demonstrate this concept dramatically. Professor Boris Klosovski (Russian neurosurgeon and neurophysiologist, Chief of Neurosurgery at the Academy of Medical Sciences of the USSR in Moscow, as described in Glenn Doman's *What to Do about Your Brain-injured Child*, p. 189) performed an experiment with kittens and puppies. He took newborn litters and divided them into matching groups, a control group and an experimental group. The kittens and puppies in the control group were permitted to develop normally, while the experimental animals were placed on a slowly revolving turntable and lived there throughout the experiment. The only difference, then, in what happened to each of the groups was that the experimental group saw a moving world, while the control group saw only as much as newborn kittens and puppies normally see.

When the animals were ten days old, Klosovski began to sacrifice the matched pairs of kittens and puppies and to measure their brains. (These stories never have a happy ending for the experimental animals.) The last pair was sacrificed by the nineteenth day. The animals on the turntable had from 22.8 to 35.0 percent more growth in vestibular areas of the brain – the areas concerned with balance – than did the control animals. In this case, the areas in the brain in charge of balance developed as a result of movement or activity. Other movements or activities can develop other parts of the brain.

We are all born with a certain amount of programming already coded in the brain. We do not have to learn crying, sucking or swallowing, all of which are complicated physical processes; we are born with the skills for these. Other skills and physical developments come to us at predictable times and in a predictable order. The appearance of teeth; the ability to sit up, crawl, walk and speak; the attainment of a certain size and level of coordination are all part of a normal pattern of human development which is 'built-in'. Some of this behavior, of course, is learned: it is an interesting question whether an infant would naturally try to walk if it were surrounded by people who crawled instead. Probably the child sees people walking, is encouraged by its parents to try to walk, and therefore initiates the series of trial-and-error attempts which eventually leads to walking. Even so, the amount of learning that can be attained at these early stages is limited by preprogrammed patterns of development. A child may learn to walk – as opposed to having an instinctual desire or tendency to walk – but it cannot, at this stage, learn to operate a forklift truck: neither its intellect nor its muscles have reached the necessary stage of development.

Even at this early stage, however, the pattern of development can be influenced and its program can be altered by the events of a person's life. For example, statistics prove that a child who is constantly encouraged to speak, is rewarded for attempts to speak, and has words repeated to her over and over and things pointed out and named for her will be very likely to speak earlier than one who is not stimulated in this way.

Brain development can be hampered as well as enhanced by life circumstances. To give an example from our own experience: Meir and his son, Gull, were both born with congenital cataracts. A cataract is an opaqueness in the lens of the eye, shutting out or obstructing visual stimulation. The brain (that is, the visual cortex of the brain, the part which is responsible for vision) is programmed to begin to respond to this visual stimulation after only two months of life; it 'expects' it and in fact needs it if vision is to develop normally. This is one excellent example of how the brain is deeply influenced by sensory input alone! If the eye is not stimulated by light, if it does not send messages to the brain about this stimulation very early in life, then the visual cortex which is programmed to receive these messages does not develop at the proper time – and having missed its cue, so to speak, never gets another chance to develop fully and properly. For this reason, Gull's parents opted for cataract-removal surgery which would allow light into the eyes and get the visual-brain development under way on time. Meir did not have such surgery until the age of four. This operation and the others that followed were unsuccessful. As a result, Meir did not begin to develop visual cortex (by doing vision exercises) until age seventeen. He has been told by ophthalmologists that, so far as they know, he is the only such case in the world. Gull, having begun to develop the visual cortex on time, has normal vision – much better than Meir's.

Everyone's development – whether of the body or of skills, abilities and so on – depends on both the programming we are born with and the events of our lives, as Gull's story illustrates. The older we get, however, the less our development depends on built-in coding and the more it depends on what happens to us, what we do or do not do. Programming gives way to conscious, cognitive learning, or training, or, if you like, self-programming. New skills may become harder to acquire with increasing age, but there is no doubt that most of us have brain capacity to spare. It is there for us to use if we want to.

It is not the easiest thing in the world, however, to get to the stage where a person really wants to learn, to change. For one thing, we are used to doing physical things in an automatic, unconscious way, and we often have a lot of resistance to having to learn, or relearn, them consciously. If you have been walking, sitting, standing, breathing, using your eyes and so on in a certain way for decades, the idea of relearning such basic skills from the ground up may strike you as tedious, irritating or even impossible. Not many people realize how much power they have to influence their body's functioning, or what an ally the mind can be in doing so.

So what motivates a person for this kind of work? The answer is usually pain, or loss of function. Athletes and dancers have shown us what miracles the human body can be trained to perform, but most people do not aspire to such achievements: they are quite content with normal (which is often minimal) function, until they develop a pain or limitation which becomes intolerable to them. What is intolerable varies, of course, from person to person. One person may be perfectly well-adjusted to life in a wheelchair, while another may feel terribly deprived if he cannot run ten miles a day. One person may be more or less resigned to the onset of blindness, while another may chafe at wearing glasses with even a small correction, choosing to put in the time and effort required for eye exercises rather than rely on artificial correction. We tend to prefer the malcontents. They are the ones who end up showing other people the amazing things that can be achieved with the body through self-programming.

Suppose you have come to the point where you know that you need to make some changes in your life. You may accept this knowledge cheerfully, perhaps even welcome the challenge. This might be true, for example, in the case of a man who has had a mild heart attack and now has a solid incentive to lose weight, get some exercise, quit smoking – things he has long wanted to do, but had no real reason to do except some rather vague assurance that they would be 'good for him'. Other people may bitterly resist the idea of change, and the effort it requires. Perhaps a woman stricken with arthritis knows that exercises can vastly reduce her pain and stiffness, but resents the fact that her illness has imposed such a necessity on her. Exercises that might otherwise be enjoyable become a burden and a chore. Feelings of pain, anger, resentment and frustration hamper the progress of such a person. The steps that need to be taken may seem to be too difficult to perform, or the person may perform them inadequately, or perform them quite well while finding them a huge source of strain, in which case the exercises may seem to the patient to be worse than the original problem. All of these problems stem directly from emotional resistance – *not* from physical incapability. In other words, here again the mind and emotions play a tremendous role in maintaining our health.

Another and much deeper impediment stems from not believing that your situation can change. We encounter this attitude most often in our work with the eyes. The notion that vision cannot improve is so strongly held by such a huge majority that even those who do not accept it, and who achieve wonderful improvements in their vision, often have difficulty believing their own results. Many of the people we see want very much to help their eyes, but simply cannot bring themselves to accept that this might actually be possible. The success rate of these people is very low.

The same is true for other parts of the body. If you have a stiff hip, have become accustomed to pain and limitation almost as a way of life, and firmly believe that the situation cannot change, then the chances are high that it will not, even if you go through the motions of stretching and loosening exercises. This is because changing the way your body functions requires the participation of both body and mind. If you do not really believe in an outcome – such as increased mobility in the hip joint – how can your brain give the motor commands necessary to achieve it? As we have said, everything that happens in your body does so because of messages carried to or from the brain by the nerves. If one part of your brain is saying, 'Lift that leg three inches higher,' and another part is saying, 'You can't be serious,' then imagine what mixed messages your nerves are carrying to and from the muscles concerned in lifting the leg. It even happens that the muscles may send a message to the brain saying, 'Actually, this isn't as hard as we thought,' but the part of the brain shouting, 'I can't do this' is so loud that it drowns out everything else. Not believing that you are able to move in a new and different way, you will unconsciously continue to move exactly as you have always done – probably in the exact way that caused the problem in the first place. When we teach shoulder rotations, we instruct people to move the outer edge of the shoulder, rather than the muscles surrounding the shoulder blade. To some people this concept seems foreign, strange – in fact, not possible – and they rotate the shoulder, forcibly, from the shoulder blade, tensing the already tense muscles instead of loosening them, and the shoulder tension remains just as it was, and the person remains convinced that the exercises do not work.

The hardest things to change are the things a person does often and habitually and has done for a long time. To some people, the way they do things can seem as ingrained and unchangeable as the color of their eyes. The only way to get around this, sometimes, is to have a person do something in a completely new way. If we are trying to help someone with a gait problem, we begin by showing that person the proper way to walk – backward. This is because trying to change the way he walks forward may initially be too difficult; he has been walking that way for too long to change it easily. He will resist the change both physically and mentally, but will be much more open to learning when he is doing something new and different. Many people have terrible reading habits which are extremely destructive to their eyes. The best way to change these habits is to teach them to read properly – upside down. And so on. **In these ways, someone can discover new abilities, new possibilities for change – and, we believe, open new neural pathways which have perhaps lain dormant all that person's life.**

Emotional resistance to learning and to change is the strongest impediment to improving one's function. Emotional resistance combines mental resistance, which we have discussed, with a strong emotion such as fear or anger or guilt. For psychological reasons too complex to explain in full here, some people experience these emotions when they try to change, or even think about changing. They create a physical tension which makes change very difficult. A person with very sick parents, for example, may experience guilt when trying to achieve perfect health for herself. If they are sick, how can she be so callous as to be well? Or a person who wants desperately to

get better may be so afraid of failure that he gets in his own way. Here again, only three things can help. The first is the breaking of old patterns by doing things in completely new ways. The second is physical relaxation, which provides an environment conducive to mental and emotional change. The body automatically equates tension with resistance, and relaxation with acceptance. The third is to work directly on the emotional problem itself, through therapy, spiritual practices, dialogue with the people involved or whatever you feel will help you most.

Trying to impose new conditions or new behaviors on your body, when your mind or emotions oppose them, automatically sets up resistance. The only thing that will disarm this resistance is experience. If you do things you have never done before, or do something in a way you have never done it before, you bring your brain and nervous system back to a learning mode, where change is possible. One of the reasons children learn so quickly and easily is that they are open to new experiences in a way that most adults are not. Children positively crave learning, development, change and novelty; most adults, on the other hand, face these things with indifference, annoyance, fear or loathing.

One way of creating new experiences is to use parts of ourselves we have neglected. There are two benefits here. One is that, if we have not used something much, we are less likely to have developed destructive patterns of use. For example, when we want to help a person develop better vision, it is often helpful to concentrate on her peripheral vision first, since this is usually an undeveloped area where the person will have fewer bad visual habits to unlearn. Second, when you use a part of your body, you stimulate the nerves which connect that part of the body with your brain, and you also stimulate the area of the brain that controls that part. When we do not use something, its related nerves and brain area 'forget' about it and themselves become dormant. As with the muscles, joints and spine, the principle of 'use it or lose it' applies to the nerve pathways as well. When we do use them, we force the brain and nerves to remember them, and to wake up. With more of our body and more of our brain awake and functioning, we are no longer forced to depend on such a limited part of ourselves.

Awakening the Central Nervous System

Once again, massage is a good place to start. Two kinds of massage are useful in stimulating the central nervous system. The first is used if you want to open as many nerve pathways as possible between the brain and the area on which you are working. When we consider nerve dysfunctions, we must remember what an astonishing number of neural pathways each of us has, and how few of these are regularly activated. Most of our emphasis, in working with nerve disorders, is in stimu-lating – 'awakening', if you will – nerve pathways which can be used in place of those which have been damaged by disease. In the case of a multiple-sclerosis patient, for example, there is usually only a minority of nerves which have been damaged, and it is often possible to 'train' other nerves to function for these damaged ones. This idea is not as strange as it may sound. Touch, and in particular the kind of touch we are about to describe, is very useful in getting the attention of dormant nerves.

Neurological Massage

Place your fingertips, including the thumbs, on the area on which you are working, and shake or vibrate your hands vigorously but without much pressure. Without actually lifting your hands off the person's body, move them very gradually up and down, left and right, in the general area you are massaging. Many types of touch can be ignored by the brain, as after a number of repetitions of those touch signals it simply shifts its attention elsewhere. You are constantly receiving touch messages from every part of your body, but most of them are ignored unless you con-sciously decide to pay deliberate attention to them. This is true even if another person is touching you, if the touch is repeated many times in a similar way. A vibrating touch, in contrast, provides a continuous stimulation that the brain is far less likely to ignore. Although the muscle being touched is passive, it is being moved in many different directions when it is vibrated: up and down, laterally, into the muscles and up toward the skin. With every sensory stimulus there is motor response. The brain learns that the muscle can move in many ways, easily. This ultimately will give you more control over movement.

We also believe that massage which aids the flow of cerebrospinal fluid will contribute to the efficient functioning of the central nervous system. This fluid nourishes, lubricates and cushions the brain and the spinal cord, pro-tecting them from blows and other traumas. If its flow is obstructed, however, this fluid can build up in a particular area and exert a pressure that may damage the delicate nerve tissue there. For this reason, it is possible that massage which helps to keep the head and neck loose and limber may also encourage the consistent flow of cerebrospinal fluid. Creating and maintaining space between the vertebrae is also crucial. Bad posture and lack of exercise often result in vertebrae which are too close together, or even fused. This damages the disks between the vertebrae, compresses the spinal nerves which leave the spinal cord between each pair of vertebrae, and, we believe, may also interfere with the flow of cerebrospinal fluid.

To increase cerebrospinal-fluid flow, refer to exercise 5–43 in the Muscles chapter, and continue with exercises 7–12 to 7–14 in the Massage chapter. The exercises for stretching the spine in the Spine chapter may very well have as many benefits for the central nervous system as for the back itself.

Visualization

Visualization is a technique which we have used over and over throughout this book to make your exercises more effective. Very often, simply by imagining an event, we produce in ourselves the physical reactions that would result if that event had actually happened. Someone with a terror of falling can acutely experience vertigo just by imagining great height. Another person can bring on an attack of vomiting by thinking about something 'sickening'. All the physical reactions of sexual arousal, up to and including orgasm, can be experienced just by thinking about sex. The response of our central nervous system to our thoughts is that powerful.

That is why thinking about, imagining, visualizing the results we want to obtain through our exercises helps to make them more effective. The tendency of the central nervous system is to help the body create exactly the situation we have visualized. Naturally, there is a limit to how much it can help, but the results of adding visualization to the practice of movement have been remarkable enough to make it standard practice in our movement teaching.

Do not let the word 'visualize' scare you. Many people have little or no ability to 'see' anything with the mind's eye, but they can work with a different imagined sense, that of feeling, and imagine how the change they want would feel. If you are actually able to visually picture changes you want to bring about, so much the better. But don't worry if you can't. Even saying to yourself that something is changing helps create the change.

6–7 To feel how visualization can work, begin with an easy motion, such as lifting your arm. Imagine first that your arm is very heavy – so heavy that it takes enormous effort to lift it. If it helps, you can imagine that you have an anvil tied to the arm. Now slowly raise your arm out to the side, as high as you can, still imagining how heavy it is. Feel how this combination of movement and visualization causes your body to react. How does it affect your arm, shoulder, chest and neck? Which muscles tighten to help the movement, which ones stay relaxed, which ones feel weak?

Lower your arm, breathe deeply, and relax for a minute. Now visualize your arm lighter than air, or filled with helium so that it will not stay down, and slowly allow it to lift again. Does the movement this time feel different?

6–8 Next, try slowly rotating your forearm. Either lie on your back or sit in a chair with broad arms, and, with your elbow supported, move the forearm in a rotating motion, making the circle as large as you can. Feel which arm muscles lighten as you do this, and notice where the movement stops being smooth and becomes rigid or jerky. Rotate the arm about ten times in both directions, and then let the arm rest completely. Now picture yourself rotating the forearm again, remembering the sensations of tension or jerkiness. Next, try to visualize the arm moving without those sensations. Imagine your muscles completely relaxed, and the movement smooth, unhampered and easy, with the fingertips describing a perfect circle in the air. You can imagine someone else lightly holding your hand by the fingertips and circling your arm for you while you go perfectly limp.

After visualizing this effortless motion for a minute, rotate the forearm again, holding in your mind that image of easy, weightless movement. Do you find your sense of the motion is now closer to what you visualized?

When you have practiced the forearm rotation and visualization once or twice, stop and instead open and close your hands very slowly, taking at least thirty seconds to fully straighten the fingers, at least fifteen to fully curl them. Concentrate on the fingers as you do this. There are small muscles in each finger. It is possible to open and close the hand without really engaging these muscles, simply by contracting the long flexor and extensor muscles which originate in your arms. The more you concentrate on your fingers, however, the more slowly you move them and the less you use your forearm, the more likely you will be to engage the small muscles of the fingers, and thereby engage nerves that you don't use often. A new part of your brain's motor cortex is being put to use.

One likely result of that is that the forearm will work with less effort. Open and close the hand at least three times in this manner, then try the forearm rotation again and see whether you find it any easier, any smoother, any more relaxed.

This is just one small example of a very important principle which underlies the whole body of Self-Healing exercises: that to use more of the body, on a regular basis, is to reduce the load of strain and fatigue on the body overall. When each part is put to use for its own appropriate and specific function, no one part has to be overloaded, strained, fatigued or worn out. When each part is put to use for its own specific function, no part is allowed to weaken, atrophy, become non-functional. When each part functions, the body as a whole functions. This has been stated throughout the book, of course. Our special point in this chapter is that the first step toward making a part functional is bringing your conscious attention to that part, becoming kinesthetically aware of it, and, with the help of your nerves, strengthening the connection between that part and its corresponding section in the cortex of the brain.

6–9   You can use the visualization process with any movement. For example, this time do it with your legs. Lie on your back on the floor, slowly lift one leg, then lower it again. Take a minute to imagine lifting it, visualizing that it is very heavy, dense and short. Lift it again, continuing the visualization, and see if the movement feels different. Do you sense a feeling of strain that corresponds with your mental picture? Now take a minute to picture the leg so light that it floats, so light that it can actually carry the rest of your body with it when it rises. Lift the leg again, with this image. How does it feel? Rest for a minute, then repeat the whole process with the other leg.

6–10 Try a similar set of visualizations while lying on your back and lifting your head with your hands. As you do so, also imagine that you are elongating your spine. Lie on your abdomen, raise the calf of one leg, and move it in a rotating motion with the knee remaining in one place on the floor. As you did with the forearm, notice how the motion feels, and whether there is any place where it becomes difficult or jerky. Stop moving, visualize the movement as it was, then visualize it as you would like it to be – smooth and effortless. When you have done this once or twice, stop, lower and relax the leg, and bend and straighten the toes of the foot. Again, let the movement be very slow, very focused in the toes themselves. Try to relax the calf completely. The relationship of the toes to the calf is very similar to that of the fingers to the forearm, and the muscles connecting them act in much the same way. Then, raise the calf and rotate it again, imagining that the toes are leading the motion and pulling the rest of the leg with them. By moving the toes independently of the calf, you may have helped the calf to relax a bit, and you may find the calf rotation smoother, more coordinated. Then bend the knee and, without moving the calf, rotate the foot, imagining that only the sole of the foot moves, and that the toes are leading the motion.

Practice this procedure with several easy movements, such as opening and closing the hands or the mouth, raising and lowering an arm, bending forward, rotating your spine, or with any movement you have come across which is no strain for you. Do the movement slowly, feeling any limitation or tension, or any other factor that keeps the movement from feeling good. Stop for two or three minutes, remember how the movement felt, visualize or imagine how you would like it to feel, experience that improvement deeply in your imagination, and then repeat the movement. We find that very often people notice a marked difference in how the movement feels to them before and after visualization. Of course, it is always possible that the difference in sensation is only imagined. This really does not matter. Whether or not you are still, in fact, tensing or tightening some muscles, the fact that you perceive the movement as easier or smoother will, by itself, make the movement easier and smoother in time. We also find that often if the movement is difficult or jerky, the visualization will reflect this. Practicing visualization will improve its quality, just as practicing movement will do.

6–11 After this warm-up, you can try a more difficult or demanding movement. This might be a Plow (exercise 20–5 in the Posture Problems chapter), sitting cross-legged and trying to touch your forehead to the floor (see exercise 4–21 in the Spine chapter), a back bend (exercise 4–37 in the Spine chapter) or any demanding lift or stretch. Unlike exercise 6–10, do not try to repeat the movement ten times before relaxing and visualizing – three or four times is plenty. Be sure to breathe deeply in and out through the nose as you move, and while you imagine the movement. Stop as soon as you feel that you have succeeded in making the movement easier, so that the next time you attempt the same movement your memory will be one of effortlessness.

Coordination Exercises

Coordination exercises are especially helpful in breaking harmful movement patterns. The more we do a movement in a certain way, the more difficult we make it for ourselves to do it in any other way. We often think of movement in very simple terms: sensory nerves carry information which initiates an action; motor nerves make it possible to carry out that action. The reality is much more complex. The truth is that, every time we move, the movement itself creates new sensory information, which the brain uses and stores. The brain has learned how that movement feels to do, and will try to reproduce that feeling along with the movement. The very first time we tense our shoulder muscles while writing, the nervous system learns to associate tensing the shoulder muscles with the other, necessary, motions of writing. Contracting the shoulders is not at all necessary for writing, but the nerves have incorporated the sense of strain into their sense of what constitutes writing, and now will automatically perpetuate it. Physical habits are very quickly formed, and not easy to break.

Coordination exercises help by 'distracting' or 'confusing' your brain in a way that breaks up your preprogrammed movement pattern. Suppose that you, like many people, have developed the habit of tightening your shoulders every time you move your head. Once it has received the information that you plan to move your head in the next microsecond or so, your brain will then think something to the effect of 'Head about to move, eh? Time to contract those shoulder muscles' and will send commands to all the appropriate motor nerves. Brains are not necessarily smart. If,

however, you decide to move your head and your hips simultaneously, your brain has to cope with several commands at once. It has less attention to give to the head movement, and it has a whole new way of thinking about head movement – that is, that head and hips, rather than head and shoulders, are to be used simultaneously. In the process of incorporating this new combination, the nerves are less likely to behave in their accustomed way.

Start with exercise 4–4 from the Spine chapter. Because most of our movements are forward, rolling from side to side not only activates muscles and neural pathways you tend to not use, it gives you a different sense of your body. Children instinctively like to roll, but you may need to let go and relax to be comfortable with this movement.

6–12 Move your head from side to side while rubbing the palms of your hands together (fig 6–12). Some people may find even this a

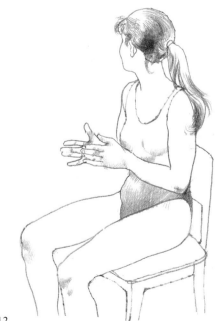

6–12

challenge. Practice it until your neck feels
loose, your hands are warm, and the movement
feels comfortable.

One of our favorite spine stretches is also a
good coordination exercise. Refer to the Spine
chapter for the three-way twist, exercise 4–24.
Some people find this exercise quite easy; if
you do, then do this one for its back benefits,
and go on to the more difficult coordination
exercises. Others find it very difficult to do all
of these motions simultaneously; these are the
people who most need this kind of movement.

6–13   Lie on your back, with your elbows on
the floor, and rotate your forearms as you
breathe slowly and deeply. Bend and straighten
your legs alternately, keeping your feet on the
floor. When you feel you have mastered that,
start moving your head slowly from side to
side.
    A variation of this exercise, if it is too easy
for you, is to open and close your jaw several
times with each movement of the head.

6–14   Sit in a chair with your back supported.
Move your feet, together, in a rotating motion.
This motion will probably be most comfortable
with a pillow under your feet. After several
minutes of ankle rotation, begin to rotate your
head at the same time. If you are rotating both
ankles clockwise, rotate the head counterclockwise and vice versa (fig 6–14). After a
few minutes of rotations, reverse the direction
of both your feet and your head, so that again
they will be rotating in opposite directions.
    A variation of this exercise is to massage
your knees by stroking them with your palms,
as you rotate your head and feet.

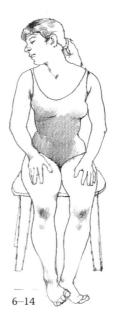

6–14

6–15   Stand, move the head in rotating
motion, and rotate the hips in the opposite
direction – for example, head clockwise, hips
counterclockwise. It has sometimes taken
Maureen several minutes and any number of
unsuccessful tries to arrive at this motion, but
the sense of release which it gives to the spine
makes the effort well worthwhile. Of course,
the difficulty of coordination exercises varies
widely. Some people may find this movement
no challenge at all, while some people really
cannot walk and chew gum at the same time.
Everyone, however, can improve coordination
to some extent.

6–16   Rotate your head clockwise and your
torso counterclockwise, and vice versa.

6–17   Rotate your head while slowly opening
and closing your jaw.

6–18   Hold your hands up before your face,
with the palms facing downward, and move
one hand clockwise from the wrist and the

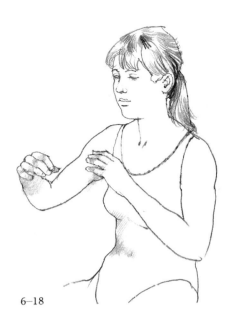

6–18

other counterclockwise (fig 6–18). Try different speeds, too!

6–19 Sit and stroke your abdomen in a circular motion while tracing circles on the floor with the soles of your feet.

A vision exercise called the 'long swing' combines coordination with sideways movement. Refer to the Vision chapter, exercise 8–19.

Walking and running backward and sideways will also improve your coordination (for running backward and sideways, refer to the Running chapter). It is always better to walk on sand, dirt or grass, rather than concrete. If you have balancing problems, it is also safer there.

Cross-Crawling

In his work with brain-injured children, the acclaimed therapist Glenn Doman developed a theory that enabled him to help children once

considered hopelessly disabled to make astonishing progress toward living more normal lives. Briefly, it was this: that every human being, in order to develop normal movement patterns, needs to make this development in stages, with each stage following the next in a specific order, since each stage makes the next one possible. If a stage is omitted, for whatever reason, the person may be unable to progress normally, and may remain trapped in the previous developmental stage.

These stages consist of (1) moving the arms and legs without moving the body; (2) crawling, which consists of moving forward with the arms and legs but with the body still belly-down on the floor; (3) creeping, which means going on all fours with the torso held up off the floor; and (4) finally, walking. These stages correspond roughly to the movement patterns of fish, reptiles, and mammals and, of course, humans. Interestingly, the human embryo passes through a similar series of developments in the womb, changing in form from a fish-like, to a reptile-like, to a mammalian, and at last to a fully human form. It seems that, in order to reach our full potential, we need to pass through each stage that our vertebrate ancestors did.

By assisting his patients in the appropriate movements, Glenn Doman found that he and his associates could often make it possible for them to progress to the next stage. If, for example, he had a patient who could crawl but not creep, the therapists would hold the child by the arms and legs and take him through the motions of creeping. This was often successful in enabling the child eventually to creep, at which point the therapists would begin to assist him with the movements of walking. What was most interesting was that if the therapists tried to get the crawling child to walk without first going through the creeping stage, they never succeeded. Each stage had to be successfully attained, and in the proper order.

We have found Doman's exercises helpful for many different people, not only the brain-injured. They are, in fact, helpful for anyone who wants to change movement patterns of any sort. By repeating the process we experienced when first starting to develop movement, we put ourselves back in our initial learning mode, back before we developed whatever harmful movement patterns we now have to deal with. If we learned a movement wrong initially, we have a chance to learn it right this time around.

6–20 For the first stage of movement, you can use exercise 6–13, or return to the three-way twist, exercise 4–24 in the Spine chapter. Or you can lie on your back and move one forearm in rotation while at the same time making large circles on the floor with the opposite foot. In short, any exercise which moves your arms and legs simultaneously while your body is at rest will work fine, and will be especially helpful if it simultaneously moves one arm and its opposing leg. If you watch an infant as she lies on her back happily flailing all her limbs, you may get some inspiration.

If you can arrange to do this type of movement in water, in a shallow pool or a bathtub, or if you can get inspired by doing it at the seashore, this is optimal. This is because at this stage we imitate most closely the movements of fish, who propel themselves by moving their fins against the resistance of water, but who do not have to contend with gravity. This type of movement can be handled by the lowest brain center, called the medulla – the highest part of the brain which the fish shares with us.

6–21 Standing, kick your left leg forward as high as you can and touch it to your right hand, and then kick the right leg up to touch the left hand. You may need to hold onto something with the free hand to balance yourself, but do at least try to do this without holding on if at all possible.

Next we come to crawling, in which we move forward using our arms and legs, with the belly on the floor. This type of movement requires the use of the pons, which is directly above the medulla, and which can be found in all vertebrates except fish – it is first seen in amphibians such as salamanders and frogs.

6–22 Begin by simply lying flat on your abdomen on a carpeted floor, or better yet on sand or in the grass. This is best done in clothes you do not really care about. Let the solid support of the floor, or ground, along the length of your body help you to relax completely, sinking all your weight into the floor. Turn your neck to one side and let your head rest on the floor; do not strain your neck by trying to hold your head up. Open your arms and legs out to either side and feel each limb sinking into the floor; relax your abdomen, back and shoulders; breathe deeply. Sometimes the pressure of the floor against your chest and abdomen will automatically make you feel like taking a deep breath. As you breathe, pay attention to where you may be holding tension in your muscles, and let it go. Stay stretched out belly-down on the floor until you feel completely comfortable and relaxed in that

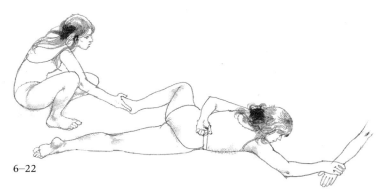

6–22

position. Imagine a cord that connects your navel with the center of the earth, so that you are rooted in place like a tree.

Before you begin crawling, we would like to warn that this exercise may be too vigorous for you if you have problems with your shoulders.

Crawling is difficult, and you may want to start with the help of two friends from your support group. Still lying prone (on the abdomen), inhale deeply, then exhale very slowly as you stretch your right arm forward, look toward it, and bend your left knee out to the side. To make sure that you are not using the left arm, rest your left palm on your back. Ask one of your friends to support your left foot, and hold on to the arm of your other friend with your right hand (fig 6–22).

Now pull yourself forward, keeping your torso on the floor as you do so. Try to use the arm and leg equally in this movement. This may at first feel very awkward, just as it does to babies who try to crawl for the first time, and you may only be able to move forward a few inches. Then stretch the left arm forward, look toward it, bend the right knee out to the side, have your friends support you at your right foot and left hand, and pull yourself forward again. Remember always to inhale before you move, then exhale slowly the whole time you are moving. Your friends can help

you a few more times, reminding you to look at your extended arm, to put your other palm on your back, to use your arm and leg as equally as possible, to breathe, and to relax. Now try to crawl by yourself. As you move, remember to imagine that your navel is attached to the center of the earth. This centering will help you put less effort into the motion.

At first, you will just stretch one arm forward, bend the opposite knee, push and pull forward, and then rest – and then repeat the same thing with the other arm and leg, and rest. When you have become comfortable with this movement, you can speed it up. As you stretch one arm, bend the other, and as you bend one knee, straighten the other, and do all of these motions simultaneously, so that you have a genuine, continuous forward motion. At this stage, you do not have to continue resting the inactive palm on your back.

This is called cross-crawling, because of the criss-cross pattern of the movement. Movement which uses the right arm with the right leg, the left arm with the left leg, is called homolateral or same-side movement. The cross-pattern of movement is used by all vertebrates from amphibians on up – including human babies from their very earliest efforts to crawl. Many brain-injured people have a tendency to move homolaterally. Cross-moving assures equal use of the two brain hemispheres during movement, since the left hemisphere of the brain controls the right side of the body, and vice versa. Since each person has a dominant side, homolateral movement would increase this tendency.

The next stage of movement is called creeping and consists of moving on hands and knees. Learning to creep requires a great deal more balance and skill from an infant than does crawling, and involves a higher center of the brain, called the midbrain, which makes its first appearance in the chain of evolution in reptiles. Although creeping is harder than crawling for an infant (at first), it is usually easier than crawling for an adult, since it is more usual for us to go on all fours than on our bellies. We often use creeping when we are working with a person who cannot walk. Since it is the stage that developmentally precedes walking, mastering it often helps the ability to actually walk.

6–23 Creeping should be done in the same criss-cross manner as crawling. Move your right hand and left knee forward simultaneously (fig 6–23), looking ahead at the hand

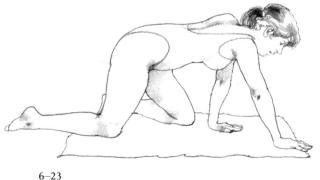

6–23

as you move. Now move your left hand and right knee.

Do the same backward. Look back toward the hand which is moving.

6–24 You have probably noticed that when people walk freely and with confidence, they tend to move in the same cross-pattern, swinging the left arm as the right foot steps out, and vice versa. The fact that we often lose this free and easy motion, because we are carrying something, have our hands in our pockets, or walk stiffly out of tension or self-consciousness, is sad, because it robs us of our opportunities to move in a way that balances the body. Suppose you have a stronger right leg, and a tendency to walk much harder on that leg. This will result in greater stimulation to the left side of your movement cortex. The tendency of the right side of the body to dominate will be gradually, continually increased. But if you swing your left arm when you step with the right leg, then the right side of the movement cortex will be stimulated by the arm's movement, and a certain amount of balance will be maintained. Without cross-moving, the tendency of one side to dominate the other increases, and so does our lack of balance. With cross-moving, we create more balance.

For this reason, we recommend swinging the arms as you walk. This motion is very natural to the body, and usually will occur spontaneously if you just allow it. If you find it difficult to do, it may be because your neck and shoulders are tense. If you practice the exercises in the Neck and Shoulders section of the Spine chapter, you can alleviate such tension.

Balance Exercises

Exercises which strengthen your ability to stay balanced and upright benefit your nervous system for the reasons we have been discussing: they distribute the 'load', or effort, of movement equally on both sides of the body (and thus on both sides of the movement cortex), and decrease the tendency of one side to dominate.

6–25 The most basic exercise is, of course, simply to stand on one foot with the other lifted. If you need to have a chair nearby to grab for support, please do, but try not to use it. Begin by lifting one foot for only four or five seconds, and gradually increase the duration to however long you can make it. You will find that in the process you will learn to relax the supporting foot, letting it flatten out on the floor; to relax your abdomen; to breathe deeply; to drop your shoulders and relax your arms. You will also find out, if you do not already know, which is your dominant or stronger side, because it will be much easier for you to stand on that foot.

6–26 Add movement to the basic exercise by sweeping the free foot forward, backward, out to its own side, to its opposite side in front of the balancing foot, and to its opposite side behind the balancing foot. You may find it easier if you stand on a stair or a box (fig 6–26).

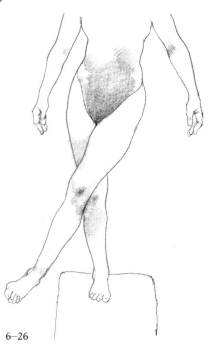

6–26

CHAPTER 7

Massage

Consider yourself a bodyworker even if you are your own client

This chapter is not intended as a massage manual – nothing can replace the full training and extensive experience required to produce a good bodyworker. We include this chapter to explain why massage is so integral to the Self-Healing method, to share our ideas on the benefits of massage as a therapy, and to share a few massage techniques which you may not have been familiar with – even if you have been doing massage for years. We hope that professional bodyworkers will enjoy this information. We also hope that we can interest non-professionals in getting into massage. Massage is a good time, a nice gift, a loving gesture and a healing tool. It can make every other health practice – nutrition, exercise, even psychotherapy – more effective. With the right knowledge, attitude and practice, anyone can do massage.

Massage, or bodywork, is an essential part of Self-Healing therapy. Since Self-Healing is foremost a movement therapy, it is made much more effective by anything which increases the range of movement, and massage is a very effective and pleasant way to do this. Like exercise, massage improves circulation, helps to break down excess connective tissue, relaxes tight muscles, and enhances breathing

and digestion. Massage has an edge over exercise in that it can be used as a therapy for stiff, sick, weak, injured or handicapped people in some instances where exercise cannot.

In the Self-Healing method, massage is used as a very important adjunct to movement therapy. Self-Healing bodywork is also a healing tool in its own right. The techniques we use are designed to:

- relax muscle spasms, so that the softened muscle fibers become more capable of free movement;
- ease the sense of constraint and tension in the body, which may be just as limiting to movement as actual tight muscles;
- increase circulation, by relaxing muscles so that blood can flow into areas that have hitherto been deprived of their full blood supply, and by promoting regulation of blood formation;
- reactivate nerves;
- strengthen weak muscles by improving circulation and nerve response;
- promote deeper respiration – an automatic result of relaxation;
- activate the parasympathetic, or relaxing, mechanism of the nervous system through

touch and relaxation and by improving respiration;

- lubricate and mobilize joints and increase their range of motion;
- enhance digestion;
- balance fluid concentrations throughout the body;
- balance and regulate body temperatures – if your hands are cold, massage will warm them; if your knees are hot, massage will cool them;
- release emotions trapped in the form of body tension;
- provide stimulation to the sensory nerves to aid in motor action – when you feel a part of your body, you can move it more easily;
- regenerate deteriorating bones;
- regenerate dystrophic muscles.

Like so many holistic therapies, massage is an ancient and respected skill whose value has been temporarily overlooked in our touch-phobic society. In Japan, China and India, and even in the colder parts of Europe such as Finland and Scandinavia, no one questions the therapeutic value of massage. Western society in general has been slower to accept it as a healing art, in part because we usually associate touch with only two things: aggression and intimacy. The very idea of touch is questionable – especially between strangers – and the idea of massage is even more dubious. Ever since 'massage parlor' became a euphemism for a place to buy sex, the word 'massage' has acquired a totally undeserved stigma. Partly for this reason, and partly because in recent years touch therapies have increased their range of techniques beyond the stroking and kneading of traditional massage, the term 'bodywork' came into use, and we like it. It implies a certain respect for the work, or craft,

of the therapist, and also suggests a workout for the body of the client, as is the case. (A thorough session of bodywork can have many of the same effects as one of exercise, including slightly sore muscles and an aftermath of pleasant fatigue.) We use the terms 'massage' and 'bodywork' interchangeably, to mean therapeutic touch, valuable both on its own merits and in conjunction with other health practices.

Acceptance of massage as a legitimate and valuable therapy began in the USA in the late 1960s and 1970s, as a part of the humanistic-psychology and human-potential movements, and people who had been perfecting touch therapies for many years came suddenly into prominence. Ida Rolf and others were recognized as authorities on healing through touch and manipulation of the body, and interest revived in past masters such as F. M. Alexander and Wilhelm Reich. It is interesting that the first therapy to gain wide acceptance was that of Rolf, which involved an extremely painful process of breaking down connective tissue. This is an effective method, but so are many other, far less painful, therapies, and it is hard not to suspect either that people were convinced that the pain proved something was working or that the pain erased their guilt over being touched. It is just amazing how many people describe a pleasant massage as 'decadent', 'self-indulgent', 'sinful'. What a shame – because here is a thing in life that really feels good and is good for you, in equal measure. Frankly, we think it should be available to everyone, on a daily basis, like food, sleep and toothbrushing.

Why is massage so necessary? Because daily life can be hard on our bodies. Sitting for many hours at a stretch stiffens and weakens our joints and muscles; then, when we do move, we bring that stiffness into the movement. Sometimes it is almost impossible to relieve stiffness through movement alone. The condition of our muscles shapes our movement. When we move with weak, tense or tired muscles, we often suffer small injuries to muscle, bone and cartilage, without even being aware of it. To protect these injuries, connective tissue will often grow and harden around them, making movement even more difficult and limited. As we age, some of our body processes begin to slow down; this makes free and easy movement even more of a necessity. Gentle, non-strenuous exercises designed to relieve stiffness may help, but how much more effective this movement is when done with muscles which are already loose, supple and relaxed. Many of the pains, limitations and fatigues we take for granted could be relieved through massage.

Many people are familiar with a type of standard massage in which the body is pummeled, kneaded, stroked and judo-chopped into a sort of warm glow of well-being. Like a hot-tub or sauna, this type of massage feels pleasant, is mildly therapeutic, and is administered equally for any body that lies on the table. Bodywork elevates this skill to an art.

The art of the bodyworker lies in having a wide range of touch techniques, and even more in knowing what kind of touch is appropriate to this particular part of this individual person's body at this specific time. Your needs change from day to day; the different parts of your body also have changing needs; and your body is unique, and should be treated as such. A client who comes in one week strong and refreshed will need to receive a very different treatment from the one she had the week before, when she came in tired and headachy. An accomplished bodyworker will know where on the body to work, how long to work there before moving on to another spot, what level of pressure to apply, which technique – palpating, stroking, shaking, stretching, passive movement – will be most helpful; and, at the same time, will be open to feedback from the client as to what helps, relaxes, relieves or hurts. The bodyworker's knowledge is largely built up from this type of feedback.

The other two important components of a bodyworker's education are the actual training he or she receives and personal experience of bodywork, which is really part of that training. We recommend any massage practitioner in training to experience as many different types of touch therapy as possible. Some may be gentle, others more vigorous; some work directly with the emotions and others more indirectly. The different aspects can be incorporated, to some extent, into any bodywork practice. Of course, in order to call oneself a practitioner of a particular method, one really has to have undergone full training in that method. However, experiencing a type of bodywork and absorbing what you find compatible in its approaches and techniques (and, of course, giving credit where credit is due when people ask you where you got that great idea) can only enrich your practice. It is not enough to read a book or attend a couple of lectures: you need to know with your own body what something feels like. You cannot guarantee that your client will feel the same things you do from a particular type of touch, but at least you will have some sense, kinesthetically speaking, of what you are doing. Meir and his students would not hesitate for a moment to send a client to bodyworkers specializing in other methods, if that type of touch or treatment came to appear best for that client.

In this chapter we will discuss some of the Self-Healing methods of self-massage and massage of others. Both have distinct advantages.

In self-massage, you do not have to go anywhere for a treatment. You are guaranteed that your therapist knows exactly what each touch feels like to you, and you can depend on your therapist to vary the touch to suit your likes. Some types of self-massage are even more effective than getting a massage from another, for exactly that reason – no one can be as sensitive to your body as you can. We especially recommend self-massage of the hands, feet, neck, chest, head, face and knees.

Self-massage is a wonderful mental exercise of self-acceptance. It is a terrific way of giving to yourself. It is also excellent training in learning to identify with the flesh under your fingers – a necessary part of true healing. Self-massage is an important part of a bodyworker's training, but, more, it is a valuable therapy available to everyone.

Getting a massage from someone else has very different advantages, and important ones. This is one of the many reasons why we so strongly recommend forming a small group to practice Self-Healing movement and massage work.

The first benefit of getting a massage from someone else is in being able to completely relax while you are worked on. The second is the exchange of energy between practitioner and client. If you have a good bodyworker, he or she will be able to transmit to you a sense of relaxation, strength and energy. (When you work on yourself, you may run into the problems of having a tense therapist.) In Meir's Self-Healing practitioner training program, students are trained to feel where a person's movement is restricted, which parts of the body need relaxation and which need additional stimulation, as well as how to guide a person toward the needed changes through touch.

Also, when allowing someone else to touch you for an hour or more with the intent of relieving your tension and pain, you come away with a sense of having been tenderly cared for, and we all need that. This sense is almost certainly based in truth: most bodyworkers do care deeply about their clients. It is extremely hard to spend any length of time touching someone you really do not like.

Group massage has all of the above benefits, multiplied by as many people as there are in the group. With more than one person touching you, you tend to lose track of whose hands are where, and so just give yourself over to the relaxing touch, creating a sensation many have described as 'womb-like'. Something about the group situation also seems to increase and intensify the feelings of acceptance, compassion and nurturing which a bodyworker feels for a client. It is very powerful to feel that much love and acceptance coming at you from so many directions at once. We feel that it could be a powerful tool in helping someone overcome feelings of low self-esteem, and so could be extremely helpful as an adjunct in psychotherapy. For some people we know, acceptance and love of their own bodies eventually made psychotherapy unnecessary. Many bodyworkers have given sessions to people who came into the session in terrible emotional turmoil but left feeling that their problems had been solved; though the problems remained, the clients felt so much better that they could approach them more effectively, with confidence and decision. We would like to see the day when everyone at a UN summit or cabinet meeting will get a good massage before going into the meeting – we strongly believe the world would be a better place for it.

Very few schools of massage emphasize the need for the practitioner to be in as good shape as they want the client eventually to be. This is probably why massage therapists are so prone to tendinitis, carpal-tunnel syndrome, cramps in the arms and hands, severe shoulder problems, back problems and general exhaustion. There is no denying that bodywork is as physical an activity for the therapist as it is for the client; it does not, however, need to be arduous or damaging. All that is needed is for you, the bodyworker, to pay attention to your own body before you go to work on your clients, and, of course, during the treatment as well. You need to be well-rested and well-fed and relaxed, with your muscles warmed and loosened by gentle stretching exercises and your energy replenished by deep, slow breathing and perhaps meditation. You need to pay special attention to your hands. All professionals understand the importance of quality tools: your hands, as well as the rest of your body, are your tools, and you can do a much better job if they are in top condition.

An essential tool for a practitioner is a sense of movement, since so many physical problems either cause or are caused by a lack of movement. You need to be able to tell when and where movement is blocked by tight muscles, excess connective tissue or unconscious holding. You must have a sense of how much movement is possible for the body in general, the average body, and also for that particular client at that particular time. At every session you should observe your client both moving and at rest; even if you just watch him or her walking into the treatment room, getting up onto the table, and settling into position for

the session, you can see enough to tell you how tense or relaxed the person is in various parts of the body. At the first several sessions, and any time the person is suffering from a serious problem or exacerbation, you should observe as many types of movement as possible. How far can your client bend, forward, backward and sideways? How far to either side will the head turn? How far up can the client raise the arms and legs? How far will the chest, diaphragm and abdomen expand during breathing? (And you will want to make these same observations about yourself from time to time as well.) The location and extent of the movement limitation should give you some clues as to where to work.

After massage, many people find movement easier, more comfortable and more expansive. Your massage work should increase the person's range of movement, but never forcibly. Never insist on moving a limb further than is tolerable for your client. Increased mobility should come about as a natural result of muscles relaxing *only*; you can stretch a limb, but never overdo it.

As we explained in the Muscles chapter, lack or limitation of movement has many bad effects on the body in general, not just on the specific area affected. Lack of muscle movement leads to slowing of every other kind of movement within the body. When muscles cannot or do not move, blood flow is slowed or blocked; nerve impulses do not travel efficiently from the brain to the rest of the body; joints stiffen because inactivity causes their flow of synovial fluid to decrease; digestion can be disturbed by tight muscles in the abdomen or lower back; excess hard connective tissue builds up around unused muscles and joints; oxygen intake decreases. Massage, like movement, can get the creaky wheels in your body running smoothly once more. Massage can make movement, and thus every other function, more possible.

The study of anatomy and physiology is extremely valuable to the massage therapist. Since you are in the business of touching muscles, it is essential for you to know where each muscle is, which organs, large blood vessels, nerves and so on either affect or are affected by its function, and which actions it controls. Knowledge of physiology will give you a much deeper understanding of your client's problems, as well as the changes which happen in your client's body during the massage session. To be a really effective therapist, however, you need, besides this knowledge, experience and the development of a sensitive touch. Massage takes years to learn, and you will find that your own work will eventually tell you as much as your study about the human body.

Self-Massage

Hands

In order to work effectively, either on yourself or on others, you must first develop strong, sensitive, flexible and coordinated hands. You need to be able to use your hands for a long time without pain or stiffness, and you need to have hands which can feel and respond to the tissue that they are touching.

7–1   Seat yourself comfortably, on the floor or at a table, with your back supported. On a hard surface – either the floor or the table-top – tap with all of the fingers on one hand only. Let your wrist be completely loose, so

that the movement of the hand is floppy; do not pound with rigid fingers. Do this several hundred times, and notice how the fingertips react. Most likely, they will first feel pleasantly stimulated, then they will hurt, then go numb, then hurt again, and then feel pleasantly stimulated again. If they just hurt, you may be tapping too hard, so ease off. When you have done this three or four hundred times, your fingers will probably be tingling, because of both an increase in circulation and an improved nerve response in the fingertips. This will make them more sensitive. Feel your face, scalp, shoulder and chest, first with this sensitized hand, then with the other, and notice any difference in the sensations registered by one hand as compared to the other. Now tap with the fingers of the other hand, and repeat the exploration.

Sensitivity – the ability to feel – is something that can be developed. The hands of blind people are famously more sensitive than the hands of sighted people, but we do not believe that this is because the blind are born with an extra dose of kinesthetic sense. This sensitivity develops in the blind because they are so constantly using their sense of touch, feeling everything they come across, seeking information through touch and paying attention to what their fingers tell them. We have a friend whose vision measures about average but who seems to be able to see much more than the average person; she's always finding things! Why? Because she uses her eyes, delights in using them, and pays attention to what she sees. You can develop this same level of awareness in your fingers, with experience, and with attention. (In Zen, it is called 'mindfulness'.)

The hand is a miracle. There is nothing like

159

it in creation for capability and versatility of function. Excluding the wrist, the hand has nineteen bones, fourteen joints, some of the strongest and most flexible muscles in the body, and so many nerves that if you made a scale model of a person based on distribution of nerves in the skin's surface the hands would look as big as the rest of the body combined. Its structure accounts, in part, for the incredible variety of things humans have learned to do with their hands. So, naturally, there are a great variety of massage techniques that you can do with your hands, to your hands.

7–2   Before you do any massage, you should rub your hands to increase their circulation, warming and sensitizing them. You can do this mainly by rubbing both palms briskly against each other, by holding one hand still and rubbing it with the other palm, by rubbing the back of one hand against the palm of the other, by rubbing the backs of the hands together, by spreading the fingers wide and letting them interlace and rub together as you rub the palms, by rubbing the fingertips with the thumb, by running the base of the palm along the length of each finger, and probably in nine or ten other ways we have not listed. Rub each palm up and down the length of the opposite arm, to increase circulation into the hands. When you do massage, you are using your whole hand, not just the palm, and so your whole hand will appreciate the preliminary warming and stimulation. Be sure, though, that you do not tense your shoulders or work too hard with shoulders or arms as you massage. Try to let the hands do all the work.

Move. The more you do bodywork, the more you will find yourself unconsciously 'knowing' about your client's body, without being told. One of Meir's students almost became convinced that muscles had subsonic voices, and would speak of the 'dialogue' between her hands and her client's body. You may have an idea about working on a specific area, or your client may try to direct you; nonetheless, your hands will wander of their own accord to the places that they feel are asking for help. This 'radar' will only develop, however, if your hands are sensitive: that is, if their nerve receptors are operating at full capacity. Massaging your own hands will help to keep their nerve receptors alive and alert.

Your hands must be loose and flexible, with a fluid and adaptable touch, for two reasons. First, they need to be flexible in order to perform the different types of touch you will want to use. Second, if they are stiff they will become tired much too soon, making you a prime candidate for problems like carpal-tunnel syndrome. Loose hands need flexible joints, and joints can be kept flexible only through movement. When a joint moves, this automatically causes the joint to circulate synovial fluid, which lubricates the cartilage in the joint and helps the bones to glide comfortably. The more frequently you move, the more constant will be the flow of synovial fluid. If a joint remains immobile for too long – for example, the hip and knee joints of a person who sits too much and walks too little – the circulation of synovial fluid will decrease.

7–3   To keep your hand joints (all fourteen of them) supple, rest your forearm against a table or the arm of a chair, take hold of the fingertips of the right hand with your left hand, and move the right hand passively in a rotating motion, with all of the right-hand muscles completely relaxed. Rotate the hand in both directions, until you feel that the right hand no longer resists or assists the motion. Now hold the right hand with the other, just under the wrist, and let the hand you are holding rotate slowly, making as wide a circle as you can without tensing your arm. Your hand and fingers should relax completely; the only movement is in the wrist itself. Repeat this ten to twenty times, and return to the passive movement. Can the right hand be moved more easily? Is it resisting the motion less? Is the range of motion larger?

Rotate each finger of the right hand, first passively, with the left hand holding the finger, then actively, and then passively again. Now do the same with each joint on each finger. Of course it will be much easier to move the joints passively, but try to move them by themselves and see how much independent movement you can get from them. Now compare how your right hand feels to how the left hand feels, in terms of warmth, sensitivity, looseness, aliveness. Run both hands over a surface – the floor, or your leg, or a piece of cloth. Can you notice any difference in how each hand responds to the surface?

Now rotate all the joints of the left hand as we have described.

7–4 Now explore the muscles of the hands. With the fingertips of one hand, palpate the muscles of the other in a circular motion. To palpate, you exert a gentle downward pressure, moving the fingertips without lifting them from the surface they are touching, until you move on to the next area to be palpated. Use your thumb to anchor your hand in place while the fingers move, and then palpate with the thumb itself; the thumb can press even more firmly, since it is stronger than the

fingers. Massaging in this way, move from the base of the hand up to the knuckles, and then along both sides of each finger. Massage each finger between the thumb and fingers of the other hand, and also with the base of the palm. You may be surprised to discover sore or tender places on your hand. The hand, arms and chest are areas which may contain numerous tense or tender places which never hurt until they are actually touched. When the tension in these areas is released, it often produces a rush of emotional feeling or emotional release.

When you have finished massaging one hand, be sure to repeat everything you have done on the other hand.

Right now is the time to begin to pay attention to your bodyworking style. As always, what you do is no more important than how you are doing it. As you press on the muscles of your hand, what is happening to the working hand? First of all, is it only the massaging hand that is working, or is the entire arm, shoulder, chest, upper back, maybe face and abdomen? You do not need that much help! If you work in that way, you will tire your whole body while failing to develop the strength in your hands that you will need both to do good work and to avoid pain, tension and other complications in the hands themselves. So concentrate your energies and attention in your hands. This does not mean pressing harder with your fingers; it means letting go of your arms, shoulders and whatever else you were using. See how few muscles you can involve in your hand motions. Be aware of the motions of each finger, the palm and the back of the hand. Visualize your massaging hand all by itself, unattached to your body, and imagine it moving independently. Breathe deeply and, as you inhale, imagine energy flowing directly into your hands; as you exhale, imagine tension leaving your arms, shoulders, neck and so on.

7–5   You will have less tendency to work with your shoulders if your fingers are individually strong. Place your fingertips on a table-top as though they are on a typewriter, and tap each finger, one after the other, from the little finger to the thumb, and from the thumb back to the little finger. Do this at first rapidly and lightly, and then more slowly, really pressing each fingertip down as hard as you can. Let all the pressure come from the fingers themselves; do not let your arms work for them.

7–6   Place your right forefinger tip over your left, with your arms held close to your body. Press down firmly with the right finger, while the left finger resists the pressure by pressing upward. Again, make the fingers work, not the arms or shoulders. Then, reverse the direction of the resistance by pressing up with the left finger while the right finger resists by pressing down. This sounds like exactly what you just did, but you will see that, if you think of one finger as exerting the pressure and the other as resisting it, the way you use your muscles will differ slightly when you reverse the situation. Do the same exercise with the left fingertip on top of the right. Then repeat this exercise for each pair of fingers.

7–7   Move each finger from side to side – right and left – and then do the same against resistance, as in exercise 7–6. Now move each of your fingers without resistance – is their range of motion any larger?

For more exercises for the hands, refer to the chapter for Musicians – chapter 10.

For massage of the wrists, refer to exercise 3–42 in the Joints chapter.

Arms

Now you will be using your strong, supple, warm and sensitive hands to massage the rest of you. Let's move on to your arms.

7–8   With one hand, gently pinch the flesh on the inside of your forearms, moving from the wrist up to the elbow, then do the same thing on the outer side of the forearm. When you pinch, take the flesh between your thumb and the other fingertips and pull it slightly away from the bone, with your thumb doing most of the work. Do not do this hard enough to hurt – even a gentle pull is enough to begin to loosen the forearm muscles. If there is enough flesh, you can also shake it as you hold it.

You may notice that some areas will redden at your touch. These are areas which have been in need of circulation; as you massage, the blood will be automatically drawn to these areas first. Areas which are not so much in need of blood will not redden as much, even if you massage the area harder. It is as though massage triggers your body processes to regulate themselves.

Repeat the pinching motion on the upper arm.

7–9   Now you can rub hard, with your palm, up and down the length of the arm, first in long strokes, then in circles, while the arm being massaged turns from side to side, slowly, so that every part of it is massaged. Next, instead of rubbing, circle the arm with your hand and gently squeeze the arm, holding the hand stable in one position and letting it move up the arm as the arm itself turns from side to side. Massage the forearm by squeezing and pressing one side of it with your thumb while stabilizing it from the other side with your other fingers.

7–10   Feel with your fingertips along the entire length of the inner and outer parts of the arm, and see where your fingers discover tense muscles. You can distinguish these places by their hardness. It might be a good idea to have a diagram of the skeleton handy, so that you will not mistake a tense muscle for a bone, since there are usually plenty of muscles in the body which feel almost that hard. When you find these spots, tap vigorously on them with all five fingertips; as always, when you tap, let your wrist be totally loose and your fingers relaxed, so that the impact is caused by the flopping of the wrist, not the pounding of the fingers.

7–11   Another good technique for loosening tight muscles is to cup your hand slightly, with the fingers held together, and tap with the whole cupped hand on the tight area. (Try this with a flat palm and you will see immediately how different it feels; the area being massaged can absorb much more impact from a cupped hand.)

Now notice how the massaged arm feels, and also how its whole surrounding area feels: the shoulders, neck, chest, upper back on that side of your body. Move your head from side to side; does the neck on that side feel any looser?

Swing your arms in circles; does the massaged one move any more easily than the other? It may not, of course, but the chances are that it will. One of Maureen's clients described what she calls 'the Igor effect', which is what happens to her body after Maureen works on just one of this client's arms. On the side which has not been massaged, the shoulder is higher, the chest more sunken, the jaw more drawn toward the neck, the upper back more rounded forward, making her feel (if not look) like Dr Frankenstein's assistant. To avoid the Igor effect, massage your other arm as soon as possible.

Neck, Jaw, Chest and Shoulders

To massage your neck, chest and shoulders, you will be most comfortable in a position where your arms are somewhat supported. You can either sit in a chair with broad arms or lie on your back with pillows under your arms; either way, try not to let your arms become tired.

7–12   Turn your head to the side and palpate very gently along the muscles which run from under your jaw, along the middle of the side of your neck, to just above your collarbone. Tap lightly with the fingertips, lingering in any especially tight area, then rub with the whole hand, up and down the side of the neck. Pinching, shaking or cupping may not be appropriate in such a sensitive area, but you can always try them – very gently – and see if they feel good. Turn your head from side to side and see if the massaged side of the neck feels any different from the other. (We recommend leaning the head against a wall while you turn it from side to side, to allow maximum relaxation of the neck muscles.) If not, keep working on it until it does. We have sometimes spent as much as half an hour massaging the neck only. Relaxing the neck is very important in improving vision, and can also help ear conditions such as infection, tinnitus and itching of the inner ear.

7–13   After you have massaged both sides until they feel looser, massage the back of your neck. Beginning at the base of the skull, palpate and rub in circles, working your way down the muscles on either side of your cervical spine. You can start by doing this with both hands at once, then try massaging the left side with the right hand, and vice versa (fig 7–13), reaching around behind the head, grasping the muscles along the vertebrae and strongly palpating them. Finish by rubbing, squeezing and tapping the muscles where the neck joins the upper back.

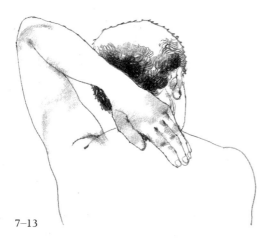

7–13

7–14   The mobility of the lower jaw influences the posture of the neck. Tighten your jaw for a moment and feel how the muscles of the back of the neck tense up. A tense jaw, therefore, leads to lack of circulation to the head – a condition you would definitely like to prevent.

Hold your chin with both hands – your thumbs underneath it and your fingers above it. Now use your hands to move your lower jaw up and down several times as you open and close your mouth. Does your jaw let your hands move it, or does it resist the motion? Try to resist less.

Let go of your chin, puff your cheeks, and stroke them with your palms in a circular motion. Relax the cheeks, hold your chin again, and move your jaw up and down as before. Does it resist the motion less?

Open your mouth widely, let your jaw drop, and tap with your fingertips in front of your ears, on the hinge joint which holds your jaw in place. You may feel soreness that you may not have been aware of; it is those tight, sore muscles that you are trying to release. Puff your cheeks again. Do they puff any more than before? Massage them again with a circular stroke, and let go.

With one hand over the other, stroke around your face – from one cheek to your forehead to the other cheek and over the tip of your chin. Use the whole palm and the fingers to circle your face several times. Now try again to move your jaw with your hands. Can you feel any difference?

Refer to the Muscles chapter, exercise 5–50, for more work on the jaws.

7–15   Now massage along the top of each shoulder. It is easier to massage the right shoulder with the left hand, and vice versa. Most people will find this area very hard and tough, so a firmer massage may be effective, but, of course, you should remain sensitive to what feels good to you. Tapping, palpating, squeezing and shaking are usually the types of touch which feel the best. It often makes the massage more effective if you slowly rotate your shoulder while it is being massaged, since this can give the hard muscles a head start on loosening up. You can also try to rotate it passively, holding the ball of the shoulder in the opposite hand. It may be a challenge for you to relax the shoulder and allow your hand to move it without the shoulder assisting the movement, but it feels wonderful if you can do it.

From here it is natural to move on to the chest. For detailed descriptions of how to massage your chest, please turn to exercises 2–2, 2–3 and 2–10 in the Circulation chapter.

Face and Head

For instructions on facial massage, which is particularly useful to people with eye problems, please turn to the Vision chapter.

7–16   To massage your head, rest your elbows on a table, place your fingertips against your scalp, and press down firmly. Now leave your hands in place and move your head up and down, letting your fingers rake along the scalp as the head moves – your hands remaining stationary.

Pinch your scalp, pulling the skin up from the head as you do when washing your hair. Press your fingertips on your scalp and shake them vigorously, moving them to different areas of the scalp. Then move the palpating fingers in rotating motion for a minute or two before lifting or moving them from their place on the scalp.

Feet

To give yourself or anyone else a great foot massage, please turn to exercise 5–2 in the Muscles chapter. Add to that exercise 2–34 from the Circulation chapter.

Back

The back is not the first place we think of when we imagine self-massage, but most places on the back can be reached if you are flexible, and many can be reached even if you are not. Most people do not have a very good kinesthetic sense of their backs, partly because the back does not have as many nerves as most other parts of the body, making it less sensitive to touch. For example, most people cannot distinguish between two points being touched on the back unless they are at least an inch apart. This makes it possible for a lot of tension to build up in the back without our noticing it and treating it in time. Massaging the back improves both circulation and kinesthetic awareness.

7–17   With your fists, you can stroke from the base of the spine up as far as you can reach, probably to the lower middle back, and also across the hips. Interlace your fingers and massage the lower back by moving the backs of the fingers across it in rotating motion (fig 7–17A); if this feels particularly needed in one area, linger there and give it a little extra massage before you move on to the next area.

You can also pound lightly with the fists on the lower back (fig 7–17B), hips, buttocks and thighs, relieving tension in the strong muscles there.

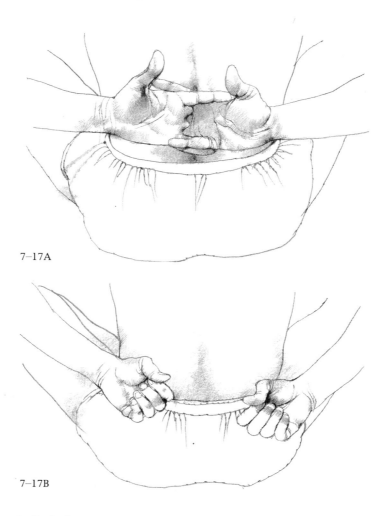

7–17A

7–17B

Sitting on tennis balls (refer to exercise 3–3 in the Joints chapter) can help relieve pain in the sciatic nerve and tension in the buttock muscles.

7–18 Bend and raise your elbows, placing your fingertips firmly on your shoulders. You can do this both with the elbows pointing forward, so that your fingertips are on the back part of your shoulders, and with the elbows pointing diagonally out to either side, so that your fingertips are on the top of your shoulders. Slowly move your elbows down and let your fingers firmly rake along the shoulder muscles as the elbows are lowered (fig 7–18).

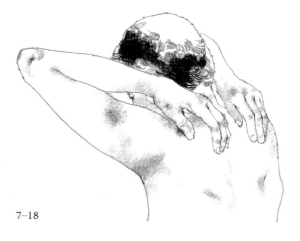

7–18

7–19 Stand with your back against a wall and your feet about a foot in front of it and hip-width apart. Let your knees slowly bend and your back slide against the wall, lowering yourself as far as you comfortably can, and then straighten your knees, keeping your back against the wall (fig 7–19).

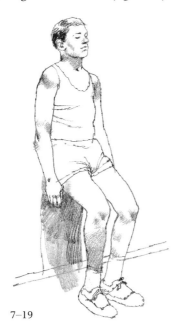

7–19

7–20 Leaning your back against the wall as before, place two tennis balls between your back and the wall, with one on either side of the spine – never pressing on the bones themselves, but rather on the erector spinalis muscles which run along each side of the spine (fig 7–20). These muscles, which hold the back upright, can become very tight and hard, along with the connective tissue which surrounds them and holds them together. Press yourself against the wall hard enough to keep the balls in place, and bend and straighten your knees slowly so that the balls 'roll' from your shoulders down to your hips, or as far as possible. Be careful not to press hard enough

to create soreness in your muscles. If you do get sore, relieve the pain with a hot towel or get a gentle massage.

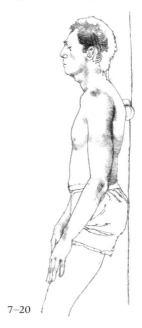

7–20

Knees

Massage of the knees is very helpful for anyone with knee injuries, and should also be done by anyone involved in active movement of the legs – including sports, dance and other types of performance – before and after exercise. The knees are among the body's most vulnerable structures, both in that they are subject to a tremendous amount of impact, especially from active people, and in that, if injured, they are slow to heal. Massage acts as a warm-up, to stretch and limber the tendons and ligaments of the knees, so that they are better able to absorb impact.

7–21 Before you massage your knees, rub your hands together with your fingers interlaced. It is best to sit in a chair, with your feet flat on the floor, and to use some sort of oil or cream so that, if necessary, you can rub fairly hard without irritating the skin. In fact you may not need to rub hard, since even a gentle massage of the knees may make them quite warm. Use the palms of the hands, especially the lower part, to gently rub in circles the areas surrounding the kneecap, including the lower thigh, the sides of the knee, and the back of the knee. Place your palms on either side of the area you are massaging, press down, and shake gently. Tap with your fingertips all around the base of the kneecap, and stroke and palpate with the fingers across the kneecap itself. Pinch all around the knees, using all your fingers and both thumbs, holding the flesh with one hand while shaking or tapping it with the other (fig 7–21).

with the whole hand. If you are going to massage your legs regularly, begin with the inner leg muscles, since these often are the most sensitive to touch, and work exclusively on these for three days before you expand the massage to include the front, back and outer sides of the legs.

When working on the back of the calf, press hard with the thumbs as you hold the front with your fingers (fig 7–22). Then do just the opposite – palpate the front of the calf with your fingers while your thumbs stabilize the hand on the back of the calf. The hand is in exactly the same position, but pressure is being exerted from the opposite side. Then repeat this same technique on the muscles of the thighs.

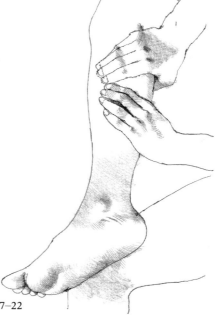

7–22

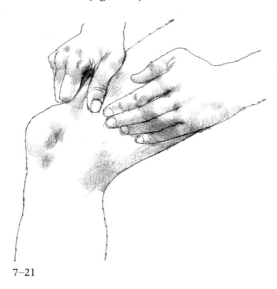

7–21

Legs

7–22 Leg-muscle massage feels wonderful, especially after the legs have been vigorously used. Massage the whole leg, from ankle to hip, in circles with the palm of the hand, then

With the base of the palm and with the fist, rub the quadriceps muscles on the front of the thigh. Massaging with the fist is best for the tough muscles of the outer thigh.

Abdomen

7–23 It is easiest to do this lying down on your back. Place your flat palms on your two hipbones and, rubbing in circles, slowly move them toward the midline of the abdomen. Stroke the abdomen with one hand moving clockwise, the other counterclockwise, letting the two hands slide over each other and pressing down momentarily as they do so. This helps relieve blockage and tension in the digestive tract. Then palpate the whole abdomen gently with all fingers and both thumbs, circling firmly but gently around sore areas.

If you find other ways and other places to massage yourself and would like to share your techniques with us, we would love to hear about them. By all means explore for them. You can be a great source of knowledge for yourself and about yourself. Use yourself as a natural biofeedback machine or guinea pig while you develop a sensitive, knowing, healing touch.

Massage of Others

Touch is one of our deepest forms of communication. The avoidance or deception possible in other types of communication vanishes during touch. If you as a practitioner are tired, in pain, uncomfortable, stressed, tense, these things will affect your performance in this work more than in most other types of work. Your first responsibility to your client is to be relaxed, flexible, strong, energetic – whatever you want to communicate to your client's body you must feel in your own. The most

beautiful music will sound bad if you play it on an instrument that is out of tune. You need to maintain your own good health, through whatever combination of diet, exercise, rest, therapy, meditation and so on works best for you. You need to get bodywork yourself, regularly, and it will help you tremendously to practice the movement exercises in this book, to keep your body flexible, energized and sensitive.

Remember that the body you touch will become like the body which is touching it. Tense hands will make tense muscles. Babies will wriggle away and cry if they are picked up and held by someone who is upset or angry or stressed, just as they will relax and smile for a relaxed, happy person. Bodies have the same innate animal wisdom that babies do.

Research being done into the electromagnetic fields which surround and emanate from living bodies may some day add inestimably to our present knowledge of healing. When we try to explain why massage is so effective, we speak in terms of muscle relaxation, better circulation, better cleansing and nourishing of the body's cells, and so on. We deal with anatomy, with physiology, even with chemistry, but perhaps it is on the level of physics – electricity – that massage, or indeed any form of medicine or healing, must be investigated. It may be that its effects are actually on a much more subtle pure-energy level, beyond our present capacity to understand or explain. We are looking forward with great excitement to the results of these studies into electromagnetism. We are very hopeful that, if anything, they will provide a better explanation of why our methods work than we ever could. For the present, we must be content with just knowing that it does, rather than how it does.

The point of the above is that, if electromagnetic fields are involved, then we are talking about the meeting and overlapping of your electromagnetism field with that of your client. Whatever is eventually discovered about electromagnetism, we know that this holds true: whatever you have, you will give to the person you are touching. To give relaxation and energy, you must first possess them.

Emotional states are transmitted from you to your client as surely as physical ones. Acceptance, compassion, nurturing, and a sense of confidence can be instilled through touch, if you feel them in yourself. If you have a feeling of anxiety or mixed feelings about the client, please think twice before massaging them.

As a practitioner, you have to do mental work on yourself all the time. What you transfer through your touch goes beyond your feelings and emotions. When you massage, visualize that your head goes up to the sky, that one shoulder goes to one side of the world as the other goes to the opposite direction. Try to allow yourself a sense of expansion. Visualize that your wrists are loose and that your fingers work independently. By doing that, you mentally work on balancing your own body, on relaxing your own muscles, and on not allowing your own emotions to take the physical form of contracted muscles. Within limits, your emotions will then not influence your touch, and you will be able to promote balance and relaxation in your client.

You can teach your client to use his or her own mental strength to benefit further from the massage. Both of you should visualize that your hands are penetrating into your client's body, softening it and strengthening it. If you both succeed in visualizing this, you will permit the needed changes to occur both in the mind and in the cells. This image should be easy, flowing and relaxing. If either of you

find it difficult or stressful, psychotherapy may be helpful in realizing the emotional blockage which is in control and removing it.

There is much in massage procedure that is really a matter of individual preference. Whether to wear clothing and how much of it to wear, whether to work on a table or on the floor, what position the client should be in, whether or not to use oil, what temperature to have the room, these are all open to question. The effectiveness of the treatment and the client's comfort are the two most important factors, and your own comfort is also essential, since you probably cannot give a good massage if you are uncomfortable. We have known therapists to insist that a client take off all his or her clothes when the client clearly was not ready for this, to insist on using thick, perfumed oils which made clients nauseous, to keep the room at a perfect temperature for their clothed selves while the unclothed client shivered, and so on. Try to be as sensitive as possible to each client's needs – and this means stay flexible. In general, your client should be just warm enough to stay comfortable, but not overly warm, since this may slow the circulation; you should be working in a totally comfortable position – have foot stools, pillows and so on around for you to use as needed; your client should remove as much clothing as needed for you to work on the areas that need it, and should be allowed to continue wearing whatever is left if he or she wants to; and you should be able to work without oil or cream, in most instances, if the client does not like it. When your fingers really need to be extremely sensitive, it may be better to work without oil, since this decreases friction and may prevent your fingers from 'reading' the client's body completely accurately. Oil is best used when you want to create warmth quickly, and when friction is created by brisk rubbing, since it helps to prevent skin irritation. It is also good to use oil when working on very weak muscles, as it allows an extremely light and delicate touch.

Your observation and your client's feedback should tell you where to begin the massage; classically, most massages begin with the back, but this may not be the best place. You must know as much of your client's medical history as possible; certainly you should know anything that might be even remotely related to the present problem (if there is one). If someone has a very tight neck, lying on the abdomen or on a very thick pillow may be uncomfortable. A person with knee problems will be more comfortable on the back with the knee elevated by thick pillows; a person with sciatica will feel better lying on the unaffected side, and so on. Ask your client what feels best, and be sure that he or she really is comfortable before you go to work. People will not always tell you how they feel – in fact, sometimes they do not even notice how they feel until you ask them. You may occasionally need to ask someone to lie in an uncomfortable position, in order to massage an important area, but always remain aware of the client's feeling and do not keep the client in this position for longer than absolutely necessary.

Sometimes you may find it helpful to begin the session with deep breathing, visualization or movement, rather than touch, if it seems that the person is not able to relax and enjoy the touch right away. If the person is very upset, touching may only produce greater agitation, whereas deep breathing and visualization can bring relaxation. If a person is tense and rushed, passive movement might encourage the 'letting go' of obligations, frustrations and so on, whereas straight massage

might meet only with resistance. A quiet voice and calm manner will also help a person to relax. However you choose to begin the session, you should ask your client to breathe deeply, to visualize the parts of the body one by one and ask each part to relax, to imagine that each inhaled breath expands the body and each exhaled breath expels tension and pain. You can use whatever other images help the client to relax and to feel his or her body. Ask your client to contribute these images, since what relaxes one person may not work for another. (Maureen remembers one hypnotist asking her to imagine herself sitting under a tree – the main sensation this evoked was of bumpy roots and bugs crawling on her.)

Above all, keep in mind that what you are really doing in massage is facilitating movement in the body. It may seem contradictory to speak of movement and relaxation simultaneously, but it is not: tension is nothing more than a holding-pattern, enforced motionlessness of specific areas. Have a sense of movement as you work, keep in mind where you want to stimulate movement in your client's body, and choose your techniques to create this movement.

It is important to listen to how your client reacts to your work, and not to have too specific expectations about his or her reaction. One person may sink into a blissful trance at the first touch; another person may need ten sessions before being able to feel anything at all.

People become numb for all kinds of reasons. An area undergoing stress usually goes through three stages of reaction: (1) pain, which may be caused by incorrect use of the body; (2) if the stress continues unrelieved, numbness will take the place of pain – the body tries to defend itself against the pain by living with the tension as if it were normal and no other options existed; and (3) if the stress continues long enough, the continued muscle tension will result in extreme pain, and possibly damage to muscle or other tissue. Sometimes massage will cause some muscle pain, and sometimes this is very good: it can mean that the layer of numbness is being removed. When you touch someone, you bring that person's attention to the area being touched, literally waking up the nerves in that area. If the area is under stress, the person's first reaction will be increased awareness of the tension and pain. This may be uncomfortable, but it is unavoidable, for how can you help a problem without first knowing that it exists? Numbness enables a person to continue with the destructive behaviors that create the problem; feeling, on the other hand, motivates the person to change those behaviors.

Massage may also cause some pain due to increasing circulation. When circulation is weak, blood vessels tend to become narrower and to lose their elasticity. Massage draws blood toward the massaged area, encouraging the dilation of contracted capillaries and the buildup of new ones. The increased blood volume may cause a feeling like muscle pain at first, though this condition is temporary.

So you cannot always expect that your client will feel perfectly splendid after each and every massage session, especially if you aim to make very deep changes over a somewhat extended period of time, using the client's increased awareness as an important part of the treatment. The type of massage done in most (legitimate) massage establishments consists of long, deep strokes all over the body. This type of massage feels wonderful while it is happening – hence its popularity – and it can be very effective with some people;

however, its effects are most often temporary, and it is not always appropriate for everyone. The client may feel that he or she had a very pleasant experience, but not have a sense of where to go from there – or what is to be the next step in healing. The type of massage that we practice and teach helps people to change their posture and movement habits, and actively supports them in their own exercise programs.

Some of the results you can look for, to let you know your massage is effective, are deeper, slower breathing; limpness in limbs and neck; increased movement of the chest and diaphragm; stomach growling, indicating that the parasympathetic, or relaxing, nervous system, has been activated and thus digestion is stimulated; a healthier color in the face, if the person started out too pale, sallow or flushed; redness in the areas you massage, showing that blood has rushed there as a result of your touch; and emotional reaction and release, whether negative or positive. If your client remains rigid, breathing shallowly or not seeming to breathe at all – in short, if you feel that what you are doing has no effect – then try another technique, such as breathing exercise, movement or passive movement. Or simply ask the client where he or she would like you to work; sometimes the feeling of being cared about and catered to will do more to relax a person than anything else.

After you complete a massage on one foot, arm, side of the back or whatever, be sure to ask your client whether there is a difference in sensation between the two sides. There may not be one, and if there is it may not be what you would expect. One client reported that the leg Meir had just massaged felt more tense than the other, but when he stood up he found that he could walk more easily and comfortably on that leg. We concluded that he was simply more able to feel the tension that had already been present. Another said that the massaged shoulder felt 'strained'. With a few more questions, Maureen found that that shoulder felt warmer, larger, longer and more alive than the other, in addition to having a tingling feeling. The 'strained' feeling turned out to be simply a sense that the shoulder had been used or 'worked' – and this client strongly associated any type of work with strain.

During the massage, you will probably want to work on any areas which are hurting, but you may not want to work on these areas first, since they may be too tense and sore to respond with anything but resistance to your touch. Bodies need time to recover from injury, and you may not want to touch an injured area until some time after the injury; if you do so, however, use a very light touch. If the left knee is injured, you may want to work first on the right leg. Your client will probably have been leaning more heavily on this leg while favoring the injured one, and so the muscles will very likely be tight and possibly sore or numb. This type of muscle tension responds quickly to massage, and as you relax the right leg the whole body will relax somewhat – including the injured knee. By the time you touch the injured knee itself, the process of relaxation will already be under way, making your massage much more effective. You may also choose to work on an area as far away from the painful area as possible, drawing the person's kinesthetic attention away from the source of pain; thus, foot massage may be a good way to begin a session for the relief of a headache.

The methods we have suggested for massage of the arms, hands, chest, abdomen and face apply just as well to partner massage as they do to self-massage. To many of them, you can add passive movement in the form of shaking, stretching and moving against resistance – that is, moving the leg, finger or arm in one direction while a partner tries to move it in the other. This last is a good technique for developing strength and for easing extreme tension.

Hands

7–24   In addition to the massage techniques for the hands which were described earlier in this chapter, here is one which will be very helpful for anyone whose hands are tight from a lot of work. Interlace the fingers of one of your hands with your client's, and stretch your client's fingers as far back as they will go comfortably. With your free thumb, 'iron' the muscles of the stretched palm (fig 7–24), pressing between the bones of the palm, from the bases of the fingers toward the wrist.

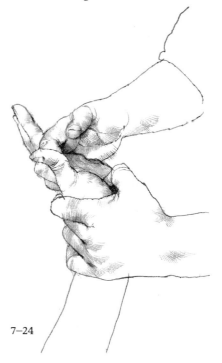

7–24

Legs and Feet

7–25 Any technique which you used in massaging your own feet (exercise 5–2 in the Muscles chapter) can be used just as effectively on your client, and you will of course be in a much more convenient position for working.

You can then rotate the ankle itself, while massaging up into the shin and the back of the calf, and downward into the heel and instep. Holding the foot at the ankle, bend it as far backward, forward, left and right as it will go without causing pain. You may find it helpful to rest the client's foot against your chest while you hold the shin with one hand and the Achilles tendon with the other, and flex the foot by pressing on it with your chest. Place your fingers between the client's toes and spread them as far as possible (fig 7–25), then, in this same position, rotate your hand, bending the toes backward and forward from

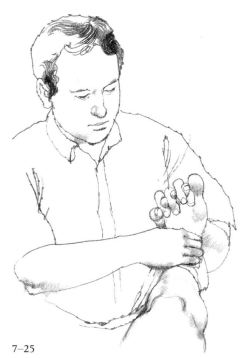

7–25

the ball of the foot as you rotate. Ask your client to move the ankle while you massage the ankle, shin and lower calf with both hands, then to move the toes while you massage the ball of the foot and the base of each toe.

You can repeat all of these techniques with your client lying on the abdomen as well as on the back.

With your client lying on the abdomen, rotate each calf, from the knee, in large circles, bringing it back so that the heel touches the buttock if possible, and keeping the foot as close to the table as possible throughout. Since the knee is delicate and easy to injure, it has to be moved slowly and carefully, and always with a great deal of sensitivity to what the client feels.

7–26 The muscles of the legs are very strong, and so can become extremely tight. Patterns of tension will vary: in an active person the calves may be tension spots, while in a sedentary person the thighs are much more likely to be contracted than the calves, particularly the hamstring muscles in the backs of the thighs. A person who spends a lot of time standing will have tension along the outer sides of the thighs, in the tensor fasciae latae muscles.

Most of the leg muscles are strong, and can often stand (in fact, greatly enjoy) a deep and vigorous workout unless, of course, there is an injury or an inflammatory condition such as tendinitis or sciatica.

As with the feet, passive movement is an excellent way to begin. With the client on his or her back, lift and rotate the client's leg. To avoid straining your own back or shoulders while lifting a heavy leg, remember to bend your knees as you lift, hold the leg close to your body, and let your whole body move with the motion as you move the leg. You can do this standing beside the table, with one hand under the knee and one supporting the ankle (fig 7–26A), rotating the whole leg from the hip joint. Bend the leg as you bring the foot near your client's body, and stretch it as you carry the foot away from his or her body.

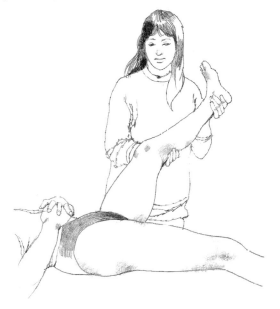

7–26A

If your client does not suffer from problems in the ankle, knee or hip joint, you can also stand on the table and lift the leg straight up (or as nearly straight up as your client's flexibility will allow) holding the ankle with both hands as you move the leg in a circle around the hip joint, pulling the leg straight up so the hip comes off the table and shaking it, then moving back a couple of steps and pulling the leg diagonally toward you.

Stand at the foot of the table and lift the leg while stretching it toward you, then rotate it from this position.

Bend both knees up to the chest, and move both in rotation simultaneously (fig 7–26B).

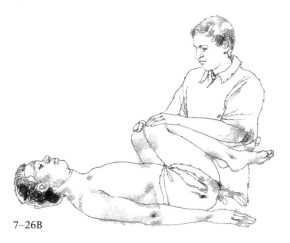

7–26B

Bend one of your client's knees, supporting the kneecap in one hand and the arch of the foot in the other. Bring the knee toward the client's chest, and move it: first bend and straighten it, then move it in rotation, then out to its own side, still bent. Now cross the leg over the client's body, until the thigh is perpendicular to the body (or as close to this as possible). Pound lightly with your fist around the hip joint, and rake your fingers along the outer thigh muscles (fig 7–26C).

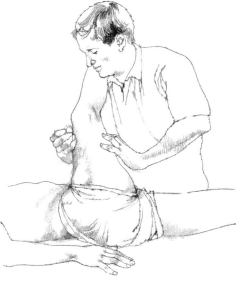

7–26C

You can lift the leg straight up, support the ankle on your shoulder, and pound lightly and rapidly with your fists on the hamstring and outer thigh muscles.

Pull the leg straight upward, and bend and straighten the knee, or do the same while holding the leg stretched out to one side. Hold the leg straight up or stretched straight out to the side and move it in rotating motion (fig 7–26D).

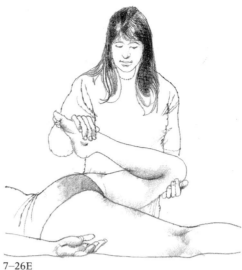

7–26E

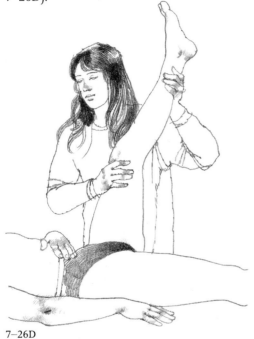

7–26D

With your client lying on her abdomen, raise her calf and rotate it from the knee; move the calf from side to side, or simply bend and straighten the leg. Though these appear to be similar movements to those done when on the back, they engage slightly different muscles and ligaments when lying on the abdomen.

For a nice stretch of the lower anterior thigh muscles, slip one hand under your client's thigh, just above the kneecap, and lift the thigh up with that hand while gently pulling the foot toward the buttock (fig 7–26E). Do

this first with the toes pointed, then with them flexed. Do not do it if it causes any pain in the back.

Holding your client's leg straight, one hand under the front of the thigh and one under the front of the calf, lift the entire leg and rotate it from the hip. Ask your client if this produces any sensation of pain or of stretch. If this sensation is in the thigh, ask the client to breathe deeply into the area while you hold and move the leg, and see whether the sensation lessens or becomes more comfortable. If, however, the sensation is in the knee, the hip or the back, reduce the amount of stretch before you move the leg again, until the position becomes comfortable. While stretching the leg, press along the muscles of the front of the thigh.

Whenever you do passive movement, encourage your client to let go of the limb you are holding. Some people, out of fear of being hurt, will resist your moving their limbs; many more will try to help you by holding the limb up for you, tensing it so that you will not be bearing the full weight. Some people are so unaware of this that they do not realize they are doing it until you take your hands away and leave the limb hanging in midair where they have been obligingly holding it for you. Sometimes simply reminding them to let go will be enough; sometimes getting them to concentrate on breathing, or to visualize a body part far away from the one you are holding, can help.

It is somewhat easier to get a person to let go of a leg than an arm, since a leg is much heavier and harder to keep in the air indefinitely. Passive movement, about five minutes on each leg, is therefore an excellent preliminary relaxation. Then, depending upon what position you have your client in, you can decide where to start on the leg.

Your massage should be a model for the change you want to create. A massage meant to relax should be gentle and soothing; a massage meant to stimulate should be more vigorous and percussive. If you want to loosen a muscle knot, work on the muscles in the direction away from the knot, stroking or palpating from the center of the tightness toward its periphery. If you want to loosen a joint, first move the limb passively, imitating the movement you would like the joint to perform by itself, then work on the muscles around the joint, massaging, again, away from the center of the tightness. In this way you train the client's body to give up the habits which have formed stiffness and pain. If your client has knee problems, begin with gentle rotations and passive stretches, then work gently from the knee area down the calf toward the ankle or up the thigh toward the groin, increasing the intensity of the pressure as you move away from the problem area (if this is comfortable for your client).

7–27   The muscles of the front, back and outer thigh can be pinched and rolled and kneaded between your fingertips and thumb (fig 7–27); pulled upward and shaken; stroked, with a varying degree of pressure, with the knuckles; pounded either lightly or firmly with the fists; and in general worked on more vigorously than many other parts of the body.

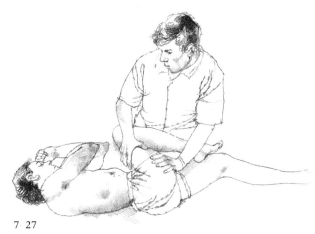

7-27

The inner thigh muscles tend to be more sensitive and may require a lighter touch, using oil and a gentle rotating motion. Placing the whole hand flat on the inner thigh muscles, press down and lightly grasp them with your hand cupped, moving the hand in circles as you do so. Or stroke, again with the whole hand, from the knee upward to the groin. Distributing the pressure in this way helps to avoid undue pressure in any sensitive spot.

Buttocks

Many people are amazed to find how much tension they carry in the buttock muscles. These muscles, principally the gluteus maximus, are among the strongest in the body, and play a major role in keeping us upright when we stand. They thus derive a natural tension from walking or standing, as well as an unnatural tension when we sit too long. Much sciatic pain is a result of uncomfortable prolonged sitting.

7–28 Palpating is an especially good technique here, pressing with both thumb and fingers to find tight or sore points, then working gradually away from those points. Pounding with the fists, especially along the outer part of the hips, also gives a great relief to the muscles. You can also press with both hands at once. This can either be done with one closed fist against the muscle and the other hand pressing down on the fist, moving the fist in rotation, or with flattened palms, one over the other, either stroking with deep, rhythmic strokes or shaking the muscle. At the top of the hip, along the crest of the pelvis, press down toward the leg; at the underside of the buttock, press upward toward the spine. Now tap from both these sides with the bases of your palms (fig 7–28).

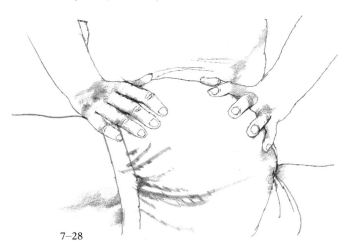

7–28

Often the client will feel most comfortable lying on one side with the upper leg bent slightly and extended forward. This allows the hip and buttock muscles to be slightly stretched while you are working on them.

Back

To work on the back, it is best to have your client lying on the abdomen. However, for many people it is uncomfortable to lie in this position for more than a few minutes. For someone with a serious back problem, it may not be a good idea to lie very long on the abdomen, as it can cause the lower-back muscles, as well as those of the neck, to tighten. Even if your table has a face-rest, a client with a tight neck may find it uncomfortable to lie on the abdomen. For such a person, you may want to begin the massage with the client lying on the back, enjoying massage and passive movement of the neck to loosen it before trying to lie on the abdomen. Be careful not to keep anyone lying on the abdomen for longer than is comfortable.

7–29 When your client is comfortable lying on the abdomen, you might begin the back massage at the lower spine, or sacral area, by placing one hand on one buttock and the other hand on the lumbar area on the other side of the back, then pressing down with each hand to pull the muscles in opposing directions, giving a diagonal stretch to the lower back. Then reverse the hands and do the same in the opposite direction.

It can also be extremely helpful to place the client in the yoga Child's pose, on the knees, with the knees drawn up to the chest and the arms either extended on the table in front (fig

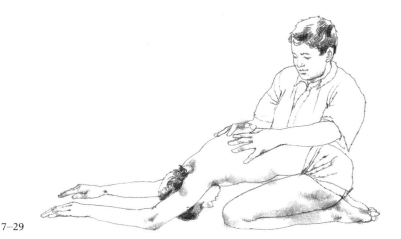

7–29

7–29) or folded so that the forehead is supported by the backs of the hands. Some people may find this more comfortable with a pillow between the calves and the buttocks.

In the Child's pose, the lower back, which in so many people is usually concave, is pulled into a convex position, stretching the muscles as you massage them. Here you can work with long strokes, from the middle of the back (the erector spinalis muscles, which hold the spine erect) to the outer side muscles (the latissimus dorsi), or make circling, pressing motions with the thumb, or place the palms flat and shake the hands on the muscle. As always, experiment to find the touches that feel good and give relief to the client. If this position is uncomfortable, you can have your client lie on the side with the knees pulled up to the chest, or possibly lie on the abdomen with a pillow under the abdomen to elevate the sacral area.

Another favorite massage technique is moving the palms or the bases of the palms in large circles, all the way from the lower back to the upper back. Keep your wrists loose, and move clockwise with your right hand and counterclockwise with your left hand, so that the pressure stretches the muscles sideways, enhancing the sense of expansion.

The back is probably the most frequently massaged area of the body, and massage of the back may seem to provide more benefits to the rest of the body than massage of any other single part. For one thing, it provides a lot of muscle area to work on, and is very user-friendly to the bodyworker, welcoming almost any massage technique. For another, the spinal column houses the spinal cord, which together with the brain contains the central nervous system. When you massage the muscles that hold up the spine, you improve vertebral posture and allow better flow of cerebrospinal fluid – the fluid which lubricates the central nervous system. When the central nervous system works better, everything works better. By causing back muscles to relax and lengthen, back massage may allow for more separation between the thirty-three vertebrae of the spine. This reduces pressure on the nerves that issue from the spinal cord between those vertebrae. Each of these nerves serves a very important function in movement. So you can see that the rewards of back relaxation are far-reaching.

Take a good look at your client's back, both while the client is standing and while lying on the abdomen. Notice the shape, posture and alignment of the vertebrae. A number of common spine problems can be easily recognized. When the upper spine is too convex, this is called kyphosis. This posture changes the position of the head and chest, limits movement in the upper body in particular, and can contribute to cardiovascular problems. When the lower spine is too concave, this is called lordosis* or swayback. This condition can tighten the pelvis and abdominal areas and affect the gait. If the spine does not run in a straight line from neck to coccyx but veers to right or left along the way, this is called scoliosis, or spinal curvature, and can distort posture and interfere with the spinal-cord functioning. If any two vertebrae seem much closer to each other than others do, the disk between them may be compressed, leading to disk degeneration or rupture. We are absolutely not suggesting that you, as a bodyworker, should attempt to diagnose a back condition, either for yourself or for your client – anyone who is experiencing severe back pain of any kind should consult an orthopedic doctor or an osteopath for a clinical diagnosis of the condition – we are only naming a few things to look for when you are deciding how to massage someone's back.

Often, the muscles on one side of the back will be stronger than those on the other, with the result that the strong muscles will pull the spine toward their own side, causing scoliosis. Massage of the back muscles eases the extreme contraction of the strong muscles, as well as bringing more circulation and stimulation to the weaker side, which in time will help to strengthen it: in short, it balances the pull which each side exerts, helping to correct the curvature. This in turn improves posture,

making the carriage of the spine straighter and more even. A person whose spine is being pulled to one side has a lot of problems: uneven pressure on spinal-nerve roots; uneven flow of cerebrospinal fluid (which may be caused by any distortion of spinal posture) and a tremendous amount of unnecessary muscle tension as the body struggles to maintain an upright posture against the pull of the stronger muscles.

7–30   To help create space between the vertebrae, pinch the flesh over each vertebra and pull slightly upward, moving from the sacrum up to the back of the neck. Follow this with long, deep strokes with both palms, then move one palm up while the other moves down, stretching the muscles in opposite directions, and shake the muscles under your hands vigorously. Another good technique is to massage with the thumbs in a rotating motion around each vertebra that you are able to feel individually, especially those which seem sunken or which stand out sharply. Have your client stand up and slowly bend forward in the spinal arch, as described in the Spine chapter (exercise 4–2), while you tap and massage the back from shoulders to sacrum.

7–31   While your client lies on his back, you can relax the spine and increase the client's awareness of it at the same time. Place your fingertips under the neck on both sides of the spine – not on the spine itself – at the base of the skull. Ask your client to press down on the area you are touching, and only on that area, while you palpate gently around the bone (fig 7–31A).

---

*The medical term for this condition is hyperlordosis.

180

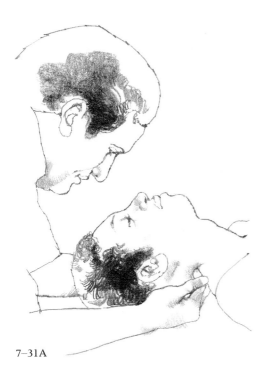

7–31A

Move your fingers to the upper back, and do the same. Repeat this for each area of the back, moving all the way down the spine (fig 7–31B).

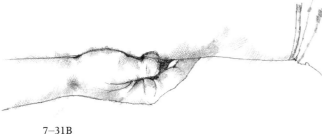

7–31B

Your client will probably not be able to isolate the movement enough so as to press down on only one vertebra, but will become more able to isolate specific areas. Ask the client to pay attention to other areas (chest, jaw and so on) which may try to participate in the movement, and to try to relax them. For some people, just to move the upper back separately from the lower back is a major triumph, used as they are to moving the spine as though it is carved

from a single block. There are Afro-Haitian dancers who can move their spines as sinuously as snakes — this massage technique is aimed toward that type of individual freedom for the vertebrae.

Shoulders

The upper back and shoulders are spanned by a large diamond-shaped muscle called the trapezius. No less than seventeen vertebrae lie below this muscle, which runs vertically from the base of the neck to the middle of the back. Tension in the trapezius can cause pain and limit movement in the neck, shoulders, arms and chest. Most people find massage of this area, especially across the shoulders and next to the shoulder blades, to be pure bliss.

7–32 With your client lying on the side, place one hand in front of the shoulder and the other behind the shoulder blade, then lift and rotate the shoulder, in both directions. Lift the arm, holding it at the wrist, and move it in a large circle. Press the shoulder forward toward the table and tap with your fingertips on the muscles between the spine and the shoulder blade; pull it back toward you and tap on the pectoral muscles where the arm joins the chest (fig 7–32A).

As your client lies on his side with his head supported, have him rotate his upper shoulder several times in both directions. Now hold his shoulder with both hands and rotate it for him in both directions. Ask him to rotate it again by himself. Is it any easier or smoother now?

With your client lying on his abdomen, place one hand under the shoulder and lift the shoulder from the table. Palpate deeply under

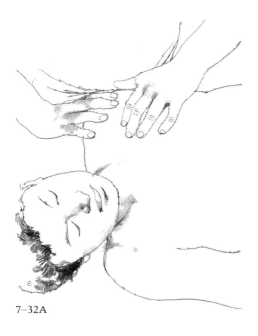

7–32A

the shoulder blade with your other hand. Massage deeply enough to cause slight, but not overwhelming, pain. Now pull the shoulder and the shoulder blade away from the body's midline while putting pressure underneath the blade (fig 7–32B).

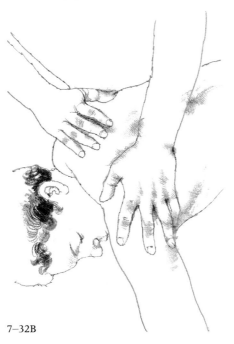

7–32B

Refer also to exercise 1–24 in the Breathing chapter.

Shoulder massage can also be very effective if done while the client is sitting up, as long as the back is completely supported. You might have the client sit on the table, with you sitting or standing behind, and lean against you as you massage. Refer to exercises 3–26, 3–27 and 3–28 in the Joints chapter.

Abdomen

7–33 In addition to the exercises described for self-massage of the abdomen (exercises 7–23), try these.

Stand at the side of your client and use long, circular strokes over the abdomen, with one hand moving clockwise and the other counter-clockwise. Put pressure only upward – toward the upper part of the abdomen. Now cup your hands and massage the abdomen with straight strokes from side to side, your left hand stroking toward you as your right hand strokes away from you. This massage was done on Meir's wife, Dror, when she was pregnant, much to her son's delight. He would begin to kick furiously as soon as the massage stopped, only to quiet down as soon as it resumed. But massage of pregnant women must be done with great care; Dror found it comfortable only when it was done with oil, and very gently. If your client is not pregnant, you may want to try light tapping with cupped hands.

Refer to the Nervous System chapter for neurological massage, which is good for everyone. Refer to the Muscular Dystrophy chapter for massage of dystrophic or atrophied muscles, and to section 18–1 in the Osteoporosis chapter for bone-tapping, which both improves circulation and strengthens bones.

We hope that you can use the ideas presented here for health, enjoyment, relaxation and improved quality of life for you, the people you love and your present or future bodywork clients. We also hope that you will explore this subject further – especially by experiencing bodywork yourself as often as you can.

The Self-Healing method includes many more massage techniques which we did not describe here. However, after a couple of years of working with the other chapters and bringing more movement to your body, massage techniques will come naturally to your hands and your mind as the need arises, because of your developed kinesthetic sense and sensitivity to others.

CHAPTER 8

Vision

Increase acuity through relaxation

Meir Schneider: A Case History

I was born blind, due to a complication of cataracts (opaqueness of the lens) and glaucoma (excess pressure in the eye). Almost immediately after birth I developed the secondary symptoms of cross-eye and nystagmus (involuntary eye movements). When I was four years old I had my first operation for removal of the cataracts, in Poland. By the time I was seven I had had a total of five operations in Poland and in Israel, but all of them proved unsuccessful. They had succeeded in removing most of the cataracts, but had left more than 95 percent of my lenses covered with scar tissue which was too thick for light to penetrate. Every doctor who examined my eyes believed that this scar tissue made vision impossible. I could see only light, shadow and some indistinct shapes. Strong light was extremely painful to my eyes.

I was declared legally blind by the state of Israel, where my family had settled, and began to study in Braille as soon as I started school. Although I was given glasses which were supposed to improve my vision a little, the truth was that they focused light on my weak eyes in such a painful way that the glasses

were worse than useless. I would try to break them at every possible opportunity, usually by throwing them on the floor and stamping on them. The frames would break, but the lenses were so thick that nothing could shatter them.

The operations I had undergone at such an early age, and the everyday traumas of being blind, left me a legacy of pain, frustration, anger and fear. These feelings, along with the more obvious physical reasons for my blindness, played an important part in restricting my vision.

Functionally blind and reading only in Braille, I nevertheless attended grammar school along with all the other kids, competing not only scholastically but in sports and games with full-sighted children. I never ceased to be frustrated by my limitations. When I entered high school and the scholastic demands got tougher, the strain of reading Braille grew greater, and many of the textbooks I needed were unavailable in Braille. I dreamed of finding some miracle surgery which would instantly correct my problems and give me a normal life. Until I was seventeen, however, the only advancement I experienced was being fitted with two new lenses. One of them had the strength of a small telescope and enabled me to read the blackboard, with one eye, from the front row of the class. The other was a monocle of microscope strength, with which I was able to read one letter at a time if I pressed my nose against the page of a book. Using either of these lenses gave me terrible eyestrain and headaches; nevertheless, I never used Braille again.

When I was nearly seventeen, I met two people who changed the course of my life. The first was an old woman, a librarian, who had become interested in health due to various physical problems of her own, and had spent much of her life independently studying movement and its effects on the body. She took a special interest in me because of my eyes, and because she sensed in me an openness to change. With her help and guidance, I began to sense the connection between my eyes and the rest of my body, and how each part affected the other. I learned how the strain in my eyes had contributed to tension in my neck, shoulders, back, stomach and other parts of my body, and how this chronic body tension in turn affected my eyes for the worse.

This woman introduced me to the second of my teachers, a boy even younger than myself. She knew that he had improved his own vision, which had been rapidly deteriorating, by practicing some vision exercises he had learned from a book. These were the exercises that Dr William Bates developed around the turn of the century, and this teenager taught me the rudiments of them. I practiced them faithfully at every possible opportunity. Though everyone around me was skeptical of these exercises, it never occurred to me to doubt or to question their value. Within several months I could see – not much, but more than I had ever seen before.

The process of gaining sight was a gradual one. The first change I noticed was simply that the contrast between light and darkness became clearer; light became brighter and shadow darker. Then the vague forms I had become accustomed to seeing began to evolve into sharper images, and then I began to notice more and clearer details within these images. Most important in preparing my eyes for sight was learning to relax my eyes, which had been constantly straining to see, and training them to accept light rather than to flinch away from it.

Within six months, I was able to read printed letters with lenses of twenty diopters. Within a year and a half, I was reading print with no glasses at all. Through my vision exercises, I had created functional vision where none had existed.

The transition from blindness to some vision was difficult. Throughout my life I had been accustomed *not* to look at things, depending on other senses and other people for the information I needed about the world around me. Seeing meant developing a whole new set of habits and skills, not simply doing exercises. I was delighted with the beauty of what I saw – and just about everything looked beautiful to me – but I was also overwhelmed by the incredible diversity of visual images. At times I almost wished I was blind again, so great was the task of seeing, and of identifying and interacting with what I saw. I was as new to seeing as an infant, and indeed I feel that in many ways my life really began when I gained my vision.

I learned much about myself through the process of working on my eyes, and not only about my physical self but my emotional being as well. I learned how deeply the eyes are affected by emotions, and by mental preconceptions too. To quote Dr Bates, the ophthalmologist whose vision exercises inspired my vision-improvement method, 'We see largely with the mind and only partially with the eyes.'

I have never stopped working to improve my vision, and it has never ceased to improve. In 1981, ten years after the whole process began, I was granted an unrestricted driver's license by the State of California. My vision is still far from perfect – it is measured at about 20/70 at its best; in other words, from twenty feet I can see what a person whose vision is 20/20 can see at seventy feet – but no one can deny that the change in it has been phenomenal.

Why should this story be considered extra-ordinary?

The real answer to this question is that we have all been trained to believe that our eyes – unlike most other parts of the body – can only change for the worse, and can never improve once they have begun to deteriorate. It is easy to think this way, because in fact the majority of people with vision problems just do tend to get worse. This, however, is only because they don't know anything about how to improve their vision.

No one can be blamed for this. Improving vision is a complex process, because vision itself is a complex process. Our eyes – and thus our visual abilities – are linked inextricably with our bodies, our minds and our emotions. Our eyes act upon every aspect of ourselves, and are in turn affected by every aspect of our lives; working with the eyes to improve vision is therefore always a challenge. In the process you may come up against deeply held physical tensions, mental resistance, emotional blocks and traumas. In facing these things, however, many people have found the strength to over-

come them, and through improving their vision have changed their lives.

By means of simple vision exercises and the development of good visual habits, it is possible to change poor vision to good vision, reverse the process of deterioration in the eyes, and completely reverse the effects of stress, overuse and other factors which contribute to poor eyesight.

Self-Healing vision improvement offers an alternative to glasses. While corrective lenses seem to offer a quick and easy 'solution', the truth is that they do not correct the cause of the eye problem for which they are prescribed. In fact, the constant use of glasses often contributes to the deterioration of vision, by forcing the eyes to function in ways which ultimately weaken them. This is why progressively stronger prescriptions become necessary over the years. Our vision-improvement exercises, by contrast, address vision problems at their source. If practiced regularly, they will not only improve your measurable vision but will make your eyes stronger and healthier.

Vision exercises have been known, in various forms, for thousands of years. The ancient societies of China, India and Tibet, for example, have included vision exercises as a regular part of their medical practice, as have various Native American cultures. It is worth noting that all of the societies mentioned have traditionally based their approach to medicine on natural healing, placing great emphasis on healthy diet; proper use of and care for the body; a balance of work, rest and exercise; and a healthy state of mind, which de-emphasizes the use of drugs and medicines.

Vision exercises are relatively new to Western society, however. The invention of artificial lenses to correct vision gave a completely different direction to the study of vision and the eyes. Research in the eighteenth and nineteenth centuries seemed to point to the conclusion that vision problems could only be corrected in one of two ways: by the use of artificial lenses or, in some cases, by surgery. The idea that vision problems could never be fundamentally cured, only artificially alleviated, gained acceptance throughout Western countries.

In the twentieth century, however, this assumption was challenged by a brilliant American ophthalmologist named William H. Bates. Dr Bates graduated from Cornell University's College of Physicians and Surgeons in 1885, and practiced in New York City. Through his extensive research into the functioning of the eyes, he developed a revolutionary approach to the improvement of vision. Dr Bates used an instrument called the retinoscope, with which he could observe minute changes in the surface curvature of the eyes and thus determine the nature and degree of a patient's vision problems. With this, he observed how eyes behave – that is, how their shape changes – when they are seeing well, and how they behave when they see poorly. Over many years, he observed the eyes of hundreds of his patients in every variety of activity, emotional state and physical condition. He noted how their eyes changed when they were doing work they enjoyed or work they disliked; in situations of fatigue, anxiety or confusion; when they were concentrated, excited, stimulated or relaxed.

Dr Bates observed how the clarity of vision changes, in the same person, from good to bad and back again, depending upon that person's physical and emotional state. He observed the simple fact that vision is not a static condition but one which changes constantly; you have

probably noticed that your own vision is better at some times, worse at others. Dr Bates was the first ophthalmologist to make a scientific study of this phenomenon. His studies show how vision defects can be created and/or worsened by the stress of daily-life situations. He also proved that these problems can be corrected by conscious and correct visual behavior.

Causes of Poor Vision

Vision problems usually relate to a lack of clarity in either near or distant vision. The physical act of seeing things close up is different from the act of seeing things in the distance. Let's think of a camera first. When light rays from the object you are trying to focus on reach the camera's lens, they need to converge so that they are focused on the film behind the lens. In order to focus, you change the distance between the lens and the film until it is just right – otherwise the object will not focus exactly on the film and the photo will be a blur. Now let's return to your eye. Like a camera, your eye needs to converge the light rays arriving from the object you are looking at, and focus them behind the lens. Rather than a film you have a retina, which is a network of nerve cells which translates the light rays into neural information to be sent through the optic nerve to the brain. The eye has a special capability that no camera has: it can change the shape of its lens. Therefore, it can focus without changing the distance between the lens and the retina. When the ciliary muscles which hold the lens in place are relaxed, the lens is relatively flat and allows for distant vision. When the object you are looking at is closer than twenty feet away, those muscles contract, and the lens assumes a more spherical shape. This process is called accommodation.

For several centuries, ophthalmologists and other authorities on the function and anatomy of the eyes have believed the eye can focus only through the process of accommodation. For a variety of reasons, however, Dr Bates came to believe that no less important than the ciliary muscles are the large, external muscles of the eyeball, which can allow focusing in a manner similar to that of the camera — by changing the length of the eyeball, and with it the distance between the lens and the retina.

There is a very important difference between the two mechanisms, because, while the action of the ciliary muscles is involuntary, the action of the external muscles can be more easily controlled. If the ciliary muscles could not produce the desired accommodation, Dr Bates believed, the external muscles could compensate. This is the truly revolutionary idea that Dr Bates introduced to Western ophthalmology — the idea that vision can be controlled, can in fact be greatly improved through conscious control of visual behavior.

Besides the factor of accommodation, the shape of the eyeball is assumed to determine how a person sees. Irregular shape of the eyeball is considered to be the cause of the two most common vision problems: myopia and hyperopia. Myopia, which is also called nearsightedness, means the inability to see distant objects clearly. Myopia results from an eyeball which is too long from front to back, making it impossible for the lens to focus the light rays from distant objects onto the retina, though it can focus the rays from close objects. Hyperopia, or hypermetropia, is also called farsightedness, and means the inability to see close objects clearly. In hyperopia, the eyeball is too short from front to back. Light rays from a distance focus correctly upon the retina, but rays from close objects are projected on the retina unfocused — they would focus *behind* the retina if they were capable of passing through it.

Dr Bates agreed completely that the shape of the eyeball is responsible for myopia and hyperopia. What he challenged was the idea that the eyeball, once having assumed a particular shape, could never change that shape. Since the vast majority of vision problems are acquired, and can be acquired at any time, the shape of the eyeball clearly can and does undergo change. Why should we assume that these changes can only be for the worse? For example, if a child born with normal sight becomes myopic, this indicates that the eyeballs have lengthened. Why should they not also be able to shorten again?

What really causes poor vision? We now have some idea of the physical, or mechanical, changes that occur in the eye when vision is bad. But what causes these physical changes to occur? The answer that Dr Bates came up with is a very familiar one to us, though in his time it was a completely new idea. In one word, the answer is stress. The eyes are as susceptible to stress as any other part of the body, and are subjected to at least as much stress. Not all of this stress is purely physical. Many of our actions and our reactions are guided by mental pictures, and much of our memory consists of mental images, including conscious and subconscious images of events which shaped our emotional makeup, and the eyes are stressed even when we are perceiving these only 'in the mind's eye'. The eye is an integral part of the brain. Because of all this, and also because we use them for just about everything we do, the eyes respond strongly to our thoughts and our emotions. Because they are such hardworking organs, they also are immediately affected by physical pain or fatigue. When we begin to work to improve our eyes, we need to approach this work from every possible angle. And in the process of doing so, we discover things about ourselves that we may never have suspected.

The Eyes and the Emotions

There has been a lot of speculation about the connection between vision and personality and between vision and past events with emotional consequences. Almost all of our clients who are working on their vision have experienced strong emotions, and sometimes powerful emotional insights, while doing so. The connections which individuals draw between their particular experience and their particular vision problems vary tremendously from person to person. This makes it difficult to generalize about *how* emotion affects vision. What can never be questioned by an honest observer is that emotion *does* affect vision, and strongly. When a person experiences strong negative emotion – whether it is fear, rage, anxiety or grief – the vision is nearly always temporarily worsened, even in people with good vision. If the experience is repeated often enough, the results may become permanent.

One way to understand how emotions work on the eyes is to look at the times in life when visual deterioration is most common, and ask what happens at those times. The first is around the age of eight, a time when children with perfectly normal sight will very often

suddenly and mysteriously develop myopia. When Maureen mentioned this fact to a schoolteacher friend of hers, the friend said, 'I'm not surprised. That's third grade. That's when they find out that all that stuff they got in second grade is exactly what they're going to get in third grade, only more and harder. In second grade everything is new and exciting, especially learning to read; they're really making major changes and accomplishments. Then they get to third grade and there it is again, all the same old junk – and you know kids get bored pretty fast. And they realize this is it: this is all school is ever going to be. Third grade is when you get the real behavior problems starting too.'

Granted, this is just one teacher's view of the situation, though as a teacher of grades one to four she is in a good position to observe behavior and attitude changes in children. However, most people could agree that the classroom is an ideal environment for the development of visual difficulties. Children are made to work indoors, often under artificial light, usually focusing for long periods on close work which does not encourage the use of their distance vision. The typical image of the bookworm with glasses is correct, but the books usually come before the glasses. If the eyes are used only for close work, the capacity for distance vision will tend to atrophy.

The two most common emotions found in the typical classroom are frustration and boredom. There can be no doubt that children suffer much anxiety about their performance in school. If they are good scholars, they are anxious to maintain their high standing and are often in fierce competition with the other 'brains' in the class. If they are poor scholars, they suffer constant humiliation and frustration – even anger. All of these emotions are experienced in the context of doing their schoolwork, which invariably requires much demanding use of the eyes. And for the student who has already mastered the lesson, as well as for the one who finds it too difficult and has given up, there is plenty of opportunity to stare blankly into space, bored to tears. Even if a teacher has conscientiously provided the classroom with a lot of visual interest, it gets memorized very quickly and the bored child's eyes lose their curiosity and their desire to look. This unfocused glassy-eyed stare can also contribute to the development of myopia, as we will discuss later in the section on 'shifting', or macular vision.

The next most common time to develop visual problems is in adolescence. In these instances one could make a case for pure emotional trauma being at the root of the problem. It is also very common to lose clear vision in the late teens and early twenties, during the stress of college and first employment. At this time, the myopia may be a mirror of the unclearness of the future toward which one is working so hard. Next comes early middle age, when many people who have enjoyed perfect vision all of their lives suddenly begin to develop presbyopia, or 'middle-age farsightedness'. The physiological factors which contribute to presbyopia are common but not at all inevitable, and can be reversed. Many doctors say, and almost everyone believes, that presbyopia is an unavoidable result of aging, but this is simply not the case, as is evidenced by the fact that many people develop the condition only in one eye.

Some of the psychological explanations our clients have found to explain their own visual problems might seem more metaphorical than scientific, but the same themes come up so often that it is worthwhile to explore them.

One is the problem of being forced to use the eyes for something they do not want to do. We have already mentioned schoolwork; sadly, for many people school is just the beginning of a lifetime of work they do not enjoy and may find really unpleasant. Some people feel that their eyes react to this by simply refusing to see clearly that which they would rather avoid. One of our clients said that her vision suffered a sharp and sudden loss when she moved from a beautiful countryside to an ugly industrial town: 'I think I just couldn't stand to look at the place.' Her vision has since returned to normal, with the help of a lot of visualization.

During times of emotional stress, two things happen which can affect vision. One is that we tend to look inward – that is, to focus more on our inner life experiences and less on the world around us. Though this is an emotional state, it affects the way we use our eyes. How many times have you come out of a deep concentration to realize that for some time you have been seeing nothing at all, even though your eyes have been open? As we have said before, this blank stare is one of the factors that help myopia to develop. It may also happen that in times of great distress we may be so unhappy with our surroundings that we may wish not to see them. At such times the eyes are used only as much as is absolutely necessary, and the tendency to look with interest at specific visual data may be lost. In other words, non-acceptance of ourselves or our lives may play a large part in vision impairment. Of course, there are many people with self-acceptance problems who can see just fine; these people will manifest their difficulties in some other way. Stress normally will leave its mark in the places where we are already most vulnerable.

The Eyes and the Mind

The British writer Aldous Huxley was a successful student and enthusiastic admirer of Dr Bates's method. After using Dr Bates's exercises to recover from a condition of near-blindness, Huxley wrote a book called *The Art of Seeing*, in which he describes seeing as a three-step process involving the eyes, the brain and the mind. He explained that seeing consists of:
Sensing: the light-sensitive cells of the eyes receive information about their environment via light rays – approximately 1 billion bits of visual data at any given second.
Selecting: the mind will not be able to deal with all of the visual data which is conveyed to the eyes, so it directs the eyes in choosing certain data to pay attention to.
Perceiving: the selected visual data are recognized and interpreted by the mind.

To improve our vision, we need to recognize that vision is a complex interaction between the eyes and the mind. We also need to learn how to make the mind work for us, rather than against us. One of the biggest obstacles we need to overcome is the belief that the eyes can never improve. This belief can keep us from recognizing or accepting it when we do have improvement, or convince us that in certain situations we simply will not be able to see and therefore should not try. (For example, Maureen assumed for her whole life that she could not thread a needle, until the day when utter desperation – no one around to do it for her – drove her to try, and succeed.)

Sometimes our vision may worsen when we expect it to, in situations where we feel our eyes are being challenged. Dr Bates describes a situation in which he had two of his patients, one with 20/20 vision and one with 20/400,

look at a blank wall. During this experiment, he monitored changes in the surface curvature of their eyes with his retinoscope. As long as both patients looked at the blank wall, their eyes remained the same. As soon as he placed an eye chart on the wall, the eyes of the person who saw 20/400 changed radically, with all the surrounding muscles contracting sharply. The eyes of the person who saw 20/20 showed only a slight, barely noticeable, change. The first one had immediately and unconsciously brought his habits of straining into his effort to see the chart.

One of our students, newly fitted with contact lenses, forgot to put them in one day. He went out, drove, shopped, read and performed all of his normal activities. Not only did he experience no difficulty in seeing, he remembers noticing especially how clear and strong his vision was on that day. Then he came home and found his lenses in the bathroom – and immediately his vision became blurry! Suddenly he had remembered that his eyes were bad, that they had to work hard, to stare and strain, in order to see anything. And as soon as his eyes began to function with that sense of strain, they lost their capacity to see details and created a blur. Anxiety about seeing can create functional 'blindness'.

The process of seeing has a lot to do with trusting that you can see and relaxing. In the early stages of Maureen's own vision improvement, she gave an eye-therapy session to a client, Charlotte, who was trying to dispense with her glasses. She asked Charlotte to take the glasses off and come out in the street with her, but Charlotte hesitated at the door. 'I don't want to go out there,' she said. 'I can't see a thing. I'm afraid I'll break my neck at the first step.' After Maureen questioned her in detail about what exactly she could see outside – from the doorway – it became apparent that she could see at least twice as well as Maureen could, if she paid attention to what she was seeing. With half Charlotte's vision, Maureen had traveled alone in Europe and the Middle East, yet Charlotte was afraid to step out the door without glasses. This is functional blindness, which has little to do with measurable vision and much to do with self-set boundaries.

To improve vision, you need to change the way you think about seeing, as well as the way you go about seeing. This is a large undertaking. Vision habits and patterns of use are among the hardest to change: we are more attached to the way we see than to almost anything else we do. Perhaps this is because our memory consists so much of visual information – once we have seen something in a certain way, we remember it that way and continue to see it as we remember it. Our dependence on sight is enormous, especially in people who see well. When these people lose their good vision, it can be really traumatic, changing their conception of themselves. In reality, these people have great resources to help them restore their vision, namely their memories of clear, sharp visual images.

Memory and imagination are the mind's most valuable tools for improving vision, and we use them in many of the vision exercises we will describe. Anything we have ever seen clearly can be used to stimulate clearer vision. We all know that it is easier to see things which are known and familiar. For example, an unfamiliar word, though it is made up of the same letters as other words, will initially be much harder to decipher than a familiar one. A thing, place or person that we already know will tend to emerge in clear focus even from the blurriest visual picture. We use visualization exercises to take advantage of the mind's tendency to associate clear vision with that which is known and familiar. We also use visualization, or imagination, to create optimal conditions. Imagining total blackness, for example, can cause the optic nerve to react as though it were in fact seeing total blackness – that is, to stop working and rest for a change.

The mind, like any other powerful force of nature, can either help or harm. It can keep us from believing that our vision can improve, or it can supply us with everything we need to improve it.

The Eyes and the Body

Throughout this chapter (and this book) we are operating under the assumption that the eyes are a part of the body. This might not seem like such a revolutionary idea, but it is one which conventional ophthalmology seems to ignore. It is true that the eyes are a very special part of the body, composed in part of tissue identical to brain tissue and very closely linked to the brain in many functions. Nevertheless, the eyes are connected with the rest of the body by way of blood vessels, nerves and muscles. They simultaneously affect the rest of the body and are affected by it.

Vision problems are very frequently accompanied by specific patterns of muscle tension and weakness. As with other types of physical problems, it is very difficult to say with accuracy, 'This tension created that problem' or 'That problem may have caused this tension.' This tends to get one involved in an unsolvable, chicken-or-egg type of discussion. Does a person have a tight neck because of myopia, or vice versa? It is not always possible to say. We have seen, however, that the two things always go together. Without even looking at the body of a nearsighted person, one can predict confidently that he or she will have pronounced tension in the forehead, jaw, neck, shoulders, upper arms and lower back, and often the calves as well. Relaxing these areas will often produce an immediate improvement in vision, and doing vision exercises will often help these areas to relax. We have found that a combination of vision exercises, bodywork and body-relaxation exercises is far more effective than simply doing vision exercises alone.

To understand the eye–body relationship, we need to experience it kinesthetically. What does seeing feel like? Most of the time we are not aware of it; we feel the effects of seeing only after the fact, in the form of eyestrain, eye fatigue, neck tension and other related problems. It is possible, however, to learn to feel immediately when we strain our eyes or the muscles surrounding them, and to stop ourselves from doing so.

A good place to begin is with the muscles closest to the eyes and most directly affected by seeing – the facial muscles. For many years we have been teaching our vision-improvement students to massage their faces, with particular attention to several specific places which seem to have an especially good effect on vision. We have just recently discovered that these are the same points used by the Chinese in acupressure massage – for the same purpose. We are not sure whether this validates their method or ours – probably both. In any case, we highly recommend facial massage, particularly as a preparation for palming, which is the first basic eye exercise we will describe in the next section. One of the most important functions of palming is, in fact, relaxation of the muscles around the eyes.

8–1 Massage of the whole face influences the circulation around the eyes. Rub your hands together until they are warm, and then massage your face with your fingertips, gently at first, and then more firmly as your muscles also begin to warm up. The pressure at first should be just firm enough to let you feel whether a spot is tense or painful, but not hard enough to make pain worse. Spend at least a couple of minutes on each separate area, noticing how your touch feels and what effect it has. You may feel a deep tension or pain, a superficial tightness, a pleasant sense of release, or numbness, which is also a sensation.

Begin with the jaw. Massage the whole area from the point of the chin outward along the jawbone, in front of and behind the ears. You can open and close your jaws while doing this, to help stretch and relax the strong jaw muscles. This may make you feel like yawning, so yawn as much as you want – it is very relaxing for your face.

Now work up from the bridge of the nose outward along the cheekbones toward the temples (fig 8–1A). From the bridge of the nose,

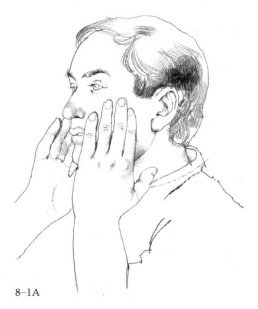

8–1A

work out along the eyebrows, massaging above, below and directly on the brow (fig 8–1B). Spend a little extra time on the point between the eyebrows; this area gathers a lot of tension from the act of seeing. Then massage in long firm strokes across the forehead and, very gently, with small circular motions, in the temple area. Stroke lightly from the temples up into your scalp, imagining that you are drawing tension away from your eyes.

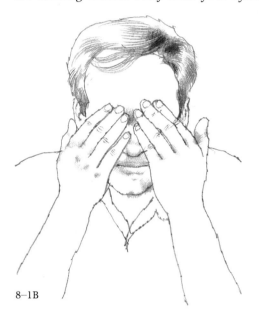

8–1B

After ten minutes or so of massage, your face will be glowing and tingling from the increased blood flow. Now you can try some eye-movement exercises. Besides increasing your kinesthetic sense of your eyes, these exercises strengthen the tissues around the eyes.

8–2   Move both eyes simultaneously in small circles. If you need to, you can hold up a finger before your eyes and move it in a circle, allowing the eye to follow it, but first see if you can move the eyes in rotation without this aid. Touch your forehead above the eyes with your fingertips.

Can you feel the muscles moving? They don't need to. Try to relax them, and practice this exercise until you can do it without working the forehead muscles. You may simply need to make your circles smaller; in fact, see how small you can make them.

Close your eyes and visualize them moving in circles, freely, with no effort. It may help to picture a wheel rolling, or a record on a turntable, or something else that turns smoothly and easily. With your eyes open, rotate them again, and this time imagine that only the pupils are rotating.

Now close your eyes and move them in rotation under the closed lids. This may be more difficult, since the movement is so much more limited. Touch your eyeballs lightly as you do this, to feel the movement. Notice whether you tense the rest of your face during this motion; if you do, try not to. You will find it much easier to do this exercise with your eyes open after this.

Eyestrain and upper-body tension are closely related. Strenuous use of the eyes can set up patterns of tension in the neck, shoulders, arms and other areas. Conversely, muscular tension in these areas can adversely affect the eyes by decreasing circulation to the head, causing a sense of exhaustion in both the eyes and the mind. Anyone whose job involves sitting at a desk, bent over their work, experiences this type of tension and exhaustion as a regular part of the job. The position in which most of us spend from six to eight hours of every workday is designed perfectly to create strain in the back and neck, and tension in the shoulders and arms.

However, reducing upper-body tension is both easy and pleasant to do. The following exercises are used by almost all of our vision-improvement students as a part of a holistic, total-body approach to healing the eyes. These exercises are best done during a break in one's working day. One of the reasons people become so fatigued at work is the tendency to work without stopping for anything but food, coffee or a cigarette. We become so engrossed in our work that we can completely ignore our physical discomfort – until we get home. People often feel pressured to work straight through because of a deadline or a backlog of work. The irony of this is that when we do take a few minutes for a break to rest, stretch, relax – a genuine 'breathing space' – we find ourselves able to accomplish more than we can when we are perpetually driven to exhaustion.

Some employers are recognizing this, and providing their workers with a place to rest, even to lie down, for a few minutes every so often. Even when Maureen worked at a cannery, the workers were given five minutes every hour to go outside on the dock, and she would use the time for sunning (see exercise 8–6) or for shoulder rotations or spine stretches. No one thought this was strange; everyone knew that the work made them stiff and uncomfortable. There is more awareness nowadays that the same can be true of sedentary jobs – particularly if they involve computers. There is a whole science, called ergonomics, which is devoted to designing workspaces which won't cripple the workers. Those of us who work at home, however, as well as those of us who do not have enlightened employers, have to look out for our own physical welfare during work.

It is preferable if you can lie down to do the next exercises – your body relaxes much more when it's not opposing the pull of gravity. Otherwise, you can do them sitting or standing.

8–3   Close your eyes and let your face go slack, especially around the jaw; the jaw area tends to tense automatically whenever you are in deep concentration. Turn your head to the side and feel gently with your fingertips along the side of your neck. The sternocleidomastoid muscle runs from behind your ear down along the side of the neck and into the shoulder and bears much of the burden for supporting the head. It can become tighter than just about any other muscle in the body, so give it a lot of special attention, since relaxing its tension is vital to the health of the eyes. Massage all along the length of this muscle, trying to follow the path of tension. (Some people have been known to mistake this muscle for a bone when touching it.) Palpate, tap and stroke it, gently at first and then more firmly as it begins to soften a little. You will probably find several very sore or tight spots. Don't dig at them, because they are probably so sore that they will only resist a deep massage. Instead, work gently on them and more firmly around them. Now turn your head from side to side, and see whether you notice a difference between the two sides. Note this difference, and then massage the second side.

8–4   When you have released some of the tension in your neck muscles in this way, you are ready to do some head rotations. It is important to relax the neck first, as doing head rotations with a tight neck can make you dizzy or nauseous. Rotate your head slowly, making relatively small circles. Most people will at first want to make huge sweeping circles, trying to shake out the tension they feel in their neck and shoulders. The problem with this is that your body, when it feels that tension, interprets the movement as strenuous and resists it, refusing to relax. So begin with small circles.

Touch the highest vertebra you can reach, where your skull and neck are joined, and imagine this as the center of the circle your head is making. This gentle motion not only relaxes your neck muscles but also releases tension in your spinal joints, making movement of the neck more easy and fluid. If you are doing this movement lying down, remember that you do not have to lift your head to make a full rotation; just imagine that you are drawing a circle with your chin or your nose, and that will give you the correct motion. Make at least 100 of these slow, small rotations, and don't forget to change direction from clockwise to counterclockwise after every ten or fifteen circles.

Shoulder rotations are wonderful for releasing shoulder and upper-back tension, since they work directly on the shoulder muscles. If you have ever had these muscles massaged, you know how tight they can get. Refer to exercise 3–16 in the Joints chapter.

You can follow these exercises with the spinal arch, exercise 4–2 in the Spine chapter, and with any of the exercises described in the chapter on Breathing. When you feel somewhat relaxed and refreshed, you are ready to go back to work, and you will almost certainly find yourself less troubled with eyestrain and fatigue at the end of your workday.

We also recommend that you do some of the exercises in this section to prepare yourself for a session of vision exercises. Working on your vision demands a high level of awareness, and it will be enormously helpful to you if you begin your vision work in a state of attunement with your body.

Basic Vision Exercises

These exercises are for everyone. If your vision is poor but your eye has not been pathologically damaged, there is no limit to how much you can improve it. If you have a pathological condition, you can see much better than you do now. If your vision is good, you should do everything you can to maintain it, and also realize that you too can improve your vision! 'Twenty/twenty' is an arbitrary measurement, used to describe what was considered normal vision when this measurement was established. It is not a definition of the best vision possible. The vision of some individuals has been measured at 20/4, which means that they could see an object placed twenty feet away as sharply as someone with 20/20 vision would see it from only four feet away. If you are enjoying good vision now, you may want to see whether you can double your acuity. In fact, it's often true that the better your vision is, the more easily you can improve it.

Like the rest of the body, the eyes have specific needs, and the reason these exercises work is because they are designed to fulfill these needs. Not many of us are living under conditions which are ideal for maintaining the health of the eyes; in fact for most of us the opposite is true – from childhood on, we are engaged in activities which are simply and purely detrimental to the eyes. This is why it is so easy to believe the eyes can deteriorate but cannot improve: we do plenty of things to hurt our eyes, nothing at all to help them, and the results are fairly predictable. This is why it is so easy to make people believe that glasses are the only solution to deteriorating vision.

Like the rest of the body, the eyes function

well under good conditions and poorly under bad ones. We are becoming increasingly aware of how to use good nutrition, exercise and rest to care for our bodies; we also need to learn to care for the particular needs of our eyes. We can speculate that the vision-exercise systems of ancient cultures, like all modern vision exercises since the time of Dr Bates, grew out of acute observation of what conditions are good for the eyes and of how the eyes function during both favorable and unfavorable conditions. What do we do to make the eyes feel and function well, and what do we do that makes them deteriorate? These are the important questions. The answers would be obvious if we had not been taught to assume that our eyes could only go in one direction – downhill.

We will now look in turn at some of the things your eyes need, and appreciate, and probably aren't getting enough of.

Rest

The eye is one of the hardest-working organs in the body, and people who use their eyes a lot become fatigued more rapidly than others. This partially explains why a typist can be as exhausted as a lumberjack at the end of a workday. We use our eyes every minute that we are awake, say about seventeen hours daily. Think about how your muscles would feel if you used them without stopping for every waking moment. And if you work, as so many of us do, at a job which requires constant and strenuous use of your eyes, then consider how your body would feel if you forced it to walk all day, every day, under the weight of a heavy burden. This is the kind of pressure we put on our eyes.

Many of our clients ask, 'Well, what about sleep – isn't seven or eight hours of rest enough for the eyes?' The fact is that during much of our sleep time our eyes are not resting enough. During dreams, the optic nerve is stimulated and the eyes are in motion under the closed eyelids; for this reason, dream sleep is known as rapid-eye-movement or REM sleep. And it has been clearly established that all humans spend several hours a night in REM sleep, whether they remember their dreams the next morning or not. In addition, many people do not relax during their sleep but maintain their tensions, particularly in the upper body and face.

What we should aim for is that improvement of vision should be achieved equally through use and through rest – both states should be equally beneficial to the eyes. Ultimately, everything we do with our eyes should be good for them. Dr Bates was often asked, 'Why should we bother to work on our eyes?' His answer was that we are always 'working on' our eyes, either for them or against them, in everything we do. And one of the most important things we can do for them is simply to counteract that abuse to which we subject them. Dr Bates warned against this more than seventy years ago, long before television, computers and video games came along to make things that much worse for our eyes. The saddest thing is how few people really understand what can hurt their eyes. For example, 'experts' are still claiming – though not so loudly as they did several years ago – that working at computer terminals produces no 'proven' damage to the eyes, while computer workers become the mainstay of the optometrists!

While practicing vision exercises, we suggest that you do not use glasses or contact lenses.

8–5 Palming the Eyes for a Total Rest The exercise of palming is one of the best ways we know to rest the eyes. Everyone will occasionally cover their eyes with their hands to give them a brief rest; in body language, it is a sign as clear as yawning that the person is tired, and perhaps a bit overwhelmed. What not everyone realizes is that the benefits of covering the eyes with the hands go far beyond a momentary rest. The benefits multiply geometrically, so that ten minutes of rest for the eyes is much more than ten times as good as one minute.

Palming is so simple and natural that many people have a hard time understanding how it can do so much good. But it is recognized as an important exercise in yoga, in Tibetan Kum Nye exercise, and in Chinese eye exercise. Eye exercise in China, by the way, is as common a fact of life as reading. Schoolchildren do it before studying, and office workers do it routinely at work.

Palming serves two important functions. First, it completely rests the optic nerve, when done properly. By shutting out all light, we can keep the optic nerve from being stimulated by outside images, and by directing our minds to imagine only blackness we keep mental stimulation of the optic nerve to a minimum. When we sleep, we have no control over the optic nerve, but while awake we can control to a certain extent what the mind's eye sees. (This is a little more difficult for people who have a tendency to think visually.) Through relaxing the optic nerve, palming affects the rest of the nervous system and relaxes it too.

Second, palming relieves the rigidity of the eye muscles which plays such a large part in restricting vision. Relaxation can have the same 'domino effect' that tension does, in that, if you succeed in relaxing a few muscles, the muscles around them may decide to relax too, so that the relaxation spreads out in concentric rings. For this reason we often recommend palming for people who have no noticeable vision problems but who need a general release from tension. Relaxing the eyes can do wonders for the whole body. This relaxation also has an important psychological effect: it teaches the brain that the eyes do not always have to strain, that they can function better and more comfortably through relaxation than through stress.

Palming can be practiced anywhere, but we recommend doing it in a dark room. The first essential is to find a position comfortable enough to remain in for twenty minutes or more. Every part of the body should be relaxed and supported. You will be covering your eyes with the palms of your hands; it is important that you neither lean forward onto the hands, which puts too much pressure on the delicate tissues around the eyes, nor hold your arms up, as this will quickly tire the arms and shoulders. Tilting the head too far backward will cut off circulation to the head. Your arms, therefore, should be completely supported at just the right height to cover your eyes without pressing on them. Part of your eye-exercise equipment will probably be a collection of pillows to use during palming. You can try sitting at a table with pillows propping your arms, or lying on your back, knees bent, with pillows on your chest to support the arms, or sitting on the floor with your back against the wall, knees drawn up to your chest and pillows piled in your lap. The actual position does not matter, as long as you can find one that works for you. You will need to experiment and use your imagination, but eventually you will find the right position.

When you are settled in your niche, first

rub your hands together vigorously to make them warm. If they don't warm up quickly, don't worry – it is truly amazing how quickly palming itself will warm the hands. But do try to start out with your hands as warm as possible. *Close your eyes* and cover them with your hands so that the palms are over the eyes, with the fingers on the forehead and extending up to the scalp (fig 8–5). Your hands should be just a little cupped so that they do not touch the eyeball but only the muscles surrounding the eye. The idea is to shut out as much light as possible without putting pressure on the eyes.

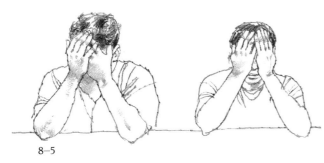

8–5

There are not many activities you can engage in in this position, but those few are extremely valuable. To begin with, you can breathe. Breathing deeply will help you to relax better than anything else. Breathe through your nose, deeply but not forcefully, allowing the air to flow into your chest, diaphragm and abdomen. Imagine that the incoming air is black, and that it fills your whole body with blackness as you inhale. Let your whole body expand as you breathe in, and release as you breathe out.

You can ask each muscle in your body in turn to relax. Imagine each part of your body, sense it, notice how it feels, and, if it is not relaxed, ask it to let go. You may be very surprised to find that you are holding tension in places you were not aware of. It is likely that you hold tension in these places most of

the time, and one of the many benefits of palming is that you become aware of this. Imagine that each of your muscles is becoming soft, warm and loose, covering your body like an old comforter.

You can imagine deep blackness. Some people have been taught that the goal in palming is to see only a perfect blackness, and they become very frustrated if they are not able to do this. The real goal in palming is to relax the eyes, and this cannot be done by straining after 'results'. Many people do not see black when they begin to palm; instead, they see flashes of light, dots, stars, masses of dark colors, or confused visual images. This indicates that the optic nerve is working overtime, flashing visual images which are useless to the eyes. This is not something which can be immediately controlled. If you cannot see black, then just imagine it. Try to call to mind a very dark place that you have been in, a place that you enjoyed – maybe in the heart of a cave when the guide switched off the lights to amaze everyone with the utter darkness, or maybe hiding under a pile of blankets as a child. Visualize large, heavy, black objects sinking into black earth at midnight. Or just imagine some other dark color that you like. Don't struggle to see black – just breathe, relax and imagine. Your optic nerve will quiet down when it is ready to. Refer to the palming meditations at the end of this chapter, which you can read onto a tape and listen to as you palm.

You can follow other meditations. Some forms of meditation call for a specific position, or must be done with the eyes open, but if yours doesn't then use this time for a dual purpose: to calm your spirit along with your eyes. It is the best time we know of for doing affirmations of health. You can listen to music, keeping in mind that you are seeking relaxation and calmness: music that makes you want to get up and dance is not recommended. Or you can simply enjoy the luxury of knowing that, while doing 'nothing', you are in fact doing something of inestimable value for your eyes.

You may experience a strong emotional resistance to palming, particularly if you palm and meditate at the same time. This is part of an overall resistance to relaxation which anxiety creates in many people. It is as though we believe that, if we let down our guard for a moment, disaster will strike from some unexpected quarter, and so we remain always on edge. Some negative emotions may be fear of the dark or restlessness with being with oneself, and the feeling may be so deeply ingrained that you cannot always overcome it just through soothing thoughts or affirmations. If you find yourself overwhelmed by negative emotion, the best thing to do is a meditative breathing exercise. This consists of ten deep breaths, drawn (as always) through the nose and deep into the abdomen. While you do this, give yourself permission to be exactly as you are. For these ten breaths, tell yourself that it is OK to be anxious, angry or impatient, OK to have blurred vision, and that whatever you think is wrong with you is not wrong, it just *is*. And then go on palming. Another very effective solution is to have a member of your support group massage you while you palm, especially when you start practicing the palming meditation.

Five-minute palming sessions are fine if you are taking a break from your work or reading, to rest your eyes. Otherwise, you should palm for a minimum of twenty minutes at a time, and if possible for three-quarters of an hour to an hour per day, either in one sitting or

divided between a few. It usually takes about fifteen minutes to rest the eyes fully, and you should have at least a few minutes – more, naturally, is better – to stay in that relaxed state and enjoy it. Don't schedule a long palming session just before you are about to rush off on a million errands, because the chances are that you will not let yourself relax fully; nor is it wise to palm when you are extremely tired, unless your goal is to fall asleep immediately. Try to find a 'between time', when you are neither exhausted nor anxious to get on to the next thing. Set aside a special time for palming, and congratulate yourself if you go over the allotted time – it's a measure of how much you have been able to relax. You cannot overdo palming. We, and some of our clients, have done marathon palming sessions of up to eleven hours, and we have had our most remarkable gains in vision following these sessions.

Light

Light is the vehicle which brings all visual information to our eyes. Light and sight are synonymous. People who spend much of their time working outdoors under bright natural light tend to have better eyesight than those of us who live mostly indoors. This is because their eyes are accustomed to, and comfortable with, strong light; they can accept and use the light fully. The more time we spend in dim, inadequate, artificial light, the less our eyes are equipped to deal with light. Normal sunlight comes to have almost the effect of a spotlight shone into the face, and eyes which have become overly sensitive to light will try to resist it. This is partly because spending most of our time indoors makes our pupils become chronically dilated, opening as wide as possible in order to take in all available light, and exposure to sunlight may be very painful when the eyes are in this condition. The muscles around the eyes will tend to tighten, squinting to shut out some of the painful light. Many people are currently walking around with sunglasses or with a perpetual, unconscious squint shielding their eyes from 'excess' light.

To some extent, squinting works temporarily. Its long-term effects, however, are very detrimental to vision. It causes the muscles around the eyes to constantly contract. It also cuts out a large part of the peripheral visual field, straining the retinal cells and forcing the eyes to stare fixedly, with effort, at a very small area. With the muscles around the eyes frozen into a squint and held there, there can be no enjoyment of seeing. Sunglasses are about as helpful to this situation as a wheelchair would be to a person with weak leg muscles: they provide temporary relief, but ultimately they serve only to further weaken the eyes' ability to cope with light.

Both of the authors of this book could be considered authorities on this particular aspect of vision. Both of us suffered since infancy with nystagmus, a condition in which the eyes move involuntarily. This condition involves a hypersensitivity to strong light, causing the eyes to move around frantically in an effort to escape from the light. Both of us spent many hours in pain due to excess light in our eyes, and both of us developed very early a preference for dark places. And yet neither of us has worn sunglasses, or wanted to, since discovering sunning. If we can manage without them, anyone can.

Of course, we are not simply saying toss the sunglasses out forever. You will still need them if you happen to be driving due west at sunset. But if you regularly practice these exercises, you will need the glasses less and less. Your eyes will accept much more light, much more comfortably. Your pupils will become more flexible, able to dilate and contract easily and quickly, making the transition from dark to light less painful. Your face will lose its squint, and your visual field will expand. You will no longer be blinded by the light.

8–6 Sunning the Eyes for More Light = More Sight. Sunning should be done when the sunlight is coming into the eyes at a diagonal angle and is not too strong. We recommend sunning at any time before 10.00 a.m. and after 4.00 p.m., but this is different in different places around the world. If you do not have fair skin, you can sun for five minutes at a time even in the hotter hours. Sit outside or at an open window (or stand leaning against a wall, or lie down, if it's most comfortable). DO NOT SUN THROUGH GLASS, **as the glass strongly intensifies the light and could hurt your eyes.** DO NOT SUN THROUGH GLASSES or **with contact lenses on.** It is also a good idea to wear a sunblock cream to protect your skin in the warmer seasons. WITH YOUR EYES CLOSED – WE REPEAT: CLOSED! CLOSED! CLOSED! – turn your face slightly up to the sun so that it shines directly onto your closed eyelids, and immediately begin to turn your head slowly from side to side. Your head should move

(1) constantly, without stopping;
(2) as slowly as possible, as though it were lazily rolling from one shoulder to the other;
(3) effortlessly – let it go a full 180 degrees if you can; if you cannot, move your upper

body with your head to allow the full movement. Imagine that someone else is holding your head between their hands and gently, gently turning it for you.

Your eye muscles may resist the light at first, even with the eyes closed. Try to notice whether you sense tension in your eyes or around them, and allow the muscles to relax. Also notice the strength of the light coming through your closed lids, and the color of the light that penetrates your eyelids, which can range from dark red through orange and yellow to a brilliant white. If you see green, it means your eyes are straining, and you should discontinue sunning for a while and try some palming before attempting sunning again.

Turn your head in this manner for two or three minutes, or about forty turns. Then turn away from the sun, rest your elbows on your knees, if sitting – otherwise, raise your hands to your eyes – and palm for a minute or two, to give your eyes a rest from the strong light. Notice the color of the darkness you see while palming.

Continue this alternation of two minutes of sunning with one or two minutes of palming and see what balance of sunning and palming feels comfortable to you. Try it for ten to fifteen minutes. You will probably notice a sense of relaxation in the eyes as they become accustomed to the bright light. You may also notice that the color you see while sunning becomes brighter, while the color you see while palming becomes progressively darker until you are truly seeing a perfect blackness. When this happens, you will know that the pupils of your eyes have become more flexible, making the change from darkness to light with greater ease. Your optic nerve will be more relaxed, able to receive stimuli more comfort-

ably and to rest after receiving them. When you have been doing sunning for several weeks, you may gradually begin to sun for longer periods, perhaps five or six minutes, between palming sessions, but it is always a good idea to break up the sunning with palming. Not only does this give the eyes a rest, it also encourages flexibility in the pupils.

There are several variations on sunning which you can do to make the exercise more effective for you. One is to place one hand on the back of your neck, the other on your forehead, making sure that the hand on your forehead doesn't block the light coming into your eyes (fig 8–6). The hand at the back of your neck should be clawed, and the one on your forehead stretched, with the bony prominences at the bases of your fingers pressing hard on your forehead. Keeping the hands stationary in this position, move your head from side to side as before, thus adding a massage of the neck and forehead to the benefits of your sunning. Do this for several minutes, to increase circulation and relaxation in the face, neck and eyes, and then palm for a minute and return to the original sunning exercise.

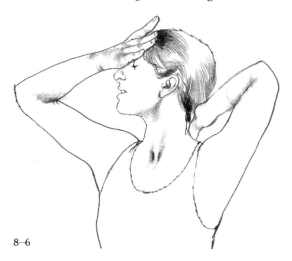

8–6

When you make a deliberate effort to see, you contract and tighten the muscles of the eyebrows (the orbicularis oculi) and stiffen the muscles of your cheekbones. When you believe that seeing is an effort, that contraction becomes chronic and permanent. Your brain adjusts your vision in such a way that you see a blur unless you tense. With time, you have to increase the tension in order to see, until you no longer see well even under tremendous tension. It is amazing how much better you can see when you give up that tension altogether. It is just like any other activity in the body: if you tense to do it, it becomes more difficult.

When you have been sunning for about ten minutes, try this variation to increase the amount of light that enters your eyes. Close your eyes and place your right index and middle fingers on the inside edge of your right eyebrow, with your hand held high enough so that it does not block light from entering your right eye. Now turn your head slowly to the left and, as you do so, slide the two fingertips on to your eyelid, pressing gently but firmly upward, exerting a gentle upward pull on the eyelid itself, stretching it, but not enough to actually pull it open. Remember, you are only touching the eyebrow, not the lid itself. The folds of the eyelid will be flattened out enough to allow more light into the eye, but the eye will remain closed. Move your head all the way to the left, then to the right, and alternate several times. Then switch hands, placing the left index and middle fingers on the left eyebrow as the head turns to the right. This may take some practice to do it smoothly; remember to breathe deeply, move slowly and relax. Repeat this motion several times, palm, and return to the original sunning.

When your eyes have become very comfortable with sunning, cover one eye, turn the head just a little more rapidly, and blink the uncovered eye with very rapid small blinks as you do so. Never look directly into the sun for more than the smallest fraction of a second. If you find this uncomfortable, try blinking only when your head is turned to the sides, and if that is not comfortable just go back to regular sunning. Be sure to palm a little extra after this variation.

You can also experiment with different ways of turning the head, allowing the light to enter the eyes at different angles. Move your head slowly in large rotations; or let the head tilt a little further backward after each turn to the side, until it is extended as far backward as your neck will comfortably allow; or move the head up and down as you also move it from side to side, so that you are nodding and shaking your head simultaneously.

Twenty minutes of sunning per day is our average recommendation, and this may be broken down into sessions of five to fifteen minutes. People who are very comfortable with the light may like to do more – some of our students do three twenty-minute sessions daily. However, it is very important to be sensitive to your eyes and avoid overdoing this exercise, so stick with twenty minutes' total sunning time daily unless you are working with a professional who feels that more would be safe for you. Don't let your eyes become tired or strained; if they do, be sure to palm until they feel good again. A cool cloth compress on the closed eyes is also very soothing and refreshing.

Take advantage of every sunny day! Don't let one go by without using it to help your eyes. Gray days are a problem, of course. Maureen moved out of San Francisco precisely because the weather there was not cooperating with her exercise regime. Some people find that going through the motions of sunning outdoors even on a cloudy day – which Meir calls skying – has some of the same benefits as sunning, and some people have used a strong lamp as a sun-substitute, with good results. Try both of these options and see how they work for you. But make sure to do your sunning every day that the sun shines, and also to spend at least an hour outdoors daily, even on overcast days. Don't let your eyes become permanently weakened by artificial light.

One additional note on sunning: we have been teaching and practicing sunning for more than twenty years, with literally thousands of students and clients. No one that we have ever worked with or heard of has ever experienced any difficulty with this exercise or damage to the eyes because of it. However, we have had clients who reported that their doctors had told them that the sun could damage their eyes, particularly in regard to the formation of cataracts. If this is of concern to you, please consult with your ophthalmologist about sunning. If your doctor objects to the sunning, inquire about studies which have been done proving the connection between cataracts or retinal problems and the sun, and, if such studies are available, take the trouble to read them yourself. If you are convinced that there is a danger to you from sunning, please do not do it. However, we believe this possibility to be minimal. We would be very happy to hear from people who have had personal experience with this issue.

8–7 Skying is a milder variation of sunning. In case you find sunning difficult at first, or if you begin to feel overwhelmed by bright light on a very sunny day, you can 'sky' for a few minutes instead. Turn AWAY from the sun and face the sky with eyes open. Turn your head from side to side as in sunning, and blink very rapidly. Meanwhile, massage the back of your head with the fingertips of one hand and your forehead with the palm of the other hand, moving the head while holding the hands stationary, as you did in the sunning exercise (see fig 8–6). You can also do this on a gray day, as even an overcast sky often has enough light to make this exercise worthwhile. The purpose of skying is similar to that of sunning: to teach the eyes and the brain to accept light comfortably, without a sense of strain.

Flexibility and Fluidity

Movement is one of the most basic factors in good vision. Eyes that do not see well tend to be fixed, or 'frozen', into a stare. Instead of making many tiny movements per second, myopic eyes, for example, tend to make large, infrequent and inaccurate jumps, or not to move at all. In their efforts to see, myopic people also forget to allow themselves to blink. Eventually the strain experienced within the eyes becomes reflected in the muscles surrounding the eyes. If you have ever been forced to stand motionless for hours at a time, you can imagine how tiring this is to your eyes, and what effect it has upon them.

Blinking   You can reverse this pattern simply by remembering to blink whenever you think of it. Blinking your eyes gives them a momentary rest from light and from the work of seeing. It gives the small muscles around the eyes a gentle workout, relieving them from chronic contraction. It massages the eyeballs.

Blinking makes the pupils continually expand and contract, and so it will eventually make them more comfortable with varying degrees of bright light. If you have been staring, it breaks the stare and gives you a chance to shift your point of focus. It can help to relax facial muscles all the way back into the scalp and down into the jaw. Forgetting to blink, like forgetting to breathe, is often caused by trying too hard to concentrate, either on what we are doing or on what we are seeing. Blinking can help both the mind and the eyes to relax. In fact, blinking can aid breathing. The eyes and the lungs are connected through the function of the sinuses, which are behind some of the muscles surrounding the eyes. Since contraction of these muscles can lead to congestion of the sinuses, relaxing these muscles helps to keep the sinuses clear, making breathing deeper and easier.

Blinking is essential in keeping the eyes moist. You may have noticed how staring can bring on a burning sensation in your eyes; this is caused by their becoming too dry. Try this experiment: keep your eyes open – not wide open, just open – and refrain from blinking for as long as you can. Naturally, you will find this uncomfortable to do while you are doing it deliberately – but it is just as hard on your eyes when you are doing it unconsciously, as most of us do for long periods daily. Blinking and palming will both help to restore moisture to the eyes.

As with all of the other exercises in this book, blinking should be done with awareness and without strain. There are many ways to blink. Maureen was recently teaching vision exercises in Israel and discovered that Hebrew has two words for blinking: one means forcefully squeezing the eyes shut; the other means a rapid fluttering blink. Unfortunately, neither of these was what she wanted her students to do. Try instead to let your blinking be effortless, frequent but not too rapid, complete but not forced. Try blinking instead of squinting when your eyes feel overwhelmed by bright light, since squinting not only tightens the muscles around the eyes but also focuses light on the eyes in a painful and harmful way. And remember to blink constantly when you are doing a lot of looking, as when driving or at a show or exhibition.

8–8   The following is an exercise for relaxing the face and eyes and relieving the strain of intensive eye-work. Lie flat on your back with your arms stretched comfortably out to the sides and your knees bent so that the feet are flat on the floor. (You can also do these exercises sitting up, but it's more relaxing to lie down if possible.) Let your head roll very slowly and gently from side to side, imagining that someone is holding your head and moving it for you. Let your head roll far enough to each side that you feel the stretch in the side neck muscles, the jaw and the shoulders. After doing this until your neck begins to relax, begin to slowly open your mouth, letting it stretch as far as it can without strain, and then letting it fall closed as you continue to roll the head from side to side. Pay attention to which muscles are moved by this exercise: where, besides the jaw, can you feel the stretch? Now, as you continue to roll the head and open and close your mouth, add a steady rhythmic blinking. This is also a great coordination exercise, because you will have your head, jaw and eyes all moving at the same time but at slightly different speeds. If it seems difficult, concentrate not on the difficulty but on the different sensations that each part is experiencing as it moves. Do this for several minutes

205

and see whether you experience a sense of relief from facial and eye tension. If not, see whether you at least experience the tension itself. Many people have this tension all the time but never really feel it, experiencing it only through its results, in the gradual loss of vision.

The above exercise may also be done while moving your head in small rotations, rather than from side to side. Don't lift your head off the floor, but move it in a very small circle, letting the floor massage the back of the skull. If you imagine that you are drawing a circle with a pencil at the end of your nose, this will give you the correct motion.

8–9 These exercises are not supposed to provide noticeable improvement of vision, but they will help you to develop a greater kinesthetic awareness of your eyes – which you will need if you are going to work on them effectively. Open your eyes all the way, keep them open, and pay attention to how this feels. Does the forehead tighten and work with the eyelids, or can it allow the eyelids to work independently? Now close your eyes, but very gradually, in stages – first one-quarter, then half, then three-quarters, and finally completely – noticing how the eyes feel at each stage. Then blink rapidly to release any strain in the eyes. Repeat this sequence several times, and see whether there is any change in the way you feel. This process should be repeated several times through the day, so that you can see how the condition of your eyes changes.

8–10 This blinking exercise should be done during palming. Palm for about ten minutes, paying attention to the quality of your palming – the relaxation, the breathing, the depth of blackness, the moisture in the eyes.

Then open your left eye, keeping the right one closed and covered, touching gently with the fingertips just under the eyebrow (fig 8–10). Begin to blink, or rather to slowly open and close the left eye. Imagine as you do so that the eyelashes are the moving force. Stroke gently along the eyelid and brush your eyelashes with your fingers. Massage your forehead. Imagine that someone is very gently raising the eyelid for you with a finger held under the eyelashes, and that gravity pulls it gradually down again – this or some similar visualization will help you to keep from blinking forcibly. At the same time, pay attention to what the right eye is doing. If it is remaining motionless, that's great, and you can simply focus on relaxing the left eye. In many people, however, the right eye will be trying as hard as it can to blink along with the left eye. As with many other parts of the body, when we strain to do something – in this case, to see – we exert unnecessary effort, using muscles which do not need to be used. This produces the rigidity around the eyes which will not even allow them to blink separately.

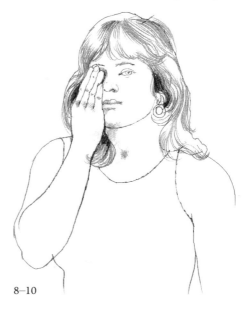

8–10

For your eyes to be able to blink separately, you must focus on opening and closing the left eye so slowly, so gently and so effortlessly that the right eye will stop trying to participate, as if it is tricked into thinking that the left eye is doing nothing. Don't worry if you can't do this at first; just practice this exercise for several minutes and then try the same thing with the left eye covered and the right eye open. Notice whether it is easier or more difficult to do so with the eyes reversed. Practice for several minutes, and then try again with the left eye open. Is it any easier this time? Now return to palming and again notice how the palming feels. Many people find that the blackness has become blacker, or that the eyes feel softer or more moist. The important thing, however, is simply to take note of what is happening, rather than to insist on particular results. Improvement will inevitably come with practice, but it will come differently for each person.

8–11 Another good blinking exercise is simply to move your head from side to side, blinking as you do so, and pay attention to the slightly different scene that is before you each time you open your eyes. This will keep you from getting fixated on any one point, and will demonstrate how blinking can help to break the pattern of staring.

Equal Use of the Eyes + Equal Use of Each Part of the Eyes = Balanced Use of the Eyes

People with poor vision commonly do two things which lead to unbalanced use of the eyes: they allow one eye to dominate, and they use only their central vision while neglecting their peripheral vision. This behavior is, of course, completely unconscious, but it can be changed by conscious retraining. Most of us are born with a tendency to have a stronger eye, just as most of us have a stronger hand. This tendency towards lopsidedness creates tension, which in turn brings on other problems. Meir has had many clients who claim that all of their physical problems occur on just one side of their bodies, so that they will have, for example, a weak right eye along with a sciatic right hip, a bad right knee, carpal-tunnel syndrome in the right hand only, and so on.

When one eye tends to dominate – and most people with myopia know about this phenomenon, because most of them will have a stronger prescription for one eye than for the other – the result is exactly the same as what happens when we use only a few muscles to do the work of the entire body. The weaker eye will be underused, and consequently will weaken further, while the stronger eye works ceaselessly until it, too, begins to lose its strength.

8–12 Many vision therapists have used patching – placing a black eyepatch over one eye, usually the stronger – to correct various vision problems such as cross-eye, double vision and amblyopia ('lazy eye'). This practice can be very helpful. When it does not produce good results, this is usually because it has been overdone. When you wear a patch over your stronger eye, the weaker eye has to do all of your seeing. This is all right for five minutes, or up to twenty minutes, but you must remember not to demand too much of the weaker eye at first, in order to avoid straining it. You also want to avoid sending your brain the message that one eye must always dominate.

The patch should be worn only for short periods of time, and never while doing any kind of strenuous eye-work. It may, however, be used frequently, preferably while walking or doing some other activity which stimulates the eye without overworking it.

While we do endorse a limited amount of patching for some vision problems, a method we prefer is working with the periphery. Most of our peripheral exercises involve blocking out the central field of vision and stimulating the periphery of each eye, either simultaneously or consecutively. When we look straight forward with both eyes, it is easy to let one eye do all the work, and to be completely unconscious of this. When we work with our periphery, however, we create a separate visual field for each eye, and so we are much more apt to notice if one eye is not working.

Besides encouraging you to use, and therefore to strengthen, both eyes, these exercises give a welcome relief from eyestrain. Intense use of your central vision can create deep tension in facial muscles, especially those of the forehead and jaw, which peripheral work can relieve. We particularly recommend these exercises for people with myopia, glaucoma, strabismus, amblyopia, tunnel vision, macula degeneration and retinitis pigmentosa, a degenerative eye disease which causes a loss of the peripheral field. Working with the periphery also helps to break the bad habits you may have established in your use of your central vision – just because you are using it does not mean you are using it optimally.

Stimulating Peripheral Vision

8–13 The first exercise is to measure your peripheral vision. You will need two dripless candles, or two flashlights, or two watches with phosphorescent dials (if you have sufficient peripheral vision to be able to see them in the dark, from the side). You will also need two small pieces of black construction paper, one about two inches by three inches for doing peripheral exercises in daylight, and one about two by four inches for doing them in the dark, each with a piece of tape on the back folded so that it will stick to two surfaces. This piece of paper is a very important piece of equipment, and will be used in nearly all of our peripheral exercises. It should be taped to the very top of the bridge of your nose.

In a completely dark room, tape the paper between your eyes and sit with the lighted candles (or whatever) held to your sides, at your shoulders, about a foot away from your ears. If you can see them there, you are doing well. If you cannot, or if you just sense the light but do not see the candles themselves, then slowly move the candles forward and toward each other, always keeping them about a foot away from your head, so that they move from your peripheral field toward your nose (fig 8–13). At the same time, shake your hands slightly so that you are waving or wiggling slightly the candles as you move them forward. (This is why they

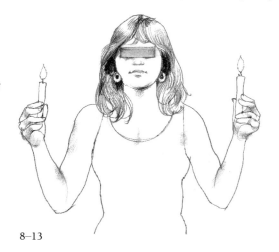

8–13

really must be dripless candles.) This wiggling or waving motion is done in almost all of the peripheral exercises, and the reason for it is that movement stimulates the peripheral cells more than anything else. It attracts their attention and causes them to work. The peripheral cells are similar to the eyes of some animals who are in fact not capable of seeing something unless it is in motion. This movement is particularly important in peripheral exercises which are done in the dark, since the rods – which are the retinal cells that you principally use in dim light can only see moving objects. Note to yourself where you actually saw the candles – you can then compare this information to a later measurement, after practicing exercises for the periphery.

When you feel comfortable with this exercise, and after you have relaxed your eyes by palming, try moving the candles from your chest area toward your chin (keeping the candles at a safe distance from your face) and from above your head toward your forehead, to measure your periphery in those directions.

8–14 To demonstrate to yourself how far your peripheral vision can be expanded, begin with the candles in front of you, and move them (always continuing to wiggle them slightly as they move) as far to the back, at the sides of your face, as they can go and still be seen. Hold them there for a minute, and then move just a little further, so that they are just slightly past the point where they can be seen. Keep them at exactly that point, close your eyes, and visualize the lights – imagine them to be placed exactly as they are, but easily visible to you. After a minute or two, open your eyes. Many people find that they can now see the candles easily, although they are still in exactly the same position they were

before. If this is true for you, then again move the candles just a little further back and slightly out of your visual field, and repeat visualization. This exercise 'stretches' your peripheral field, and may stimulate some hitherto unused peripheral cells. It is not at all unusual for people to expand their peripheral fields by as much as several inches in a very short time by using this exercise. We have had clients who were incapable of peripheral vision in daylight who responded very well to this exercise.

Always remember to periodically stop, rest and visualize the lights moving in your farthest periphery. If you find this exercise helpful, it may also be done in a dimly lit, rather than pitch-black, room.

Remember that, though this exercise may be very relaxing and refreshing for your eyes, it may also tire them, as may other peripheral exercises, since you may be using new and untried cells.

8–15 Peripheral exercises may also be done in full daylight. With a black paper, two by three inches, taped between your eyes, sit and move your head from side to side, slowly. Look straight ahead at the paper, while waving your hands or wiggling your fingers on each side of your head – close to the ears to stimulate your peripheral cells (fig 8–15).

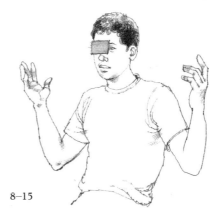

8–15

Now close your eyes and visualize your hands waving and the room swiveling slowly from side to side, as it appears to do when you move your head from side to side; try to imagine that it is indeed the room, rather than your head, which moves. Then open your eyes again and repeat the first part of the exercise. Vary the movement of your hands, moving them in circles, up and down, and out to the sides, always imagining that your peripheral field expands.

Since you are doing this in daylight, there will be more visual data to attract your attention than in the dark; your eyes may therefore fall back into their old habits of letting one eye dominate and do all the work for both. To make sure that you are using both eyes, always remember to pay conscious attention to what each eye is seeing, and occasionally close your eyes and visualize that both eyes see fully and clearly in the periphery.

Remove the paper from between your eyes, cover your right eye with your right hand, and, as you look forward, stimulate the periphery of your left eye by wiggling your fingers all around your visual field: the periphery of your left eye is not just to your left, but also above and below your face and to your right. Repeat this with the other eye. The importance of this exercise is also in keeping your stronger eye from dominating; even with the paper between your eyes, you may 'forget' to let the weaker eye see, but a moment or two of working on its own may remind it to wake up and work.

Return to using both eyes simultaneously, with the black piece of paper between them. Whenever your eyes begin to feel tired, stop and close them, resting them and imagining blackness until they feel strong again.

Now move your head slowly up and down,

imagining as you do so that the room, not your head, is moving, and that it is moving in the opposite direction from how you are moving. Thus, as your head moves downward, imagine that the room is moving upward; as your head comes up again, imagine that the room is moving down. Do the same while bending your whole upper body up and down. Another variation is to move the head in circles.

8–16 A very simple and effective peripheral exercise is the following. With the paper between your eyes, hold up the forefinger of each hand in front of your eyes, so that the hands are about a foot apart from each other and a foot in front of your face. Now begin to move the hands in circles, first with both hands moving in the same direction, then with one hand moving clockwise and the other counter-clockwise. Be sure that both eyes are working, with the right eye following the movement of the right hand, the left eye following the left hand. Gradually let your circles become bigger and bigger, but only as big as you can make them and still be able to see each finger – don't let the movement of the finger take it out of range of that eye's visual field. In this exercise, as in most peripheral exercises, it may help to wiggle the finger as well as moving the hand, since increasing the movement increases the stimulation to the peripheral cells.

8–17 Riding in a moving vehicle can be an excellent peripheral vision exercise. The motion of the vehicle creates an automatic stimulus for the periphery, the same kind of stimulus you are trying to create with the movement of the head and hands in exercise 8–15. It is most effective to look straight ahead while at the same time paying attention to the scene rushing past backward on either side of you. As long as you are not the driver, you can make the ride a better vision exercise by taping a black piece of paper on the bridge of your nose. Look straight ahead at the paper; your brain will be bored with it quickly, and will pay more attention to the moving scenery at your sides. If you are on a train, try sitting so that you are facing the direction opposite the one in which the train is going; this will make you even more aware of the movement.

8–18 When you read, write or do any kind of work which could tax the central vision, it is very helpful to stimulate the periphery by waving or wiggling the hands to the sides of the eyes; this motion genuinely seems to take the strain out of reading. We have many opportunities to overwork the central vision and neglect the periphery: crowded city streets, narrow freeway lanes, computers, documents covered with tiny print and incomprehensible data – all these seemed designed to promote tunnel vision and narrow our horizons. Peripheral exercises are one way to counteract this problem.

8–19 Long Swing Stand with your legs far apart, hold one forefinger up before your eyes, about two feet from your face, and focus on it. Then move the finger as far to each side as you can, following it with your eyes, moving your head so that the finger is always in front of your nose. As you look at your finger, see all of your surroundings moving in the opposite direction.

After moving your head from side to side several times in this manner, continue the motion while allowing your body to follow the movement of your eyes. As you turn toward the left, turn far enough to actually bring the

right heel off the floor; as you turn to the right, the left heel will lift (fig 8–19A). The purpose of this exercise is to increase the sense of movement while you look.

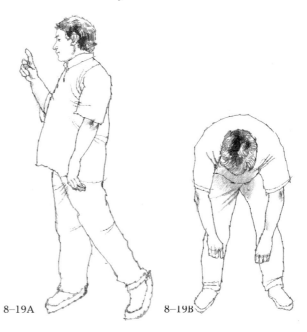

8–19A   8–19B

The third stage of this exercise is to increase the swinging of the body and include bending the upper torso when you are looking forward (fig 8–19B), then stretching upward at the sides (fig 8–19C and 8–19D).

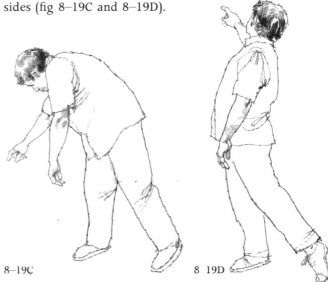

8–19C   8 19D

Shifting – Seeing What There is to See

The normal eye makes many tiny movements per second. These are known as saccadic movements, after *saccade*, the French for jerk. You may have noticed that the eyes of people with exceptionally good vision often have a sparkling or a piercing quality. This appearance is caused by these constant small movements of the eyes, which produce not only this special brightness but also the clarity and sharpness of vision which accompany it. The movements themselves are not visible, neither when the eyes shift automatically nor when you consciously direct them to shift. Even when you practice shifting exercises, no one looking into your eyes would be able to detect the movements. The most they would notice would be that your eyes look alert and alive.

The purpose of these movements is to engage the central part of the retina, which is known as the macula and is the part of the eye solely responsible for sharp, detailed vision. In the center of the macula itself is a spot called the fovea centralis, and it is at this point that the eye sees with its greatest clarity. When we see with any part of the eye other than the macula, we lose most of our capacity for detailed vision. Because it is small in size, the macula can see only very small portions of the visual field at any one moment, though it sees these portions in very fine detail. For this reason, the normal eye will make constant, small, rapid movements, and with it the macula will move from point to point and receive a constant stream of visual information. If you imagine the images on a television screen, or a dot-matrix computer printout, or the paintings of Seurat – all of which present a picture composed of tiny bits of color and shape – and then imagine deciphering these images dot by dot, you can understand how the healthy macula works.

One of the things which happens when a person's vision begins to deteriorate is that these saccadic movements will become slower, larger and less frequent. Vision becomes blurred, as details lose their definition or are lost altogether. We speak of this process as the 'freezing' of vision. It can happen as the result of physical or emotional causes – or both – but either way it is the beginning of the loss of good vision.

'Shifting' exercises are designed to restore the natural free movement of the macula. As the name implies, these exercises all involve shifting one's point of focus from place to place, in imitation of normal saccadic movement. Though this movement must be consciously practiced at first, with time it becomes an automatic and effortless process, as it is for the healthy eye.

Shifting is, as we have said, the natural state of the eye. Curiosity and interest naturally cause people to shift, unless they have developed a habit of staring or have lost the confidence that comes with a belief that they are seeing accurately. When we look at something which we enjoy seeing, the eyes will want to move from detail to detail. Boredom, fear and loss of curiosity or confidence will stop us from shifting and cause us to freeze our vision into a stare. So will constant use of our near vision, if it is not balanced with use of our distance vision. It is an integral precept of our work, and one which applies to every part of the body, that the less movement you experience – the more you freeze – the worse you will function. This is true of muscles, joints, lungs, nerves and digestive organs; it is also true of the eyes. To encourage appropriate movement is to promote optimal functioning.

Our perceptions and sensations can also 'freeze', if we allow ourselves to become insensitive or numb to what we see, hear or feel. We can and often do turn off the flow of information from our environment. We can selectively turn ourselves off, and are most likely to do so when we don't like what our senses are telling us, or when we have lost interest in it. The act of emotionally or mentally distancing ourselves from our surroundings can be as effective in deadening our perceptions as though we had actually, physically, left. Thus, we spend a lot of time 'seeing without seeing'. We may miss even things which can easily be seen, simply because the eyes and the mind are not working together. Rest is very important for the eyes, but there is a big difference between rest and disuse. Allowing your eyes to remain open in a dull, unfocused stare is not a good way to rest them. Shifting, on the other hand, is a restful use, a functional rest. Shifting is conscious vision.

When you practice shifting, the key to success is to look with a 'soft' eye, by which we mean that you allow yourself to see whatever you can see, without straining or forcing yourself to see anything in particular. You should not demand from yourself that you will see this or that detail with clarity. Instead, you allow your eyes and your mind to take in every detail which is available to them, without straining after the details which are not yet available. For anyone who wears glasses, no matter how strong or how weak the prescription, this is especially important. You have been accustomed to using your glasses to bring you whatever detail you want to see, and you must become willing to give this up, at least temporarily. You must give up the need to see

before you can improve your vision. Looking with a 'soft' eye is similar to taking a walk for the pure pleasure of moving your body, without scheming over the calories you are burning or the muscles you are toning. 'Soft' eyes absorb the world, rather than trying to capture it. Having a 'soft' eye really means that your eyes rest while you look, rather than striving. While your ultimate goal is of course to improve your sight, your immediate goal in shifting is the shifting process itself, the creation of lively, enlivening movement in the eyes and increased perception in the brain. Don't try to see anything in particular, because as soon as you try, you strain. You will then become fixed on the point you are trying to see, your vision will freeze, shifting will stop, and you will be back where you started.

If your eyes become tired during shifting, this is not because the shifting itself is strenuous but because you bring into the shifting your old habits of straining to see. When this happens, it will be helpful if you close your eyes and visualize random and beautiful patterns of movement, such as waves rolling in, seagulls wheeling, a shower of autumn leaves or petals from a flowering tree, or clouds blowing across the sky. Let your mind's eye move with these images for a minute or two, and then try to continue this graceful, easy flow of movement when you open your eyes and look again.

8–20 Begin with shifting this way: for one week, just shift. Whenever you remember to, move your eyes from point to point on whatever it is that you are looking at. Instead of looking at 'a tree', look at the individual parts that make up the tree visually, and then move from larger to smaller details of those parts. Remember to blink and breathe as often as possible, because both of these actions will help your eyes to move more freely and easily. You may be surprised at the amount of detail you will see. Without any measurable change in your vision, you will be seeing better simply because you are seeing consciously.

8–21   You can then continue this process and refine it, now taking note of those details which you cannot see clearly. For example, you may be able to clearly distinguish a tree, a branch on the tree and an individual leaf on the branch, but not be able to see the veins and markings on that leaf. Let your eyes roam freely over the leaf, noting whatever you can of its shape, color and so on – anything you can notice, without worrying about forming an exact picture of the leaf. Just look and look, like a child, or like a visitor from outer space who is seeing earth things for the first time. Don't force yourself to see; just allow yourself to *look*. Then close your eyes, recall whatever details you can, and picture them as being in sharp contrast to their background. See the leaf as bright where the background is dark, in color where the background is white, and coming toward you as the background recedes, or whatever will most sharply distinguish between them.

8–22   Next, bring fine details closer to you, making them more accessible. Take a picture that you like, and hold it close enough for you to see every detail clearly without straining, and then shift from point to point. If you are looking at a face, take one eye and look at every separate eyelash, every separate spot of color in the iris. Take the forehead and divide it into quarters, then divide each of those quarters into eighths, and so on until you are looking at the smallest possible unit of detail.

Close your eyes and recall those details you have seen, then open them again and look for new details. After a while you may notice the distinctions between separate details growing sharper. For some people, this change can happen almost instantaneously, while for others it may take months. The time factor is not important. Learning to see details is.

8–23   Look at faces. If even the thought of it makes you uncomfortable, it is even more important that you do. Looking at faces, studying their details, is something which has become unacceptable in many social situations, being considered impolite or even aggressive. Because for many of us faces compose a great part of our daily scenery, we end up avoiding much of our surroundings, being careful not to 'stare'. This habit is detrimental to vision. We deliberately do not focus on faces, learning to look 'through' them – in elevators, on trains and buses – and we end up losing much of our ability to focus altogether. You may find it more comfortable to practice this exercise in the company of friends or of your support group. Sit at a distance where you do not see your friend's face perfectly, and shift from detail to detail. Don't be judgmental; just take your time shifting, whether trying to locate the nose and eyes or counting the hairs on the eyelashes.

8–24   Shifting can also be done with things seen at a distance. In fact, this will give you very good practice in looking without insisting on seeing exact details, for the simple reason that you won't be able to. Find yourself a place, preferably a pleasant place, from which you can see well into the distance. The top of a hill or any other high place is especially good. Look all the way to the farthest horizon, and let your eyes move from point to point, as though you are sketching the outlines of what you see. You will probably be able to distinguish only general shapes, colors and degrees of brightness at this distance. Let your eyes enjoy playing with these as they might enjoy looking at an abstract painting. Then focus your attention slightly closer, and keep your eyes shifting from point to point. Perhaps the details you see may be a bit more distinct, but remember not to become fixed on them or try too hard to see them. Just enjoy them, keeping your eyes soft and receptive. You can repeat this process, bringing your plane of focus a little closer to you each time, until your eyes are shifting on the area immediately in front of you, whether it is on the window-sill, a heap of leaves on the ground, or your feet. At this point, look for the tiniest details you can possibly distinguish. Always remember to blink and breathe as you do this and all eye exercises. Blinking is in itself a form of shifting, as it keeps us from seeing the same picture constantly; it keeps the light waves upon the retina in constantly changing patterns.

When you begin to work on your eyes, you should set aside at least twenty minutes a day specifically for shifting exercises. Your aim is ultimately to make shifting an automatic function, and the best way to do this is to shift all the time, whenever you remember to, and you will remember more and more often as you continue this practice. It is, however, necessary at first to spend time concentrating entirely on the shifting process, since it is one of the most important things you will do to change the way you see. When you begin to find yourself shifting automatically, you will

know that your eyes have become more relaxed and that your vision is on its way to improvement.

Palming Meditation

Read the following meditations very slowly onto a tape, or have a friend with a deep, soothing voice read them onto a tape that you can listen to as you palm. It will be even nicer if you record soothing music in the background. The reading should be very slow. Whenever you see a *** in the text, pause for thirty seconds, and keep the music going. In the text there are a few notes for the reader, not to be recorded; these are written in [ ]. This dictation will prepare you gradually for the full meditation sequence on the third day.

A Meditation for Your First Palming Session

Relax your lower back and imagine that it is light. Relax your chest and imagine that it is light. Visualize that your hands are warming your eyes. Now breathe deeply, counting to six as you inhale and to nine as you exhale. Inhale one two three four five six. Exhale one two three four five six seven eight nine. Inhale again and feel how your abdomen is expanding, and exhale feeling how your abdomen is shrinking, six seven eight nine. ***. Inhale and imagine your lower back expanding with your breath. Exhale and feel it shrinking gradually six seven eight nine. Inhale one two three four five six. Exhale one two three four five six seven eight nine. Inhale and imagine your chest, ribs and upper back expanding, and exhale letting them shrink four five six seven eight nine. Inhale again and imagine your whole body expanding as you inhale, shrinking as you exhale. Count ten such breaths. ***. ***.

A Meditation for the Second Day

Repeat the meditation for the first day and continue with this:

As you continue to breathe slowly, imagine that your head is expanding as you inhale ... and shrinking as you exhale ... Imagine that your neck is expanding as you inhale ... and shrinking as you exhale ... Imagine that your shoulders are expanding as you inhale ... and shrinking as you exhale ... Imagine that your arms are expanding as you inhale ... and shrinking as you exhale ... Imagine that your elbows are expanding as you inhale ... and shrinking as you exhale ... Imagine that your forearms are expanding as you inhale ... and shrinking as you exhale ... Imagine that your hands and fingers are expanding as you inhale ... and shrinking as you exhale ...

Think of your eyes as soft, big and watery ... Imagine that your eyes are expanding as you inhale ... and shrinking as you exhale ... Imagine that your back is expanding as you inhale ... and shrinking as you exhale ... Imagine that your chest is expanding as you inhale ... and shrinking as you exhale ... Imagine that your abdomen is expanding as you inhale ... and shrinking as you exhale ... Imagine that your pelvis is expanding as you inhale ... and shrinking as you exhale ... Imagine that your buttocks are expanding as

you inhale ... and shrinking as you exhale ... Imagine that your thighs are expanding as you inhale ... and shrinking as you exhale ... Imagine that your calves are expanding as you inhale ... and shrinking as you exhale ... Imagine that your feet are expanding as you inhale ... and shrinking as you exhale ... Now imagine that your whole body is expanding as you inhale, and shrinking as you exhale.

[Use the above palming meditation three times on the second day.]

A Meditation for the Third Day

[On the third day, repeat the first two segments and continue with the following. (If you are uncomfortable with the color black for whatever reason, replace the word 'black' with 'dark' or 'darkness' or 'dark blue'.)]

Visualize that you are seeing black, but do not try to force it. Imagine a starless night ... Imagine movement in that blackness ... a train running on a mountain ... a white sailboat on a black sea, a black river flowing [Note to the reader: describe any image or place which will be pleasant and easy to remember, and paint it black. The thought of movement and the contrast of colors in the mind can greatly relax the optic nerve] ... If the image disappears, it is all right – don't try to force it back ... Imagine that your whole room is black. Think of every object in your room and paint it black ... *** Relax your jaw, inhale through your nose, exhale through your nose, and exhale further through your mouth with a sigh. Feel completely relaxed. ***. ***.

Part Two

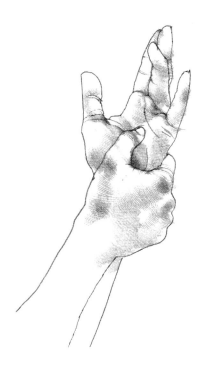

The reason why we have divided the *Handbook* into two parts is that each part serves a different purpose. The purpose of Part One is, ideally, to make the second part unnecessary – its goal is prevention. Part Two is here mainly to help you if you have already developed a specific problem.

In other words, the first part of the book was written for anyone who is interested in developing a better relationship with his or her body, in developing the ability to listen to and to feel the needs of the body, and to respond to them. The exercises in it are designed for anyone who is interested in moving, using, developing and studying his or her body, in recognizing one's abilities and limitations and accepting oneself as one is.

In the second part of the book we offer programs for more specific needs. If you have an ailment that needs addressing, you will want to start here, and we will refer you to Part One for exercises that are relevant to your condition. If you are generally healthy, you will benefit more by using Part One to develop your kinesthetic awareness, and by only later focusing your work on a specific area – such as your running, your back or your vision.

The purpose of this book is not just to help you rid yourself of symptoms, but to develop your intuition and creativity in taking care of your body, your health and your life. You may start by targeting one particular improvement, and end up developing a new sense of your body, a new understanding of it, a feeling of increased engagement with it. At that point the book will have had the effect we hope for. The deeper involvement and the ability to invent is at a level of understanding which is not only physical or mental, but spiritual too.

To make this book an effective guide for years to come, it is not enough to flip through the pages, understand some concepts and work with them. It is not even enough to be open to change. What has most importance is your belief in yourself: belief in your physical, emotional and spiritual strength and resources. Those of you who worked with the first part of the book have an idea as to how many resources your bodies have that you have never tapped, how many more you have which you can use, and how much healthier and more vital your bodies may be if you keep learning to live in them better.

If you do not find your specific problem addressed in this book, please do feel included anyway. The scope of this book is not large enough to describe all that we could suggest, but we believe that, whether you find yourself in Part Two or not, you have enough general material to start with.

Many of the exercises can be used to meet a great variety of needs. Even if you have found within this book exercises which address your specific condition, this may be only the beginning. It may well be that after experimenting with them you will use your newly developed kinesthetic awareness to devise others which work even better for you.

We recommend that you keep a daily diary of your achievements and your difficulties, so that after six or nine months you can assess your improvement. Use this book, use your friends, use your intuition and any input from teachers of this or other therapeutic methods to learn more about what you can do to better your body.

We hope Part One is what you will work most with to increase your health. But if you do need the help of Part Two we urge you to work under professional – especially medical – supervision. Conventional medicine has been extremely important and helpful to many millions of people in understanding the body, in overcoming infections, in removing obstructions, in giving life to people who would otherwise lose theirs – but it has never taught people to strengthen the vital force of life. When you increase your awareness, your mobility and your overall strength, when you learn of your capabilities, then you can become less dependent on the external intervention of medicine.

We would like to suggest again that you work with a small support group of people who gradually become more and more familiar with you and your capabilities and may help you in your development.

You may intuitively sense that there is a time to work by yourself and a time to work with a group, a time to work with a therapist and perhaps a time to work with a different therapist. One client who exhibited this understanding was Danny, a muscular dystrophy client whose story is chronicled in Meir's book *Self-Healing: My Life and Vision* (Routledge & Kegan Paul, 1987; Penguin 1989). Danny exchanged the helplessness and passivity of a nearly wheelchair-bound invalid for the confidence and dedication of the jogger and cyclist he became. At a critical point in his treatment, Danny sensed that it was time to work very intensively on his own. He thought of himself as a sculptor, building his own body. After three months, and with much stronger muscles, he felt prepared to resume therapy. Like Danny, what you need is the discipline and commitment to work on yourself, and to follow what is best for you. We are here to support you.

Every step you make is an opening for the next. You never know what your next step will be. The exercises will lead to new exercises — those which your body, as it develops, will demand. But be careful here: we have met many people who thought they knew their bodies, but moved and lived with overwhelming rigidity and tension. Your support group, therapists or friends will help you evaluate your condition. What are some of your criteria? (1) That your movement is smooth. (2) That you are at ease. (3) That you are breathing deeply at all times. (4) That you have a sense of spaciousness in the joints and lengthening along the spine. (5) That your body and mind are working together for one goal.

The major goal of the *Handbook* is to help you work with your body in a sense of union — never with a feeling of struggling against yourself, or in spite of yourself, or in order to prove something. Whenever you work on your spine, nervous system, breathing, vision or any other system, you are almost bound to encounter your limitations. As you try to relax, you may realize that you are tense or restless. When you try to move more fluidly, you may realize how stiff you are. When you challenge the way your central nervous system functions, you may be frustrated by how fixed your patterns are. Recognize the resentment you may have toward working on your body. The wrong thing to do is to give up. You may get lazy or feel bored, but remember that boredom or lack of discipline are not the causes for your not working with yourself: they are just other forms of resistance, of limitations you have imposed on yourself, which have underlying, subconscious reasons. It is, in a way, much easier to keep your limitations than to break your boundaries. The danger is that you may find yourself quitting work on your body just when you begin to see improvement.

However, if you recognize this process as your own, do not fight against it, do not resent yourself for resisting, because anger will not get you anywhere, and anger at yourself constitutes resistance to change. Be happy with the recognition, because it is an important step toward healing. Consult your support group or a good therapist, receive nurturing and support, and keep working. Try to keep the word 'should' out of your dictionary, and have instead a sense of purpose. Working toward relaxation, mobility and fluidity is much healthier and more effective than forcing yourself into any of these. Overcoming these limitations will allow you more liveliness, more energy and a greater sense of well-being.

CHAPTER 9

Running

Running can be the best or the worst form of aerobic exercise, depending on how it is done. On the plus side, it can improve all of your body processes, beginning with the most vital ones of circulation and breathing and extending even to digestion. On the minus side, runners can and do injure their muscles and joints, sometimes so severely that they are forced to give up running. One of our most popular workshops is one exclusively for runners who want to learn how to run without hurting themselves or, to take it a step farther, to run so that they reap all the potential benefits of running.

Running not only doesn't have to hurt you, it can actually help you to be more relaxed and pain-free overall. Our interest in running began with one of our practitioners who has been a runner since junior high, had developed sciatica partly as a result of the way she was running, and had spent two years rehabilitating her body and her running habits so that she was able to return to regular running without fear of sciatic attacks. It grew as Meir adopted running as a form of exercise and meditation, exploring its possibilities as a Self-Healing tool.

Reaping the full rewards of running means stronger muscles, healthier joints and bones, better circulation, deeper and more regular breathing, a great feeling of accomplishment and satisfaction, and – most of all – a sense of overall well-being that encompasses body and mind. If you injure yourself, however, not only will you lose that glow of well-being, you may decrease your running capacity with time. Many – perhaps even most   injuries that result from running happen simply because people push themselves too long or too hard, or are insensitive to body signals like pain and fatigue. In other words, most of these injuries are preventable, and what can best prevent them is a self-nurturing attitude.

Most likely, you run at least partly out of a real desire to have a healthier body. If you make this desire your first concern, your body will reward you. Often, though, people have other concerns: trying to make their bodies more beautiful, testing their endurance and strength, competing with other people, or simply trying to live up to some self-imposed challenge. Or someone may be trying to strengthen his heart, meanwhile forgetting that the rest of his body has to be considered at the same time. Whenever any of these becomes more important than overall health, running may become a potential hazard. It is then that people injure backs, hips, knees, ankles and feet; or develop tendinitis, shin splints, and a host of other joint and muscle problems – or die of a heart attack in the middle of running.

Try to take the attitude, then, that you are doing this for yourself, and for your body, so that *all* of you will feel better and function better. If you are the kind of person who needs pain and strain and genuine prolonged suffering in order to feel that you have really accomplished anything (and a lot of runners fall into this category), here is an opportunity to let go of this approach for a while. Often, people will run precisely because they believe it requires tremendous effort, and they believe that only tremendous effort gets any results. You will find that this is not necessarily so. You can learn to run for its own sake, without challenging or pushing yourself; you can learn to run with *no effort* – and you will see that the rewards will be even greater than when you ran with maximum effort. Try to put your emphasis on nurturing, rather than challenging or competing – with yourself or anyone else.

Almost all of the exercises we have suggested so far in this book have been non-vigorous in the extreme. (There are plenty of books available on vigorous exercise already.) If you have tried our other Self-Healing exercises, you may have found that at first you have been straining to make even the simplest, most undemanding movement. Most of our exercises have been designed for practice in giving up such a sense of strain, and replacing it with a sense of effortless ease. It is relatively easy to do this with non-vigorous movement. We now invite you to carry this sense of effortlessness into a more strenuous activity. Begin with the idea that running is easy, pleasant and fun,

and that you don't have to run one step further than you really want to. After all, there is no need for you to be doing this. Most of us have little need to run, either to or away from anything. Running must once have been a required activity for everybody, and it certainly is an enjoyable one, once you get used to it. But your life doesn't depend on it anymore. So make sure that it is a pleasure for you, not an ordeal. The less you challenge, push and criticize yourself, the more you enjoy and nurture yourself, the more beneficial your running will be.

The first thing to consider is finding a good place to run. Most runners know how harmful it is to run on concrete, and do it anyway. One of the most baffling sights here in the San Francisco Bay area is that of runners jogging along on sidewalks near or next to busy, heavily-trafficked streets, breathing in deep draughts of car and bus exhaust as they batter their joints against the concrete. Quite often we see them on just such a street which borders Golden Gate Park, where there are miles of dirt paths and acres of trees expelling oxygen. We have never been able to figure out what they are doing outside the park when they could be inside. Or why anyone would run on concrete when there is for most people a park or a schoolyard within easy reach, with paths or a track to run on. In the Joints chapter, we explained that, while plenty of vigorous exercise is essential for the health of the joints, repeated sharp impacts or shocks to a joint often cause osteoarthritis to develop. Running on concrete definitely produces such impacts.

By far the best place to run is a sandy beach. It allows you to run barefoot, which lets you use many more muscles in your feet and legs than does running in shoes. It gives you the choice of running on hard-packed or on soft sand, which are two completely different exercises. It also gives you the chance to breathe sea air, and to run in the water if you like. Running with your feet in the cold water can, in fact, help to take away any swelling in your legs which you might experience as a result of running. If you are lucky enough to live close to a sandy beach, take advantage of it, and do your running there. If not, think carefully about the places that are available to you. Hiking trails, paths in city parks, empty lots, woods, or playing fields at schools — almost everyone can find some flat place that hasn't been covered with concrete. And if finally you can't find anywhere to run but the street, try to find a quiet street. It will also help you to have two or more different pairs of running shoes. These will tend to wear out at different rates, so the wear patterns inside the shoes will be different and will distribute your weight slightly differently. This may make your muscles adjust slightly when you change the shoes from day to day, and help to keep the impact of running from landing on the same part of every joint each time. Wearing heavy socks will also absorb some of the shock if you are running on the street.

The next question is how far to run. This varies widely, of course — the main question is: are you being considerate to your body? We know one runner who set himself the arbitrary standard of nine miles a day. On this schedule, he steadily lost weight from an already thin body. He became so 'wired' that he could not sleep more than four hours a night, and went about his daily life in a fog of fatigue, ultimately endangering his job. He developed tendinitis in both knees, which he steadfastly ignored. This sounds like an extreme case, but in fact such behavior is not unusual at all. We all know people who endanger their health by fanatic devotion to their work. Fanatic devotion to excellence of *any* kind can take the same toll in physical or emotional strain.

So, when you are deciding how far to run, pay attention to how far you are already running, and how it is affecting you. This sounds elementary, but many people, like the runner in the preceding paragraph, don't do it. If you pay attention to your body, it will tell you everything you need to know. If you are a new runner, take it easy and build up slowly. Your muscle strength and lung capacity will increase a little each time you run, so you may frequently add a little distance, such as twenty-five yards or so, so that your muscles are being constantly, but not overly, challenged. You will have to decide for yourself what constitutes a 'little' distance. For a strong muscular person in good shape, it may be another 100 yards each time; for an absolute beginner, it may be another fifteen yards. Pay attention, and see what feels right to your whole body. Stay with your new distance until it is easy for you, and then add to it again. You don't need to add distance every time you run, but do it as often as it is comfortable. And don't be a slave to some arbitrary idea of how far you need to run each day. Again, be sensitive to yourself. You may have been running four miles each day, but if you are stiff and tired and achy and what you really need is a rest, don't insist on being up to your usual performance. It is how you run, much more than how far, which will ultimately improve your well-being.

Massage is an excellent preparation for running, especially if you have problems with muscle or joint stiffness. You can massage your feet, ankles, legs and knees to warm and loosen them. If you would like some tips on this, see the Self-Massage section in the Massage chapter.

Part of the reason Meir loves to run is that running and vision exercises supplement and support each other.

9–1   It is an excellent idea to do some palming (see exercise 8–5 in the Vision chapter to learn about palming) as a preparation for running. It relaxes the eyes along with the whole upper body, letting you go into your running feeling calm and refreshed. It also prepares your eyes for some exercise; there are a number of vision exercises that are easily done while running. Blinking the eyes frequently will relax them and break their habit of straining and staring. Another useful exercise is to shift your gaze back and forth between the ground in front of you and the farthest point in the distance. One of the healthiest things for the human eye is to look far into the distance – especially for nearsighted eyes, or for eyes which have been strained by too much close work. Running gives an excellent opportunity to look into the distance. When you begin to run, direct your gaze toward a point as far into the distance as you can see. Some people look only at the path in front of them, which can give the sense of being on an endless treadmill. If you look far into the distance, it can give you a sense of having already arrived at the point you are seeing. Visualization of this kind can reduce fatigue. (One of our clients imagines, while running, that someone is standing at her finishing-point holding a rope and pulling her along with it.) It also tends to keep your posture more erect, which will make running easier on your back and allow you to breathe more fully. You can also try picturing yourself running in the opposite direction – that is, if

you are running south, imagine yourself running north.

Now we come to breathing. If you have read the previous chapters, you already know how to breathe: deeply, fully, slowly, inhaling and exhaling through the nose *only*, and making sure that your exhale is as long and as complete as your inhale. (If you have not read the rest of the book, please be sure to read the Breathing chapter. Learning to breathe properly is the best preparation for running you can have.) Breathing through the nose will probably slow you down at first. Most of us have become mouth-breathers to some extent, and our nostrils are not used to taking in enough air to keep us going in vigorous exercise. Breathing through the nose takes more time, but it gives you a much deeper breath, and ultimately gives you more oxygen, since it allows more time for the exchange of carbon dioxide for oxygen within the lungs. So have patience.

The more you breathe through your nose, the more you will be able to, and eventually you will not need to breathe with your mouth even while running at top speed. The day Maureen felt she had really learned to breathe was the day she found herself actually panting through her nose instead of her mouth – it can be done. Ideally, of course, you don't want to be panting at all, but breathing evenly and fully. Make sure that your whole torso expands when you inhale. You should feel your chest lifting, your ribs moving further apart, and your abdomen and lower back stretching out. If you need to, slow your running speed for a while to allow your breathing capacity to expand gradually. Breathing deeply while running is the best way to ensure that you will stay relaxed both during and after running.

You don't need to hold your arms stiffly as you run. Many runners either hold the arms tightly, with the shoulders and elbows rigid and the fists clenched, or else pump the arms back and forward, working as hard with them as they do with their legs. This, obviously, is unnecessary and fatiguing, particularly if you run for long periods of time. Your shoulders have enough opportunities to get tense – this should not be one of them. Practice running with your arms hanging loosely at your sides, moving only with the motion of your body. If you do want to raise your arms, keep your shoulders down and your hands relaxed.

9–2   You can use your hands to massage and relax different parts of your body while you run. Massaging your chest will help you to breathe more fully. Stroke and tap along the sides of your neck. Place your palms on each side of your head and pull upward to stretch the neck muscles. Pound with your fists and pinch with your fingertips – very lightly – on your thighs, hips and lower back, to keep the muscles loose. Massaging your scalp is also very relaxing, especially if you work your fingers under your hair and lift the hair slightly as you massage; this not only relaxes the scalp but also cools off your head.

9–3   Concentrate on your feet. Many runners have an image of the torso, especially the lower back, lifting and moving the heavy legs, with the feet dragging along behind, and this visualization by itself can be exhausting. Think instead of your feet as the propelling force, as if they have a life of their own and are carrying your body along with them.

Your front knee should be bent as the foot touches the ground, and should then bend even further. It straightens gradually as the foot pushes against the ground and the other knee comes forward. This will give you your best forward impetus, and will also protect your knee joints from the impact that would result from hitting the ground with the knees locked or stiff.

9–4   Fatigue often comes from a feeling of fighting gravity. Visualization can help you here. You can visualize that your body is utterly weightless, a balloon on a string attached to your feet, being blown along by the wind. Or you can go with the pull of gravity, imagining yourself firmly planted on the ground, with the earth itself carrying you forward. Picture the revolving motion of the earth, and imagine that it is this force which carries you forward. You will be surprised to find how much your imagination, or attitude, can change the way you feel. One of our clients used to have to carry two full, very heavy water-buckets on a wooden yoke across her shoulders every morning, but said that she actually liked this because she imagined the weight of the buckets forcing her tense shoulders to drop and her tight neck to lengthen. When she felt that her body was being helped by the hard labor, and let her muscles work with the pressure rather than against it, it actually felt good to her. If you constantly give your mind images of effortlessness, lightness and ease, the strain on your muscles will be eased dramatically.

One of the greatest things about any vigorous exercise is that it can help us to strengthen new sets of muscles, and so balance our use of our bodies. But if we exercise with a sense of strain, we'll find ourselves falling back on the same old muscles we use all the time for everything. If you are in the habit of making your back work for the rest of your body – that is, contracting the back muscles when it is really some other set of muscles that needs to work – then you will find yourself doing the same thing during running, especially if you begin to tire. Unconsciously, your back will tighten to take some of the burden off the rest of you. However, this does not decrease your fatigue – just the opposite is true. The only reason the body does this is because it is in the habit of doing it. Because it senses you are under stress, it starts to call on the aid of 'backup' muscles which really should only be used in an emergency. This is one of the reasons why we so strongly encourage cultivating a sense of relaxation in running: it will allow you to develop new muscles and new ways of moving, whereas a sense of strain will inhibit you.

As you can see, most of the above instructions and suggestions have to do with breaking existing patterns and habits of movement and attitude. Most people will run the same way they do everything else in their lives. If they tense their shoulders at work, they will do so while running; if they breathe shallowly, squint and strain their eyes, walk stiff-legged, land more heavily on one foot than the other, tighten the abdomen – whatever – they will bring these habits into running. Because running is more strenuous than other activities, the bad effects will show up faster, in the form of injuries to muscles, tendons and joints. This is why we encourage people to be aware of everything they are doing while running – and to change or vary it, if possible, in order to create a more balanced use of the body. The sole purpose of the following exercises is to help you break your movement patterns and experiment with new ones.

9–5 It is important to vary the height of your steps while running. If you lift your feet exactly the same distance off the ground each time, you are forcing exactly the same muscle fibers to work, and placing a sharp impact on exactly the same part of each joint. Lifting your legs a little more or a little less will distribute muscle use and joint impact much more evenly. If you run at the beach, you can do this automatically by switching from the packed wet sand to the soft dry sand; if you run on a path, it helps to run on one where the ground is slightly uneven and forces you to make the adjustment. If your path is mostly smooth and even, then it will be up to you to remember to vary how high you lift your feet. It may seem more of an effort to lift them higher, but in fact you may actually be reducing your fatigue, since you will be using many different muscles rather than overworking a chosen few. Be sure, however, that you keep the center of your body at more or less the same level from the ground – you are trying to lift your feet higher, not your whole body.

One day Meir ran ten miles, a goal he set for himself though for him it was then an unusually long distance. Finding that he was only able to lift his feet about a foot off the ground, he tried to lift them higher and found that his body would not cooperate with this request. His muscles had fallen into a pattern of movement and would not budge from it. If you come to such a point, the best thing to do is to take a break and do some exercise which will 'confuse' your muscles and thus help them to break out of their pattern. One such exercise is crosscrawling, which is described in more detail as exercise 6–22 in the Nervous System chapter. This movement imitates the kind of movement you did before you learned to walk, 'reminding' your brain and nervous system of a time when your coordination was just beginning to develop, before you had developed imbalances and uneven stresses in your movement and posture. It allows your brain and nerves to 'think' about movement as easy, balanced, coordinated; and allows your muscles to respond accordingly. After cross-crawling, Meir returned to running and found that he could now lift his feet higher, and with less effort. With the movement pattern broken, he could use different muscles – muscles which had not already been fatigued by prolonged use.

9–6 Working some other exercises into the running also helps to break up movement habits, and adds a lot to the benefits of running. If your balance is good, you can turn your head slightly from side to side while running, or bend the upper body slightly forward, then slightly further backward. These movements stretch the neck and upper back and keep them from tensing as you run. You can bend forward very gradually with the whole torso, beginning with the shoulders and working slowly down the spine, then gradually straighten the body, then bend it backward, tilting the head first and letting the shoulders and back follow, then again slowly straightening. Extending your arms to the sides to balance yourself, you can tilt your body slowly first to one side, then to the other. These bending exercises will help keep your spine from stiffening. You can run with your toes turned inward, and then outward, which will increase the flexibility in your hips, knees and ankles.

9–7 Interlace your fingers behind your back, and then lift your arms up as high as you

comfortably can. Running forward with this stretch can be very effective in loosening the whole back, particularly the lower back.

9–8 To change your body's conception of how to run, the best exercise is to run backward. Try it and see how different it feels from running forward. Your back and abdomen are held differently, your arms move differently, your legs are lifted differently. Your head tends to be carried more erectly, since there is nothing to be gained from craning your neck forward as so many runners do. You will not be able to run as fast or as far backward as forward; the main value of running backward is to change the habits you may have developed while running forward. For example, there is more of a tendency to relax the abdomen while running backward; if you practice this enough, you will find yourself relaxing the abdomen during your regular running, along with your neck, your lower back and your quadriceps. At the same time, you are building up a completely different set of muscles from those used in running forward, making your overall body strength more balanced. Meir normally runs four miles, and out of that he will run at least half a mile backward.

9–9 If you can do so without losing your balance, turn your head slowly from side to side while you run backward. Not being able to see where your body is going may cause you to tense instinctively, and this head movement will counteract that, as well as letting you see a little of what is behind you. This head movement, whether running backward or forward, is also a good vision exercise. Moving the field of vision, whether you do this by moving the eyes or moving the head, stimulates the part of the eye which is responsible for sharp vision. Blink as you turn your head, and let your eyes shift rapidly from point to point.

Without turning the head, you can also stimulate your peripheral vision simply by focusing on a point in front of you so that your peripheral, rather than your central, eye cells have to work to see what goes by on either side of you. The tendency to allow the peripheral eye cells to work is stronger when we are going backward, because all the new visual information which the brain is interested in is provided by the peripheral, rather than the central, vision. If you have ever sat on a train facing backward, you may have noticed that you are much more likely to pay attention to what you can catch in the corners of your eyes.

9–10   Next, try running sideways. Again, you are using a different set of muscles. There are two ways to run sideways: you can either move one foot to the side and 'slide' the other foot to meet it, without crossing one leg over the other (fig 9–10A), or you can run so that

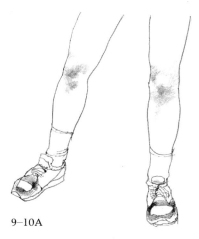

9–10A

one leg crosses the other (fig 9–10B). Both of them will use new muscles, and will relax your hip muscles by moving them in a more expansive way.

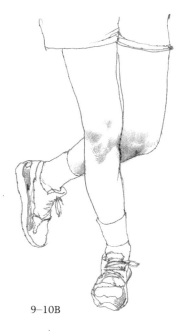

9–10B

For most people, running is not an exercise which makes them more flexible, loose or relaxed: its main purpose is to strengthen and build, which can also tend to stiffen and tighten, some parts of the body. Some runners do know how to run and stay relaxed, and that is what we try to teach people to do; nevertheless the chances are good that if you are a runner now, whether beginning or advanced, your tendency is to tighten your muscles while running. It can take years to overcome this. This is why a session of stretching and cooling-down exercises should follow every run. Relaxing your muscles after working hard with them will not erase any of the benefits of your exercise; it will only increase them. And it will reduce your chances of developing muscle or joint problems through going back into your daily life with your muscles still contracted as in running.

9–11   You may want to take special care to stretch out your back after running. If there is one area that we unconsciously tighten more than any other, it's the back. Exercises which stretch both the back and the lower body will be very helpful. One good one is to sit on the floor, with both legs on the floor and both knees bent and pointing in the same direction, so that if both knees are bent and pointed to the left, the left foot will be positioned near the right knee. In this position, slowly twist the body from side to side (fig 9–11).

Other excellent stretches are given in the Spine chapter in the sections titled Sideways Stretches for the Lower Back, Sitting Stretches and Rotations for the Lower Back, Spinal Arch, Spinal Flexion, and Loosening the Hips and Pelvis. Try all of these exercises and find which ones feel the most effective and pleasant for you, and then make them a regular finish to your running.

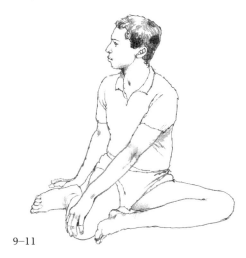

9–11

CHAPTER 10

Musicians

Our work has brought us in contact with many musicians – so many, in fact, that we have designed for them a special workshop, entitled 'You are the Instrument', to address the special needs of the musician. These needs vary widely, of course. A pianist, a violinist and a flautist all have specialized problems to deal with; they all use their hands differently and adopt completely different postures while playing. Yet there are some concerns common to most instrumentalists. We don't have enough room in this section to describe exercises relating to each instrument, but we can describe tools for awareness and relaxation which have helped every musician we have worked with. These have included harpists, violinists, fiddlers and violists, bassists, cellists, pianists, drummers and other percussionists, flautists, guitarists and electric guitarists, an accordion player and singers.

Before working with this chapter, work with the first six chapters of this book. Pay special attention to the coordination exercises in the Nervous System chapter (exercises 6–12 to 6–19).

All people who work for long periods of time with their hands are at some risk of developing pain and tension, not only in their hands but throughout the upper body. Many musicians have the added difficulty of needing to maintain an awkward or tiring position while playing: the violinist or flautist with the head twisted to the side, the harpist with arms held up unsupported, the saxophonist who has to hold up a heavy instrument. The range of problems includes tendinitis, muscle cramps and spasms, arthritis, headaches, facial pain and eyestrain, and aches and pains in the chest and shoulder muscles. Perhaps the most common problem is carpal-tunnel syndrome – an inflammation that causes pain, burning and numbness in the forearms, wrists and hands.

These problems do not arise simply because you are using your hands a lot. As bodyworkers who sometimes use our hands for many hours a day, we have proven that it is possible to do so without pain. These problems happen as a result of using your hands and arms through tension, that is, using them while their muscles are continually tight and contracted. Some of this contraction is unavoidable, a part of the process of holding and playing the instrument. Much of it, however, is completely unnecessary. By becoming aware of it, you can eliminate it. This will not only reduce your pain, it will also vastly improve the quality of your playing.

There are three main elements to improving your musicianship: relaxation, strengthening and awareness. Relaxed muscles are more flexible and more mobile, allowing you to play with the precision, speed, tone and expression that you desire. Strong muscles tire less quickly, making it possible for you to practice for extended periods without fatigue. Most important of all, however, is awareness. The first level of awareness is simple body awareness. Many musicians lose this, intent as they are upon notes, pitch, timing and other technical aspects of music. Much of a musician's physical pain comes from forgetting, during playing, that it is the musician who is the real instrument and must be kept finely tuned. This includes awareness of how you are holding or moving, tensing or relaxing, your entire body while you play. Awareness of how you touch your instrument and how it responds to your touch, awareness of the sound you are making, is the second level of awareness. The exercises we have included in this section will both relax and strengthen your hands and upper body; their main focus, however, is on awareness – of you and of your music.

Relaxing the Body

You may not be aware of any practice-related pain or problem in your body. If this is the case, we nonetheless recommend that you do two things. First, visit a massage therapist, chiropractor, kinesiologist or other person who knows bodywork, and take your instrument with you. Have the practitioner watch you play, and ask that he or she tell you of any noticeable tensions or posture misalignments, or anything else that might eventually cause a problem. In this way you may be able to avoid future pain. Not all therapists have a gift for this kind of analysis, so explain what you want when you make the appointment. Second, be sure to make some form of relaxing exercise a part of your practice, whether it is Self-Healing work, yoga, stretches or t'ai chi. People often come to us very confused with a pain which they say 'developed suddenly'. In our opinion, the pain may *manifest* suddenly, but it *develops* through years of unconscious abuse.

If you do have a practice-related pain or tension, we recommend that you first comb this book for all of the exercises related to the particular problem area. Refer especially to the Nervous System chapter. Work daily on the exercises for your problem area, thinking of this exercise as a part of your musical practice – which it is, since it will certainly improve your practice for you to be pain-free. You may find that the problem will disappear, or you may find that it will shift. For example, a hip pain may in fact originate in a lower-back stiffness, and as you release the hip you may begin to feel the problem more in the back where it began. If so, then shift to the exercises for that area.

Another thing to remember is that you should take time during your practice period to do some stretching and relaxing exercises. You may tend to become stiff during practice, though we hope that as you increase your awareness you will be able to stay relaxed and comfortable. In either case, some body movement will be good for your energy level and sense of well-being, and will counteract the sedentary nature of playing. The following are a few exercises we recommend most.

Refer to the Spine chapter, exercises 4–2, 4–5 and 4–11, which is a very nice release from the tension of sitting still and a gentle stretch for the lower back and hips.

Refer to exercise 2–11 in the Circulation chapter. Let your hands flop against you as you turn, feel how the movement stirs up a slight breeze, and imagine that your arms are floating on this breeze. Try also exercise 2–15 from the same chapter, and then exercises 1–10 and 1–13 from the Breathing chapter.

10–1 Position yourself so that your hands and the toes and balls of your feet are touching the floor, keeping your heels in the air (fig 10–1). Move your hips up and down, so your middle body bends toward the floor and then pulls away from it. If your lower back is stiff this movement may be very limited at first, but its range will increase.

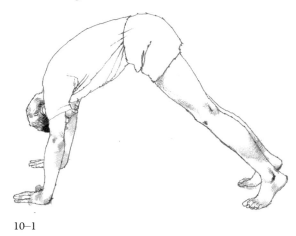

10–1

10–2 Stand with your back to the wall, feet slightly apart, and lean all your weight against the wall. Raise one knee as high as you can, and then take it in both hands to lift it up further; try to pull it up to your chest if possible. Hold it there for five or six seconds, then lower it and raise the other knee. Repeat this ten times, always alternating the knees.

Exercises for the Hands

We have two important recommendations for the exercises for the hands, wherever applicable:

(1) After moving the hand or finger or wrist as described in the exercise, stop and visualize yourself performing the same movement smoothly and without any effort. Move again, and see whether the movement has indeed become smoother and easier.

(2) Exercise one hand, and then compare it to the second hand before exercising that. Is it warmer, lighter, more flexible? This will help you to learn the effects of each exercise, and is therefore important especially while familiarizing yourself with each exercise.

10–3 Sit, and support one forearm on your lap, or on a table or the arm of a couch. Open and close your hand very slowly. Visualize that your fingertips are leading this motion, as though by their moving they pull the fingers, then the palm, along with them. Try to feel the movement of bones and muscles and tendons under your skin. As you open and close the hand, feel the muscles running through your forearm and hand. The area may feel tight and the muscles rigid. Imagine them relaxing completely, becoming loose and flexible. With your thumb pressing on the inner side of your forearm and your forefingers on the outer side, massage gently and firmly up and down the forearm (fig 10–3); then tap with your fingertips, especially on the places where the muscles feel tight. Continue to do this while opening and closing the hand. Repeat the exercise with the other hand, and then with both simultaneously.

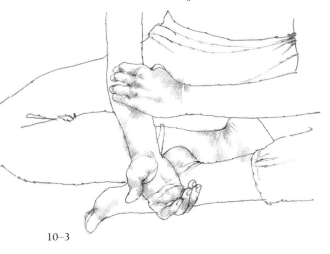

10–3

Fill a deep basin with warm water, and repeat this exercise with your hand immersed. If you have a problem with swelling in your hands, add some salt to the water.

10–4   Hold the bases of your palms against each other, and tap the fingertips of one hand against those of the other hand (fig 10–4A and 10–4B). Let your wrists and fingers be loose. Imagine that the tips of the fingers are leading the motion, and that no muscles of the arms, wrists or hands are involved in the motion.

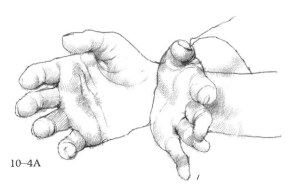

10–4A

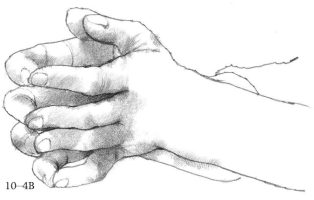

10–4B

10–5   Hold your hands about six inches apart, with the palms facing each other. Imagine that there is a current of energy that runs between them (we feel that there is). Imagine this energy moving in different directions – drawing the hands together like a magnet; pushing the hands away from each other; connecting each finger; expanding and contracting as it flows; growing warmer and more electric as you play with it.

Refer to exercise 7–1 in the Massage chapter, which is probably the most effective exercise for increasing sensitivity in the fingers. Continue with exercises 7–2 to 7–7. Massage doesn't just relax your hands and relieve pain: it will make your hands more sensitive, increasing your ability to get just the sound you want out of your instrument, to put just the sound you want into your music.

Continue with the Circulation chapter, exercises 2–17 and 2–21 to 2–24.

Now you are ready to continue with some advanced hand techniques, many of which combine massage with movement to simultaneously relax, strengthen and sensitize your hands.

10–6   Close your eyes and imagine each finger separately expanding and contracting. First visualize the fingers doing this by themselves; then imagine that your breath flows into them, expanding the fingers as you inhale and shrinking them as you exhale.

10–7   Massage each joint separately. There are fourteen finger joints as well as eight small bones that make up the wrist. Imagine the spaces between the bones in each joint, and visualize your massage making these spaces a little larger. The freer your joint movement, the easier and smoother will be your playing. As far as hands are concerned, you are a dancer, and you need a dancer's flexibility.

10–8   Place your palms together, interlace your fingers, and rotate the hands from the wrists, ten times in each direction. First, use the muscles of your forearms to push the hands; next, imagine that your wrists are the moving force; then your fingertips. Then move the hands in rotation by allowing one hand to relax while the other pushes for the first half of the rotation, then switching for the second half of the rotation.

10–9   Clasp your hands, with fingers interlaced. Flex the right wrist backward, with the back of the hand toward the arm, so that the movement causes the left wrist to passively bend (fig 10–9). Now let the right hand pull the left down and to the side, away from you, then toward you. Repeat all of these movements with the left hand actively moving the passive right hand.

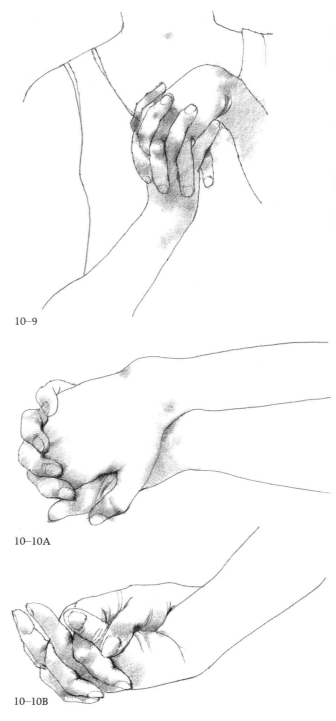

10–9

10–10A

10–10B

10–10   Cross your arms, turn your palms face-down and then facing each other. Interlace the fingers of both hands in that position (fig 10–10A), and now pull one hand to give the other wrist a stretch (fig 10–10B).

10–11   Spread the fingers of your right hand as far apart as possible. Place your left hand between the little finger and the third finger of the right hand, and, by slightly spreading the left-hand fingers, push the right-hand fingers as far apart as possible. Do the same between the third and second fingers (fig 10–11), the second and first fingers, and the first finger and thumb. Place your hands on a flat surface and compare how the two hands feel. Does the stretched one feel bigger? Switch hands and repeat the exercise.

10–12   Now stretch two fingers as far apart as you can, while bending the other three fingers toward your palm (fig 10–12). Do this with each pair of adjacent fingers.

10–13   Push your right thumb into the middle of your left palm, trying to feel the 'center' of the hand. Bend each finger in turn toward this center, without moving the other fingers as you do so. Do the same bending only the middle knuckles. Last, try to bend only the fingertips toward the center, so that the joints which move are the joints furthest away from the palm (fig 10–13). Repeat with the other hand.

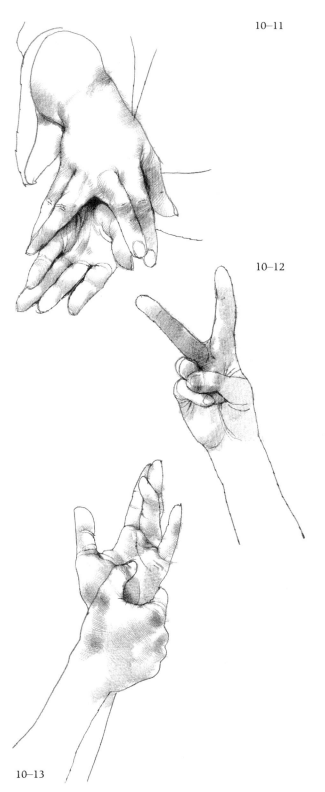

10–11

10–12

10–13

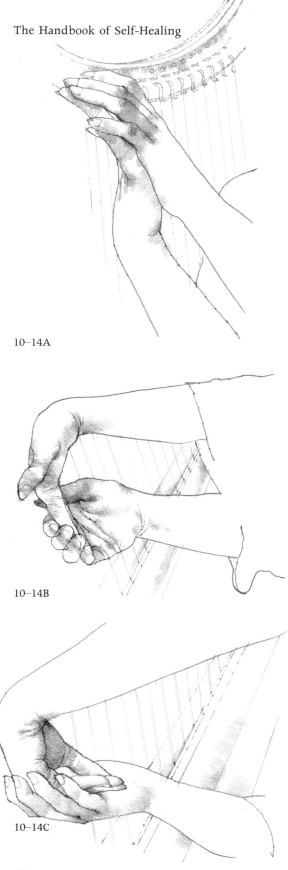

10–14A

10–14B

10–14C

10–14   Your fingers curl naturally toward the palm of your hand, and most hand movements emphasize this inward curl. This hand position, however, can turn your hand into a cramped, arthritic claw if you use your hands through tension. To reverse this tendency, gently bend your fingers backward by pressing on them with the fingertips of the other hand (fig 10–14A). Now bend each joint of each finger in turn backward, as far as it will comfortably go, and move it left, right and in rotation while stretching it backward.

Stretch the wrist backward and forward by pulling on all fingers (fig 10–14B and 10–14C).

10–15   With one hand, massage the space between the base of the little finger and the third finger of the other hand. Massage with your thumb on the palm side and your fore-finger on the other side of the hand, pressing from each side. As you massage, bend the little finger toward the center of the palm, without moving the other fingers. Now massage the space between the third and second fingers, and bend the third finger toward the palm. Do this in turn with each finger, and then switch hands.

10–16   Interlace your fingers, turn your palms so that they face away from you, and then stretch your arms straight out in front of you (fig 10–16). Hold this position for a count of five, breathing deeply, and allow your hands and wrists to stretch fully. Bend your arms slightly to ease the stretch, and then straighten them again. Repeat this five or six times, and then try this variation: interlace the fingers, turn the palms away from you and then *upward*, facing the ceiling. It may help to tuck the hands under your chin – the little fingers

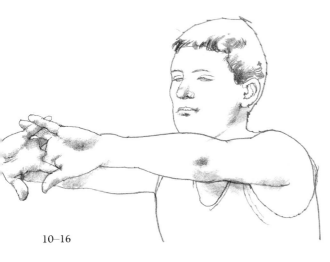

10–16

will be nearest your throat — so that they use the chin to push against as they turn upward. This variation stretches the forearms and elbows as well as the hands and wrists.

10–17 Stand on all fours, and rotate your forearms outward until your fingers point toward you and your little fingers are near each other (fig 10–17). To increase the stretch in your elbows, shift your weight by bending your knees as much as you feel comfortable with.

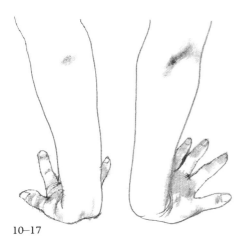

10–17

10–18 Rest your right elbow on a table while your left hand, holding all four fingers of the right hand, moves the right hand in a circle, rotating around the wrist. Now hold the right forearm with your left hand while the right wrist rotates itself. The first is passive movement; the second is active. When you are passively moving the wrist, let it relax completely; when it is actively moving, visualize that you are still moving it passively, and try to keep it equally relaxed. Rotate the wrist passively again. Does the movement feel any smoother?

Now move the wrist actively in a slow rotating motion; this time, however, hold the wrist itself instead of the forearm, and massage the wrist as the hand turns. Try not to let the pressure of your massage influence the movement of the hand, but massage as deeply as is comfortable, trying to feel the bones of the wrist and the spaces between them.

10–19 Massage with your fingertips, in a circular, palpating motion, beginning with the palms of your hands and moving up the inner forearm, the upper arm, the armpit area and into the chest. Then massage in the same manner, moving down the outer upper arm, the outer forearm and the back of the hand. Breathe deeply, and visualize your breath expanding and energizing your arms and hands.

10–20 Sit at a table. Tap your fingertips lightly on the table; then tap with the knuckles farthest from the palm; then with the middle knuckles; then with the knuckles nearest the palm; then with the inner side of the wrists; next with the outer side of the wrists; and last with the elbows. Tap from thirty to fifty times each.

10–21 Bring your arms to your sides with your elbows slightly bent (fig 10–21A), then bring them together so that the fingers meet (fig 10–21B) and bounce away from each other. Keep your wrists loose, and feel the motion of the air as your hands move toward each other. Repeat this motion thirty times.

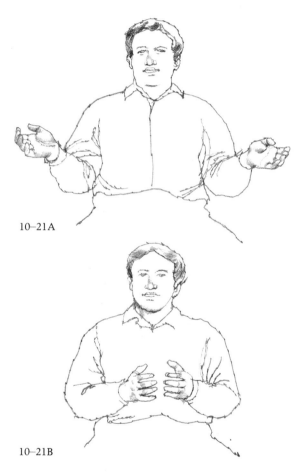

10–21A

10–21B

In ancient times, blind people were often trained as musicians and as masseurs. Lacking the sense of sight, they were well-known to have exquisite sensitivity, as well as unerring precision, in their sense and their use of touch. No doubt the lack of vision also helped them to develop finer hearing as well.

10–22 If you tend to look at your instrument when you play, then try playing your instrument in the dark. This will help you to develop your touch and your 'ear'. Take a simple exercise or passage that you know by heart, and practice playing it in the dark. You may make many mistakes at first, but you will probably be amazed at how fast your fingers learn to find the proper string or key or hole. Your kinesthetic sense will take over the work of your eyes. This creates a stronger sense of connection between your instrument and your hands.

When you feel that you are able to play a passage smoothly in the dark, continue playing while putting your awareness – that is, consciously trying to feel your sensations – in each joint, in each finger, on both hands, as you play. Conscious concentration on a particular area improves the nerve function in that area. Each part of your body has both sensory nerves (nerves which feel) and motor nerves (nerves which direct movement) and these nerves work together. When you pay attention to the messages from the sensory nerves, you are better able to direct the impulses of the motor nerves. Feeling what your hands feel (rather than ignoring it, as we commonly do) will help you to fine-tune their movement.

10–23 This is another exercise which can be done in the dark or with the eyes closed. Move your hands playfully and randomly over the keys, strings or holes of your instrument, without trying to play anything in particular or trying for any specific sound. Be aware of the sensations in your fingers, hands, arms, shoulders and chest as your hands assume various positions. Touch the instrument in ways that feel good to your body. If certain positions feel uncomfortable, try to find out why. Can you make them more comfortable by breathing, or dropping your shoulders, or stretching part of your arm or hand a little differently?

10–24   Sound is vibration. When we hear music, we are really feeling sound waves striking our eardrums at different frequencies. As the player, however, you can feel the sound in two different ways: not only by hearing it but also by feeling the vibrations which travel through your body whenever your fingers produce a note. For this exercise, concentrate at first on the latter sensation. Produce a series of notes – either specific or random – and feel the vibration of your touch against the instrument as it travels through fingers, hands, arms, chest and wherever else in your body you can feel it. See whether you can in fact feel it throughout your body; if not, try at least to imagine the vibrations traveling from your fingers throughout your body. Now pay attention simultaneously to these vibrations – the sound you feel through your hands – and to the music itself – the sound you feel with your ears. Imagine the two sets of vibrations meeting inside you.

10–25   You are now beginning to have a sense of 'feeling' sound. In order to enhance this sense, practice playing very slowly, lingering over each note in order to feel the vibration of that note traveling through you. From time to time, stop at one note and play it a number of times, perhaps ten or fifteen, altering your touch so that the note sounds different. Don't try for any particular tone color; just see how changing the intensity of the touch, the position of your finger, hand or arm, or even the thought in your mind, can alter the quality of sound that you produce. In other words, feel

the relationship between the nature of your touch and the nature of the sound it produces. Again, do all of this very, very slowly and pay attention to vibrations as you did in 10–24.

10–26   One of your ultimate goals is to make your playing effortless. You can bring yourself closer to this goal by learning to release your *sense* of effort. Practice playing as lightly as you possibly can. Imagine that your arms are weightless, your shoulders and head are floating, and your hands are boneless and light as silk. How lightly can you touch and still produce a sound?

10–27   Much of your sense of strain may come from trying too hard, playing too forcefully, and using muscles which are not at all needed for the motion. Hold your hands with the palms facing each other, and tap just the fingertips of both hands together, about 100 times. When the fingertips feel warm, tingling and stimulated by this tapping, play a short piece, trying to play with your fingertips *only*. Imagine that the rest of your hand, arm and so on is completely limp, and that only the fingertips can move. This exercise will strengthen your hands by encouraging you to relax your forearm muscles, which sometimes work too much for the fingers, and will also increase the sensitivity of your fingertips, which are after all the parts which have the most contact with the instrument. It will also encourage the rest of your body to relax while you are playing.

10–28   Nothing will relax you as much as will full, regular breathing. We believe also that directing the inner rhythm of your body can improve your rhythmic sense while playing.

Select a piece you know by heart, and play it at the slowest possible speed, while coordinating it with your breathing. Inhale; play a note; exhale; play a note; inhale; play a note; exhale; play a note; and so on. This part of the exercise is not only to help you to coordinate your breathing with your playing, but also to get you to breathe in the first place, since many musicians become so caught up in the mechanics of playing that they forget to take a real breath for minutes at a time. When you have established the rhythm described above, play your piece, still very slowly, this time coordinating your breath with the phrasing of the piece, rather than with every other note — for example, you might inhale for the space of two measures, and then exhale for the space of three measures. Keep your breathing in time with your playing.

10–29   When we play music, we use both hands simultaneously. Since each of us has a dominant hand, the weaker hand may not always receive the attention it needs to develop fully. This exercise will help you to concentrate on each hand, and is also a coordination exercise which strengthens your central nervous system. Play something relatively simple, and as you do so, focus strongly on what just one hand is doing. If you are focusing on your left hand, tap your right foot in rhythm with what the left hand *only* is doing. If you are focusing on your right hand, tap your left foot in time with what the right hand *only* is playing. Do this for two or three minutes, and then switch to the opposite hand and foot.

10–30   Play once again with your eyes closed, and try to create a mind's-eye picture of the patterns of sound you are making, whether it is a single line of sound going up and down and in ripples, or several interweaving patterns. Now open your eyes and watch your fingers move, imagining that they are creating the patterns you have visualized.

10–31   Play your piece again, slowly, and this time focus on the spaces of silence between the notes. Listen intently to this silence, and see how listening to it affects the feeling of the piece.

10–32   Play a short piece at normal speed, once. Then sit and hear yourself playing the piece in your mind, trying to recall how every individual note sounded. Repeat this five or six times, and see whether your recollection of your playing deepens or changes in any way, or whether you have any trouble holding the memory of the sound in your mind. Repeat this with the same piece, then try it with another piece.

10–33   If at all possible, change hands. Try to play a few notes holding your instrument in the opposite direction. You can do this with a guitar, an accordion, a violin and many other instruments. If you cannot, then try to place the instrument in a different position: lean your harp or fiddle on the opposite shoulder, for example. It will feel very awkward, but it is great exercise for the central nervous system. Playing normally again may feel easier than ever.

You can also exercise your central nervous system by playing or working with one of the exercises while doing other motions, such as rotating your head and opening and closing your jaw.

Visualization

Your central nervous system cannot always distinguish between a thought and an actual event, and it will often cause your body to respond to a thought with exactly the same reactions as it would have to an actual event. This is one of the reasons why visualization is such an important part of our work. Sometimes we can bring ourselves closer to our goal just by creating a mental image of what we want to achieve. If we imagine that our fingers are long and light, it can help them to behave — that is, to play — as though they are in fact long and light. If we imagine that we are one with our instrument, it can help us to produce a sound that reflects that. The following are a few meditations/visualizations that can help to give added quality to your playing.

10–34   Imagine that your fingers are very long. Do this first while holding your hands loosely in your lap, eyes closed and breathing deeply. Imagine that your fingers grow longer with every breath you take in. Then begin to play, holding the image of long, graceful fingers. Next, stop playing, close your eyes, and imagine that not only your fingers but your arms are very long, very graceful, very flexible. Play again, holding this image. Stop, and now see not only your arms and fingers but also your spine and your neck as long, graceful, flexible. Play while holding this image of your body.

10–35   Touch your instrument, imagining energy pouring forth like radiant light or heat from your fingers, from your whole hand, and coursing down your arms from your chest. Breathe deeply, and imagine that the ultimate

source of this constant, strong flow of energy is in your heart.

10–36   Begin some simple familiar piece, and, as you play, imagine that your fingers don't just touch the instrument but actually pass right through it, penetrating it and becoming a part of it.

10–37   Conversely, play the same piece and imagine that, instead of you lifting your fingers after playing a note, the instrument actually pushes them off – every time you hit a string or a key or cover a hole, imagine that the instrument pushes your finger away. Next, imagine that when your fingers land on the instrument they bounce off it, as though they are rubber.

10–38   Imagine that your body, like the body of your instrument, is a hollow space, filled with resonance and vibrating whenever a note is sounded. Play, and imagine that it is your body, rather than your instrument, which is producing the musical sounds. Many musicians speak of a feeling that their instrument is playing them; use your imagination and feeling-sense to visualize that this is *literally* so.

10–39   As you play, visualize the sound waves circling your fingers, and imagine your fingers being guided and directed by these vibrations, as though every note is a little wind that carries your fingers effortlessly on to the next note.

10–40   Place your hands as you would to play a note, and inhale deeply, imagining that not only your whole body but the body of your instrument is filling and expanding, becoming larger and lighter. Then play the note as you slowly exhale. Do this with the entire chromatic scale.

10–41 Close your eyes, and once again play your easy, familiar piece, while imagining that you are a guest at your own concert. Picture yourself playing as you listen, and really observe what this musician is doing. This is a technique musicians have used to get over stage fright. Distancing yourself a little can help to ease emotional tension and give you more objectivity about your playing. It may also help you to enjoy your playing more.

CHAPTER 11

Computers and Office Work

This chapter is for anyone who spends most of the day working at a desk, and particularly for those who spend more than an hour or so a day working – or playing – with a computer, for those whose job compels them to sit at a computer terminal and for those who just can't tear themselves away. The computer is one of the most useful tools and entertaining toys ever devised. Unfortunately, though, it is also becoming the leading health menace to the white-collar workforce. Almost as long as computers have played a major role in the workplace, the people who use them have complained of a host of physical problems which stem directly from extensive computer use. These conditions include eyestrain and deterioration of vision even temporary blindness – headaches and migraines; and severe, debilitating pains in the neck, shoulders, wrists and back. There is even evidence that miscarriage is more common among women who work at computers, though whether this is a result of radiation from the monitor screen or just of too much stress on a pregnant body is not known. In any case, if you work at a computer we don't have to tell you about these problems – you, or your co-workers, will know all about them.

There are many things, most of them quite simple, which can make your working environment better. Adjustable-height chairs, keyboards and terminals are absolute essentials. If you are going to be doing something for hours at a time, your posture and position must be as comfortable and natural as possible, to avoid damaging strain on your joints, muscles and eyes. You must be able to sit so that your back is straight and totally supported, while your hands and your eyes are at exactly the right level for you, not for someone else. There should be plenty of light – preferably natural light (make every possible effort to avoid fluorescent light) – but it should not be projected directly onto the screen or it will create a glare that can hurt your eyes. Terminals should be equipped with glare reducing screens. Almost all screens are made this way now, and we hope that eventually all companies will be using them. The print or numbers displayed on the screen must be large enough and clear enough to be read easily, or they will ultimately damage your eyes. If the print is small or muddy, find out whether the problem is with the monitor or with the software, and try to change it.

Most important, however, is that you take frequent short breaks from your strenuous activity, and that you have a space, away from the workplace, where you can go and sit, stretch, exercise or lie down during your breaks. These are the minimum considerations a computer worker needs. And that goes double if your employer is yourself – a lot of people are more demanding, more abusive, less considerate of their own health than any employer could be! It's great to love what you are doing with the computer, but not when it makes you forget what you are doing to yourself.

After you have done the best you can with your working conditions, the rest is up to you. Every job carries with it some great perks and some major drawbacks. You happen to have a job which is hard on your whole upper body and harder still on your eyes. One obliging company took upon itself the responsibility of paying the cost of new eyeglasses when it saw how rapidly and how often its workers were suffering loss of vision. If you want to avoid the health hazards associated with computers, there are many things you can do both to prevent and to alleviate these changes. And, like one of our arthritic clients, who, through movement exercises, had a more flexible body after recovering from arthritis than she had ever had before her illness, you may find yourself treating your body better than you ever did before.

Of course, if you have a very specific, chronic or severe problem due to your work already, you may find it best to begin by working with the part or parts of your body most affected. The Spine chapter, the Vision chapter, the Joints chapter, the Circulation and Nervous System chapters, all have exercises which are relevant for you. This chapter contains more general guidelines for office work – and recovery from it – on a daily basis.

You have to be ready for your work. Perhaps you have trouble preparing yourself for it emotionally. Some of this emotional stress may stem from the physical demands of your job, without your being aware that this is so. If this is the case, there are many things you can do to feel better physically and thus start your day with a better mental outlook. For example, many people wake up stiff and don't get a chance to loosen up before they lock themselves into position at their desk for the whole day, at the end of which they are too tired to have much enthusiasm for flopping their spines or muscles or joints into flexibility. You will be doing your body a big favor, and improving the quality of your whole day, if you will take just a few minutes to limber up before you start work. (Of course, if your problems with work are on a more truly emotional basis, we strongly recommend that you do whatever you can do to remedy your situation, relationships and so on. Just as physical discomfort can darken your mental picture, emotional stress can contribute to all sorts of health problems.)

In Japan, businessmen are beginning to die for no apparent cause – not even a heart attack. They just go. And no one is mystified by this phenomenon. They see these men shoot out of bed in the morning, take five minutes to eat some rice and miso – standing up, dash out the door, run for the train, ride clinging to a strap and hemmed in by hundreds of others for up to two hours, and after this ordeal fling themselves into their workday without a second to calm down. The rest of their typical day is no more conducive to health or happiness, but somehow it is this harried beginning above all that seems to set the pattern for a totally frenetic life. Does your own day start off anything like this? Is there anything you can do about it? Like, for example, give up the last half-hour of television at night, so that you can have that half-hour in the morning to do a few minutes of stretching, take a few more minutes with breakfast, and arrive at work just a couple of minutes earlier to palm your eyes (exercise 8–5 in the Vision chapter) before you harness them to the video screen? Could you take a bus instead of your car to work, so that you could spend the time doing breathing exercises, palming, or massaging your hands and wrists? It really takes very little effort to make a big difference in how you will feel throughout the day. Think of your preparation as similar to the warm-up exercises of a dancer or athlete.

It is not so much what you are doing at the computer but how you are doing it that is the problem. It's true that there are some very non-optimal conditions built into the activity itself. You are looking for hours at something very close to you, and near vision is much more of a strain on the eyes than distance vision. You are sitting still, and the body craves movement. You are performing the same motions over and over again, when varied and balanced use of muscles is what your body really needs.

However, these factors are not the only ones which cause problems. Much of our unconscious behavior makes things worse than they need to be. Computer workers, typically, do the following things:

- squint at the terminal screen, which tightens and hardens the muscles surrounding the eyes;
- stare fixedly at the screen, forgetting to blink;
- never look away from the screen to something more distant;
- ignore their peripheral vision, looking only at what is directly in front of them on the video display;
- allow their shoulders to round forward, and hold them high, near the ears, for no reason;
- tense their shoulders, chest and arms, contracting and 'working' these muscles when all they really need to move are their fingers;
- let the head sink into the chest, and the chest cave in upon itself;
- sit so that the lower back caves in, forming a swayback, or with legs crossed, encouraging low-back pain;
- become so absorbed in their work that they forget to breathe deeply for hours at a time;
- neglect to go to the bathroom, leading to pelvic tension.

These are all things that you can avoid, once you become aware of doing them, and avoiding them is the best preventative measure you can take.

A Healthy Workday

You really should get up early enough to allow for a little limbering-up exercise, an unhurried breakfast and a couple of minutes at your workplace before you begin work at the desk or terminal. Try to take a few minutes before you get out of bed to do some deep, slow, relaxing breathing. Many people, especially those with demanding schedules, don't relax completely while they sleep; they may wake up with tense face and neck muscles, from grinding their teeth while they sleep, a stiff neck or back from sleeping in uncomfortable positions, or general tiredness from tossing and turning or dreaming anxious dreams all night. If you sense that your sleep has not really rested you, don't be mystified – this is very common.

However, any amount or quality of sleep does some good, and you can often recover fairly quickly from the effects of a restless sleep. Taking ten or fifteen long, complete breaths, in and out through the nose, will relax and energize you. If your neck feels stiff, lie on your back without a pillow and turn your head slowly from side to side, then move it in rotating motion (without lifting it – imagine that you are drawing a circle with your nose). Clasp your hands and stretch your arms behind your head. Pull your knees up to your chest to stretch your lower back, and move them in rotation. Stretch your legs out, and point, flex and rotate the feet. Think of how a cat stretches when it wakes up, or how you used to stretch deliciously when you were a child on a Saturday morning, and your body will begin to expand itself naturally. This whole process need not take more than five minutes, but it will put a different face on your day.

Another ten minutes to do slightly more vigorous stretches will also help your stamina tremendously. Wait until you have been up and moving around for a few minutes, giving your muscles a chance to loosen up naturally and your blood a chance to start circulating. You should choose five or six stretches and do each one for about two minutes, selecting those which best suit your needs. You may prefer yoga asanas, or have some favorite stretches of your own.

A very short word about breakfast: eat it. We can't tell you what to eat; we are not nutritionists, and, besides, everyone's nutritional needs are different. You need to pay attention to how different foods affect you, and choose accordingly. You should be aware, though, that almost everyone is affected similarly by sugar and caffeine. Both of these things will give you a strong feeling of energy and well-being – *temporarily*. How long this feeling lasts will be determined by your particular metabolism, but it will almost certainly be followed by tiredness, nervousness, irritability and reduced effectiveness. If you have a tendency to be hypoglycemic (this means that your blood sugar gets used up more quickly than other people's), this change can happen as quickly as half an hour after that café mocha or glazed doughnut. Other people may be able to keep themselves pumped up by constantly replenishing their sucrose or caffeine supply. These people are often the ones who function beautifully at work, then come home exhausted and may be irritable for the rest of the day. There is absolutely nothing to be gained from sugar or caffeine, and much to be lost, so we strongly suggest that you discover those foods which will give you a sustained feeling of steady, calm energy, rather than a fast and fleeting burst of it. Your breakfast may consist of eggs or other proteins, grains, vegetables, dairy products or fruit, depending on what works best for you. Try different foods and different combinations until you find out what keeps you going the longest and the best. This will be different for everybody; don't let anyone else tell you what ought to work for you. The right breakfast will affect your sense of well-being throughout the entire day.

When you arrive at work, give yourself a few minutes to settle in and relax, especially if you have a nerve-racking commute between home and work. Take at least five minutes to palm. You may want to stretch your lower-back, hip or hamstring muscles. If your co-workers are curious, you may want to let them in on what you are doing, and why – it can help them too.

In the Circulation chapter, we have included a section called 'Sitting', in acknowledgement of the fact that many of us have to do a lot of it, especially at desks and terminals. Please read this section, and use whatever you can from it to prepare your body for all the sitting it will do during your workday.

Your Eyes

We recommend that you read the Vision chapter to understand the basic techniques and principles of eye exercises.

Sit at a distance at which you can read comfortably. This sounds so obvious, but many people come to realize that for months they have been squinting and straining to see, without being conscious of it. Make sure the light is good. It should not be in front of you, shining directly into your eyes, nor directly behind you, reflecting into and glaring off your screen. If possible, plentiful but indirect natural light is the best. And, if at all possible, place the computer where you can look up frequently to gaze at something more distant – near a window would be perfect, but you could even place it so that you could glance down a long hallway (put up a picture at the end of the hall so that your eyes will be attracted toward the distance, if possible). By 'frequently', we mean at least every five minutes.

Palming should become an intrinsic part of your work and your life. There simply is nothing as effective as palming to help your eyes recover from the strain they are under-

going. Stop at least every fifteen minutes to palm for two or three minutes. You don't even need to get up from your workstation – just close your eyes, cover them with the cupped palms of your hands, breathe deeply, relax your body, and imagine that you see a deep soft black. Once an hour, take a slightly longer break of five minutes or so. During lunch, try to find ten or fifteen minutes to palm and breathe deeply. Does this sound like a lot of palming? Think about how much and how often you would need to rest if you were walking briskly along with a heavy load on your back. This is roughly the equivalent of how much computer work stresses and tires your eyes. The amount of rest we have suggested is an absolute minimum, in either case.

You should also palm for twenty minutes or so either before or after work. You can combine the palming with meditation, or with listening to some relaxing music, or just consider it as the brief rest you would have needed anyway to recharge yourself after your workday. It is truly the most refreshing rest you can have, not only for your eyes but for your whole body. The Vision chapter gives much more complete information on how palming helps, and how it should be done (exercise 8–5). Please be sure to read this section. If you never do anything else for your eyes, this one thing will still benefit them enormously.

Blink constantly – not rapidly, not hard, but frequently. This will help you to break the pattern of staring fixedly which contributes so much to eyestrain and tiredness. Blinking moisturizes your eyes, gives them a momentary massage, helps to reduce tension in the muscles around the eyes by breaking their holding-pattern, and also encourages your eyes to move from point to point by interrupting your staring. If you have experienced dry or burning, inflamed or itching eyes, the simple act of blinking will go far toward alleviating these conditions.

Blinking will help to give your eyes a sense of movement. The whole problem with computer work, for your eyes as much as for the rest of your body, is that it tends to create rigidity. The tightness you feel in your neck, shoulders, arms or back is also happening in your eyes, where it may be more difficult for you to feel it. Exactly as moving and stretching relieve stiff muscles, fluidly moving your eye muscles and your point of focus will keep them from tightening, and therefore from tiring.

Resting your eyes is one important part of keeping them healthy. Learning how to use them without strain is the other. There are two basic types of eye-movement exercises. The first, and simpler, type involves movement of the muscles around the eyes. Chinese workers and students routinely do eye-movement exercises to stretch and tone their eye muscles. We highly recommend these exercises, especially before work, to increase blood circulation in and around the eyes.

11–1 With your head held still, move both eyes in a circle, in the same direction (either clockwise or counterclockwise). Move them three times in this direction, and then three times in the opposite direction. Do this slowly, blinking once per second, and make sure both eyes are moving equally, at the same speed, covering the same amount of ground. The best way to make sure of this is to really look at what your eyes are seeing, rather than going unconscious while your eyes make an aimless sweep of the room, pay close attention to every detail they come across. Don't try to see anything in particular, but be aware of all that

you do see. Repeat this same exercise moving your eyes from left to right, from up to down, and from one diagonal corner to the other – upper right to lower left, for example. These exercises can also be done with one eye open and the other covered, especially if you have one eye that tends to dominate. In that case, cover the dominating eye more frequently.

Refer also to exercise 8–2 in the Vision chapter.

The second type of eye movement is much more subtle. It involves a constant shifting of your point of focus from one small point to the next, so that you are constantly moving your attention from one tiny detail of your visual field to the next, and the next. This type of movement uses and strengthens the part of your eye which sees detail most clearly, the spot called the macula, at the center of the retina. It is within the macula that the clearest and sharpest images are received by the eye. The other side of the story is that the macula can only see small bits of visual data at any given time ('time' meaning a tiny portion of a second). So, in order to form a clear picture of what is seen and send this image back to the brain, the macula in a healthy eye moves continuously from point to point, forming a total picture out of many tiny, sharply detailed visual bits. We believe that poor vision results at least partially from a slowing-down of this macular movement. This can happen when, as a result of boredom, a person becomes uninterested in her surroundings, does not bother to look at details but instead 'spaces out' and looks at nothing. It can also happen as a result of anxiety, which can make people frantically try to take in every visual detail at once, which the macula simply is not equipped to do. This might happen, for example, if you were searching wildly for some necessary information, and forced your eyes to try to take in entire paragraphs at one gulp, so to speak. Or it can happen as a result of staring fixedly, which discourages the natural movement of the macula.

All of these tendencies are easy to develop at the video screen. We counteract them by a process called shifting, which is nothing more complicated than moving the eyes from point to point in a way that imitates the macula's natural tendency. You create strength in a weakened muscle by encouraging it to do what muscles do, optimally – that is, contract and relax, contract and relax. If your vision has lost its macular clarity and sharpness, you encourage your mind to engage with the macula in doing what it does best: moving frequently and fluidly from one small point to the next.

This process is exactly the opposite of what is taught in speed reading. If you have ever learned speed reading, please, for the health of your eyes, try to forget that you ever knew it. Speed reading is very good for what it is designed to do, which is to make it easier for you to take in large amounts of printed information in a relatively short time. It teaches you to read several sentences almost simultaneously, skipping over much of what you see. This type of reading hampers the action of the macula, ignoring its natural tendency to look at small areas and many details and to make a continuously flowing movement consisting of very small jumps from point to point. If you make it impossible for the macula to function, it will eventually become inactive, and the result will be the gradual loss of your ability to see with sharp, clear detail. 'Use it or lose it' applies to the macula as to any other body part. We believe that this type of eye

use may contribute to a condition known as macular degeneration, which is now the leading cause of adult blindness.

The plus side of working with the computer is that there is in fact plenty of movement and detail to give your eyes a healthy, instead of an exhausting, workout. You can follow the movement of the data as it appears on the screen, or the movement of your fingers as they type. Be aware of each letter, number, figure, picture on the screen as a visual form, not just as a piece of information. Look at letters, and spaces between letters, rather than at words. As frequently as you can, take a moment to 'trace' around the shape of a letter or a number with your eyes, rapidly moving from point to point on the outline of that letter. Move your eyes slightly from left to right, or up and down, as you did in exercise 11–1, tracing the shapes of all the letters in a row, at least once per page. This will not take more than a minute, and will eventually train your eyes to move in this way automatically. In our vision-improvement courses, we always suggest that people look at moving things, such as ocean waves; when these are not available, we have to create the movement by ourselves.

While concentrating on the rush of information on the video screen, it is very easy to completely forget about our peripheral vision. In this way the central-vision cells of the eye become overtaxed – a dangerous situation which may contribute to glaucoma as well as to loss of clear vision. Stimulating your peripheral cells will provide some rest for the central cells. The simplest way to do this is to hold up your hands to the side of each eye, look straight forward, and wiggle the fingers or wave the hands vigorously so as to attract the attention of the peripheral cells, which are best able to see things which are moving. This exercise is most easily done by people who work alone – if you do it in the office, you are going to have to explain it to people. There is no doubt, though, that it gives a feeling of rest to tired eyes, so maybe you can get your co-workers to try it. Another, less obvious, way to stimulate your periphery is simply to remind yourself to become aware, every so often, of your side vision, paying attention to it without actually taking your eyes off the screen. You are actually seeing quite a lot with your peripheral cells as you keep your eyes on the screen, but most of the time are not aware of it.

You can wake up the peripheral cells using exercises 8–15 to 8–19 in the Vision chapter. These exercises can be done before working, to activate the peripheral cells so that they will stay active while you work. They can also be done during and after work, to give your central cells a rest. **If you look away from the screen and toward your sides, you are only changing the location of your central vision, but if you keep your central vision occupied with the screen and simultaneously pay attention to what you see to each side, you are genuinely using your peripheral cells.**

The lens of your eye has a different shape when it looks at something close than it does when it looks at something in the distance. When looking into the distance, the lens remains relatively flat; when you must look at something closer, the lens 'accommodates' to this by becoming more curved or convex. It costs something of an effort for the eye to maintain the lens in this position, which is one reason why people who do a lot of close work tend to suffer loss of vision more than people who continually look at the distance. Since

you are spending so many hours doing close work, you will need to protect your eyes by making, as often as possible, the shift from near to distance vision.

For people who work on an upper floor and have access to a window, the simplest solution is to go to the window several times each hour and let your eyes sweep out to and along the farthest horizon that they can see. If you wear glasses, take off your glasses while you do this. Remember to look out the window or at a picture down at the end of the hallway, as often as you can. If you have no other alternative, just look up and around the room, to the ceiling and the farthest corners, as often as possible, and let your lens flatten for just those moments before you go back to work.

On your breaks, and on your way to and from work, remember to refresh your eyes by looking at distances whenever you can. Driving can actually offer a good opportunity to do this, just by looking as far down the road as you can see. At the top of a hill, look to the farthest horizon. When you walk, keep your eyes focused at the end of the block and beyond, or let them slowly sweep from the spot directly in front of you out to the horizon and back. Don't insist on seeing clearly in the distance, especially if you are nearsighted, just let your eyes move from point to point on whatever they can see – even if it is just a mass of shapes and colors – and, of course, remember to blink frequently. The very best rest for your eyes is to take them to some beautiful place which offers a faraway, broad horizon as well as lovely, soothing things to look at, such as the beach, an open field or the mountains. One of the reasons people feel so good when they get out into nature is that she is very kind and healing to the eyes as well as the rest of the body.

Another way to help your eyes is to keep your face relaxed. Strain in the eyes and in the muscles around the eyes can radiate to the entire face. There is also a tendency, during intense concentration, to clench the jaw muscles – particularly if you are frustrated or angry. The combination of eye tension and jaw tension can lead to a common condition called TMJ, or temporomandibular joint syndrome – a very painful facial neuralgia.

Tension in the face is actually fairly easy to relieve. Yawning frequently is one of the best and simplest ways; it stretches the jaw, moisturizes and relaxes the eyes, and reminds you to breathe. Opening and closing your mouth as wide as you can will also relax the jaw. Massaging and tapping on the jaw area will relax your whole face. You may be amazed to find out, through touching this area, how tight and sore it really is. For some ideas on relaxing the jaw muscles, turn to the Muscles chapter, exercise 5–50, and to exercise 7–14 in the Massage chapter. Refer to exercise 8–1 in the Vision chapter for a massage of the whole face in a way that will be especially helpful for your eyes, using acupressure points which have been known for centuries to help the eyes.

11–2   Let your whole face go slack, and blink rapidly. Tense every muscle in your face simultaneously, as hard as you can, and then let them all relax at once. Repeat this five times.

11–3   Applying hot and cold moist towels to your face, holding each one over the face for a minute or so, is extremely refreshing and relaxing to a tense face and tired eyes.

Your Body

There is a recognizable pattern of upper-body tension which can be found both in computer workers and in people with eye problems. In both groups, we almost always find tight jaws, extreme tension in the side neck muscles, and tightness of the upper trapezius and other shoulder muscles, as well as the muscles of the chest, sides and arms. There is a question as to whether this pattern of tension causes eye problems or whether eye problems cause this tension, and the question is unanswerable; each seems to cause the other. In any case, you can help either condition by relieving the other. Relaxing and strengthening your eyes with the eye exercises and practices we have described will definitely reduce your upper-body tension, and relaxing your neck, shoulder, arm and chest muscles will, in turn, benefit your eyes.

11–4   The first thing you can do to relax your upper body is to breathe deeply. Close your eyes, inhale deeply through your nose, and feel this breath expanding your chest and upper back. Drop your shoulders, let your arms rest comfortably at your sides, and relax your elbows and wrists. Now begin at the top of your head, and get in touch with your tense areas. How does your scalp feel? Your forehead? Your eyes? Your jaw? Your throat? Your neck? Your shoulders? Your chest? Your upper back? Your arms? Your hands? Allow each area in turn to relax. Ask each area in turn to expand as you inhale, and to shrink as you exhale. Try to really feel each area. You may be holding one shoulder higher than the other, or clenching one hand, or even expanding one side of the upper back more when you inhale. Learning to feel your tensions and the way you habitually use your body will help you to become more aware of things you may do to make these patterns worse, and will help you to stop doing them. You will find it helpful to repeat this exercise often during the day, checking in with your body to see how it's doing.

You may have developed frequent or even chronic pain or stiffness in one or several of these upper-body regions. If so, the following exercises will help to relieve it. If not, practicing them regularly will help to prevent problems from developing in the first place.

For a few exercises for neck tension, refer to the Breathing chapter, exercises 1–10 and 1–23; to the Circulation chapter, exercise 2–18; to the Joints chapter, exercise 3–26; to the Spine chapter, exercises 4–2, 4–21 and 4–26 to 4–28; and to the Nervous System chapter, exercise 6–15.

For shoulder tension, refer to the Breathing chapter, exercise 1–9; to the Shoulder section in the Joints chapter; and to the Muscles chapter, exercise 5–40.

For tension or pain in the arms, turn to the Breathing chapter, exercises 1–8, 1–10 and 1–13; to the Circulation chapter, exercises 2–12, 2–16 and 2–18; and to the Muscles chapter, exercise 5–44.

For tightness in the chest, refer to the Breathing chapter, exercises 1–5 and 1–18; to the Circulation chapter, exercises 2–2, 2–6, 2–10 and 2–13 to 2–15; to the Joints chapter, exercise 3–4; and to the Nervous System chapter, exercise 6–2.

For back problems, you will find it helpful to read the entire Spine chapter, trying each of the exercises which seem to apply to you and selecting those which work best for you. If needed, refer to the Back Pain chapter.

Your Hands

Your hands are kept very active in your work, second only to your eyes. This activity can be very good for them, if you use your hands in a relaxed, fluid way. It may even prevent arthritis in the fingers, since proper use of the joints keeps them healthy and lubricated. The problems that computer workers, typists and other keyboard users encounter are usually not with their fingers but with wrists, arms, shoulders, backs and necks. This is because, instead of developing strength and agility within their fingers, they contract other muscles – particularly those of the shoulders – and force them to work for the fingers. This is ultimately an exhausting effort for those muscles which are being needlessly tightened. Even worse than fatigue, though, is the effect upon your circulation. When your shoulders, neck and chest are constantly contracted, they inhibit the blood supply to the head and to the arms. If you have cold hands, you can often trace it directly to upper-torso contraction. If you often feel tired, confused or irritable, or just find it difficult to concentrate, you may have a tight neck that is limiting circulation to the brain. We believe that this may contribute to strokes, which are often caused by a temporary shut-off of blood to the brain.

11–5   The best thing you can do for your entire upper body is to remember that it is your fingers which should be working. Sit down at your keyboard, place your fingers on the keys, and begin to type, paying attention now not to the words on the screen but to what your muscles are doing. Imagine the top of your head stretching up toward the ceiling, your shoulders moving far apart from one another, your back and hips relaxing against your chair, and your arms at rest; let your jaw and your abdomen go slack. A tight jaw can tense neck muscles all the way into your shoulders, while a tense abdomen can paralyze your chest muscles and restrict your breathing. Visualize that no muscle except those in the hands is moving at all. When we focus mentally on a particular area, we are then more likely to use the muscles in the area we are concentrating on, and less likely to 'use' – that is, needlessly contract – muscles we really don't need. For example, we don't need to contract our shoulders, jaws or buttocks in order to type – but an amazing number of people tighten them anyway.

Continue your typing for five or ten minutes, and you will almost certainly see what we are talking about. You may find it very difficult to keep your body relaxed, your breathing deep and full, and your movement concentrated in your fingers. Notice which areas of your body want to try to work for your hands – these are probably chronic tension spots for you, and you may want to do some special relaxation work with them.

You may also feel your hands becoming tired, since they are working harder than usual. You cannot create aliveness, strength, flexibility and sensitivity in your hands just by remembering to work with them while you type – though doing so will go a long way toward that goal. You will reach it a lot faster, though, if you work on your hands with massage and special hand and finger exercises. These will stimulate the nerves of the hand, making it easier for them to work, and will also prevent conditions like tendinitis and carpal-tunnel syndrome which can stem from using your hands in a tense or rigid way.

The Massage chapter has a section which describes how to massage your own hands, either in preparation for using them for work, or to relax and soothe them when they are tired (exercises 7–2 to 7–7). A friend can help you with exercise 7–24. We have recommended these exercises for massage practitioners, but they are equally helpful for anyone else who works for hours with the hands, such as a factory worker, a musician or you. These exercises can and should be done before and after work. Even if you never have any trouble with your hands, these exercises will benefit you by strengthening your hands and focusing your attention on them. Practice also exercise 2–21 in the Circulation chapter, either lying down or sitting with your elbows supported.

Special exercises for the hands are described in the Circulation chapter, exercises 2–17 and 2–19 and the section on Hands; the Joints chapter, the Wrists section; and the Musicians chapter.

Co-Worker Massage

If you have a friendly atmosphere in the office, ask someone to give you a little massage on your shoulders, neck, scalp, arms or hands. A few companies have begun to employ massage therapists to give ten- or fifteen-minute massages to their employees on a regular basis, which is wonderful, but you don't need a professional practitioner – just offer a little neck and shoulder massage to someone who seems congenial. In working on your friend, you can show him how to work on you, if he likes. Once a person gets the feel of it, massage is easy to do. You can read the Massage chapter for techniques on massage of the shoulders, neck, face and head, hands and arms, or wherever seems appropriate.

Some good techniques are: to rub with both thumbs, in rotating motion, along the spine from the skull all the way down the back; to squeeze the trapezius muscle where it runs along the top of the shoulders; to gently but firmly hold the head and rotate it in each direction; to do the same with each shoulder in turn; to tap firmly with the fingertips along the length of each arm; to take hold of the hand, pull the arm gently out from the shoulder and shake it; to place the thumbs and fingertips on top of the head and shake the scalp vigorously; to palpate with the fingertips along the sides of the neck, from behind the ears down into the shoulders and chest. Ask your partner to breathe deeply, with closed eyes and relaxed muscles, while you massage, and remember to do the same when someone works on you. Wouldn't this be a nicer way to spend a break than having a cigarette or another cup of coffee?

After Work

Your workday may end at four or five, but that doesn't guarantee instant relaxation. You may already know that you need to cool off and slow down gradually after a heavy workout. After running, for example, you should walk for a while, not just plop down. In aerobic dance classes, the jumping and pumping exercises are always followed by slower, gentler ones before the class is over. Just as you need to warm up gradually before vigorous exercise, in order to avoid a shock to your system, you need to cool off gradually afterward, for the same reason.

If you apply this philosophy to your workday, you will enjoy your after-hours much more. Throughout this chapter, we have been using the premise that work at a desk or terminal is a heavy stress on your body, as indeed it is. To be consistent, you need to cool off after work as you do after other strenuous activity. Don't leap up from your chair, grab your things and hurl yourself out into the commuter traffic. Take at least five minutes to relax. If you just sit, you may be so tired that you'll never get up again, so a much better idea is to stand up and do some spinal stretches, leg swings, neck and shoulder rotations, or whatever; or do a few lower-back stretches if you are lucky enough to have an area where you can lie down. Drink a glass of water, take ten long breaths, palm a little and *then* head out.

As you walk, drive or take the bus home, keep in mind what you have learned about caring for your eyes. If you are on a bus or train, you can palm, or you can rest your central vision and stimulate your periphery by (1) placing your palm between your eyes so as to shut out your central vision, looking straight ahead at your palm, or (2) looking straight ahead (remembering to blink) at any fixed point, letting your peripheral cells be stimulated by the constantly moving stream of visual data that will flash by on either side of you as the vehicle moves.

If you are walking, you can practice 'shifting' exercises, constantly moving your focus from point to point on whatever you see, and blinking each time you shift. You can also practice changing from a close to a distant focus, looking from the sidewalk at your feet to the farthest horizon, following the parallel lines of the sidewalk or street until they converge and then back again to your feet. Try to take your time, breathe deeply and enjoy your walk. If possible, go home by varying routes, and make a game of noticing new things each time you walk down a familiar street. You may be amazed to find how much you have been ignoring.

If you are driving, remember to blink and to shift your eyes as often as you can, and to focus on the distant horizon whenever possible. Breathe deeply; relax your shoulders, chest, abdomen and jaw; and palm as soon as you get home.

Another ten to twenty minutes of exercise, similar to your morning session, will give you more energy for your evening activities, and help you sleep better. The ideal time to do these is between coming home and dinnertime. After eating, your body is using much of its energy to digest your food, so this is not a good time to exercise. Some people like to do some gentle stretching just before bed, but more vigorous exercise could keep you awake. So before dinner seems the optimal time. Be considerate of your body. If you are exhausted or aching, choose exercises that let you lie down on your back and unwind slowly before you try anything more demanding. After that, if you do have the energy for something more aerobic, by all means go for it. Stimulating your circulation and stretching your muscles after a sedentary day, infusing your blood with endorphins after a frustrating day, being purely and enjoyably physical after a day of mental labor, all will help to break up unhealthy patterns which otherwise tend to rigidify your body and your life.

CHAPTER 12

Asthma

When Tony first came to see Meir, he complained that he had been suffering from asthma for twenty-six years, he was dependent on four different drugs, and he used his inhalator six times a day. Tony was sick and tired of the drugs and their side effects, but was not very optimistic about alternative therapy. After his first session, Tony gave up the drugs and reduced his use of the inhalator.

The first thing that Tony learned was that he did not need to struggle in order to breathe deeply into his chest; all he needed to do was breathe slowly into his abdomen and lower back. The first exercise Tony tried was standing, breathing deeply while bending forward and curving his whole back. In that position he could feel the movement, or lack of it, in his lower back, but at the same time breathing to his chest was limited. He found that in that position he could use his breathing to expand his lower back and abdomen. He asked whether, in doing so, he was perhaps simply compensating with the lower back for his difficulties in breathing into his chest. Meir's reply was that this was not a compensation but an expansion of the areas into which he could breathe.

An asthmatic's two worst enemies are (1) the fear that he or she may not be able to take another deep breath and (2) the constant tendency to try to breathe heavily into the chest. True deep breathing fills most of the upper torso: the abdomen expands, the ribs and shoulders rise, the upper and lower back expand. Chest breathing is shallow, as it utilizes only a small portion of the lungs. Breathing into the lower parts of the lungs allows more oxygen to enter the blood.

For an asthmatic, exhalation is more difficult than inhalation. This may indicate a very tense and anxious personality. In fact, if you have a harder time letting go of the air than breathing it in, you may be more prone to asthma than others, even if you have not had asthma, and you may benefit from the following exercises too.

One of your major goals would be to breathe 'into' areas which you normally do not use.

12–1 Kneel and bend forward, resting your forehead on your knees, and stay in that position. Close your hands into loose fists and tap on your lower back. You will find yourself encouraged to breathe into your lower back, now that your chest is somewhat blocked while your lower back is expanded. Breathe very slowly, without making any effort to breathe very deeply, imagining your lower back expanding as you inhale and shrinking as you exhale.

When you feel the need to use the inhalator, you may sometimes find that just placing yourself in this position will help you breathe more deeply. This will work only if you do not panic – if you do, you may as well use the inhalator – and if you already have experienced improved breathing in this position and are confident that it can help you.

You will also benefit from kneeling in this position and having someone tap on your lower back for a few minutes at a time while you experience breathing deeply to expand your lower back, in and out.

The next exercise we recommend is the first one that Tony tried: the spinal arch, exercise 4–2 of the Spine chapter. This blocks some of your chest-breathing capacity but allows you to explore other breathing areas which you are less familiar with. As you bring your chin to your chest, you can feel your middle and lower back. As you bend further down, you may feel only the lower back. When you straighten up and stretch backward, you will feel your chest and abdomen. You want to use all of your lung capacity, and therefore expand and contract in all directions.

Continuing with the same exercise, when you bend down toward your right foot, feel your left side expanding as you inhale, shrinking as you exhale. Then bend toward your left, and be aware of the expansion and shrinking of your right side.

Another very effective exercise to increase

breathing is exercise 6–5 of the Nervous System chapter.

Refer also to exercise 3–10 in the Joints chapter. As you sit with your knees pointing outward, have a friend push your knees down toward the floor very gently and very slowly, to help you increase the stretch. This stretch opens up the pelvis and is very helpful in improving breathing. Breathe deeply as your legs are pushed down and imagine that you are breathing into your pelvis, then release the stretch. To help a person during an asthmatic attack, Meir uses this type of stretch combined with a hot wet towel on the client's chest.

It seems to us that often people tend to develop asthma because they live in congested cities. You may have a weak breathing apparatus in the first place, but you can help yourself by living in more favorable surroundings, if possible. A warm climate can be helpful, at least temporarily. Sitting and looking at very pleasant views for long periods of time is very relaxing and very effective. This is not an exercise which brings instant relief, but it is well worth your while.

Exercises 2–6 to 2–9 of the Circulation chapter along with exercise 6–2 of the Nervous System chapter are all very appropriate for asthmatics.

We suggest that, in addition to the exercises mentioned so far, you receive two massage sessions per week from a friend, and if possible from a professional therapist.

After two months of work with the program suggested above, work with all of the Breathing chapter. We recommend especially exercises 1–5, 1–13 and 1–14.

After four months of working with the Breathing chapter, turn to the Nervous System chapter, the section on cross-crawling. Several sessions of crawling can help you breathe into your abdomen and chest with less tension, but practice crawling only if you do not have rheumatic heart problems in addition to your asthma, and if your physician does not object to it. Not all asthmatics are capable of vigorous exercise, because their breathing limitation increases the load on the heart; however, if you can practice crawling, you will find that it is a wonderful exercise for both the heart and the lungs.

CHAPTER 13

High and Low
Blood Pressure

High Blood Pressure

When you have your blood pressure measured,
what your doctor is measuring is the force
that the blood exerts against the inner walls of
your arteries. Two measurements are taken:
one of the pressure while the heart pumps
(systolic) and the other just afterward, when
the heart rests (diastolic). High blood pressure
occurs when the blood flow encounters
greater-than-normal resistance within the
blood vessels; this condition is also known as
hypertension. Naturally, this condition impairs
circulation and causes a tremendous number
of health problems, such as heart disease,
circulatory insufficiency and stroke.

Diet plays a major role in causing and in
controlling hypertension. Salt and fat are the
worst culprits, and eliminating or reducing
your intake of salt and fatty foods can prevent
or vastly improve high blood pressure. There
are numerous books on this subject, and most
heart specialists understand the significance of
diet and will be happy to advise you. If you
have high blood pressure, we urge you to
consult a cardiac specialist, both on the subject
of diet and also regarding the exercises in this
chapter – you should not attempt these or

other exercises without your doctor's approval.
If your condition is severe, you should check
in with the doctor frequently, to be sure that
the exercises are not having any adverse effect.
If the condition is not severe, you should still
be in touch with your doctor, but probably
will not need to do so as often.

Many factors affect blood pressure. Among
these are posture, the degree of contraction or
relaxation in your muscles, and the activity of
your autonomic nervous system (for more
details on the role of the nervous system, please
consult the first part of the Nervous System
chapter). All of these are factors which you
can influence, to a surprising degree, by the
way you move your body and by learning to
relax. Emotional stress and physical tension
can cause contracted muscles, through which
blood cannot easily flow. Stress also activates
your nervous system to produce such changes
as increased heart rate and increased blood
viscosity, both of which put an added strain
on your vascular system. Therefore, one of the
best ways to reduce your blood pressure is
through relaxation. One of the quickest routes
to relaxation is through meditation. Meditation
may take many forms, but its essence consists
of quietly sitting, breathing deeply and

regularly, and focusing your attention, pref-erably on things which calm and ease you.

Conscious breathing is itself a meditation. Physiologically, increasing your oxygen intake improves your blood circulation, taking the strain off your heart; emotionally, deep breath-ing centers, calms and focuses a restless mind. Thus the benefits of breathing for your heart are twofold. At this time we suggest that you turn to the Breathing chapter and practice all of the exercises described there; begin with exercise 1–15. Devote half an hour each day to this and the other breathing exercises.

Walking can also be a form of meditation, and in fact is used as a meditation by some Buddhists. Walking is one of the most relaxing forms of exercise, both physically and men-tally. Doctors recommend long walks for heart patients, and we have found that they work like magic. While you walk, pay attention to how you are using your body; this is good for its own sake and also to focus your mind on constructive self-awareness. Please refer to the Muscles chapter for a discussion on how to improve your walking. Try walking backward and sideways, and observe how these unfa-miliar movement patterns influence the way walking feels to you – you may find it even more relaxing to move in novel ways than in accustomed ones. Walking improves cir-culation in a gentle and gradual way which is less likely to strain your heart than more vigorous exercise.

Having begun to relax and to regulate your blood flow, your next goal is to increase cir-culation to your hands and feet. Exercise 10–3 in the Musicians chapter has been helpful in regulating circulation to the hands.

13–1   Sit and rest your elbow on a table or the arm of the couch, and rotate your forearm.

Imagine that your fingertips are leading the motion, as though there are strings attached to them that someone gently pulls to move the forearm. Next, rest the elbow in the same position and rotate your shoulder. Both forearm and shoulder rotations should be done slowly, at least twenty-five times in each direction, while breathing fully and regularly.

Rest one hand in your lap, and, with the other hand, take hold of each finger in turn and move it, passively, in rotation. Then allow one finger at a time to move actively, by itself, while you hold onto the other fingers. You will feel more blood coming to your fingers.

Be sure to do all of these exercises with both hands. At first, it will be best to run through the entire sequence – forearm, shoulder, passive and active finger rotation – on one side before working with the other side, so that you can compare the feeling of one hand to that of the other.

Refer to exercise 5–2 in the Muscles chapter for a detailed description of massage for the feet. Refer to the Circulation chapter for exer-cises to increase circulation to the feet (exercises 2–25 to 2–34). Practice the exercises mentioned above for the hands and feet for a month before continuing to the next exercise.

13–2   Stand with your back against a wall. Alternately swing your arms up and down, touching the wall above you with the back of the hand when the hand is raised and with the palm when the hand is lowered. Move your hands up and down rapidly, but do not strike the wall forcefully. You may want to pad your hands or the wall so that you can move your hands quickly without fear of bruis-ing them. Imagine that your fingertips are leading the motion. This exercise is both helpful for stiff shoulders and increases blood flow to the hands. Now practice the same alternation away from the wall.

At this stage, work with all of the Circulation chapter.

Low Blood Pressure

Low blood pressure is considered healthier than high blood pressure, but it does involve problems. It can cause dizziness due to insufficient circulation to the head, and a feeling of low energy. You don't need to increase the stress level of your life or the junk food in your diet in order to increase your blood pressure: there are exercises which can help. But be sure to get your physician's approval of your exercise program, especially if the low blood pressure is a result of a heart problem.

Vigorous exercise increases blood pressure, but may cause other problems, such as injury, if you exercise when you are tense and your energy is low.

13–3 Running in water is a helpful vigorous exercise. The resistance of the water makes it hard work, but also slows you down and cushions each step. If you are a good swimmer, try running from shallower water to deep water, and then treading through the water with your arms and legs. If you are not a good swimmer, do not do this beyond chest-level depth. In both cases, move both your arms and your legs throughout the whole run. Running twenty or thirty yards will be a good workout for your heart — enough to raise your blood pressure without causing excessive stress.

Any kind of exercise in cold water is helpful, since the blood is drained from the surface and remains mostly in the larger inner vessels, increasing the pressure in them temporarily. Cold showers may be helpful, as may swimming in cold water, whether it is an ocean, a lake, a river or a pool. If the water or the weather is very cold, however, be sure to warm your body with exercise after your swim, even if it is just a short, brisk walk or jog.

The following three exercises may be somewhat of a challenge, but they will quickly increase your respiration and heart rate. Refer to exercise 1–14 in the Breathing chapter.

Practice exercise 1–16 from the Breathing chapter, and then exercise 6–2 from the Nervous System chapter.

13–4 Stand with bare feet, bend your right knee slightly so that only the heel comes off the floor (fig 13–4, right), and, as you straighten the leg again to hit the floor firmly with the heel, bend the other knee to raise the other heel. Alternate for both feet for a few minutes.

Now do the opposite — flex your feet alternately, bringing only the front parts of your feet up and keeping the heels on the floor (fig 13–4, left). This part of the exercise is harder to do and takes longer, but notice how it brings warmth to your calves and ankles

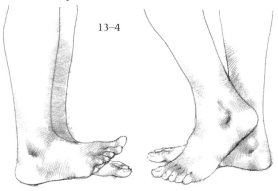

13–4

A good exercise to improve circulation to the feet is sitting, holding each ankle with one hand, and rubbing the soles of the feet together. (See also exercise 2–34 in the Circulation chapter.) It is no wonder that we recommend the same exercise for people suffering from high blood pressure – like many other exercises, this one helps regulate and balance the blood pressure, which is beneficial in either case.

Massage can also help increase blood pressure, particularly if done after exercising. Refer especially to exercises 7–9 and 7–22 in the Massage chapter.

Work with the exercises mentioned above for at least four to six months.

CHAPTER 14

Heart Problems

Heart disease is the number-one cause of early death in the United States, and a ruthless killer in many other countries as well. Naturally everyone has to die sometime, of something, but many of these heart-attack victims die thirty or forty years sooner than they had to. The number of these deaths which could have been prevented by a change in lifestyle is so high that it is staggering to contemplate. This is very sad for those who are gone, but it is wonderful news for you if you have heart trouble now. It means that, by making your habits healthier, you can preserve your heart — and your life.

Most heart problems are not the result of genetic or congenital problems alone. Even if you are born with a weak heart or a tendency toward heart disease, heart problems may never manifest themselves if you care for your body and keep it in good health. Similarly, a person born with a naturally strong heart may nonetheless suffer a heart attack if his or her habits of eating, smoking, alcohol and drug use, exercise patterns and working are bad enough. In general, heart problems come from the way people live, rather than from how they are built — through function rather than through structure, in other words.

A few of the main causes of heart disease are known to virtually everyone. Anything which reduces the amount of oxygen in the blood, or impairs the flow of blood through the vascular system, makes the heart work harder *without increasing its efficiency*. This is an important distinction. Exercising also makes the heart work harder, but this extra work benefits the body by sending more oxygen and nutrients to the cells via the increased blood flow. When the extra oxygen is not there to be sent, or the increased blood flow meets resistance inside the blood vessels, the heart is working for nothing, and this exhausts it.

Smoking reduces the capacity of the lungs to take in oxygen. When blood passes through the lungs of a smoker, it doesn't get the oxygen that it needs to supply all of the body's cells. The cells, starving for oxygen, trigger the body to circulate blood more vigorously, to make up for this lack. In order to create this increased circulation, the heart must overwork, and it must do so while itself suffering from the same lack of oxygen. Smoking causes the muscles, including the chest muscles, to become more rigid, interfering further with circulation and heart movement. And, lastly, smoking narrows the blood vessels throughout the body, so that not only does the heart have to pump blood more often, it must struggle to force it through narrowed channels.

Alcohol damages the liver, which, among other functions, has an important role in producing many blood proteins, and it may also cause damage directly to the heart itself.

Probably as dangerous as chemical abuse is eating irresponsibly. Worst are foods rich in fat and cholesterol, such as red meat, eggs and cream, which cause clogging and stiffening of the arteries. Malnutrition is also a problem, since it creates blood poor in essential nutrients. Malnutrition doesn't just happen to poor people: it happens to anyone who doesn't eat a balanced diet. Many people eat only refined, starchy foods with little nutritional content, and don't realize that this, too, strains the heart. Even people in poorer countries may be able to change their diet to include more fruits, vegetables and whole grains; in North America and Western Europe we certainly can do this.

We recommend that fruits, vegetables – particularly those in the cabbage family (broccoli, cauliflower, cabbage, Brussels sprouts) – and whole grains should be the basis of a heart-health diet. Some people may choose to add a small amount of chicken or fish, but in moderation. Tobacco, any alcohol besides a very occasional glass of wine or beer, and coffee should all be viewed as the poisons that they are, especially to the vascular system. Caffeine, which is found in coffee, black tea, chocolate and cola, speeds up heart activity and stresses the heart; white sugar does the same. Both caffeine and sugar affect the nervous system, causing it to increase your heart rate. It should be obvious that if you eat so as to let your blood vessels remain unclogged, and allow your nervous system to regulate your pulse and circulation undisturbed by nicotine, caf-

feine and alcohol, you will be increasing your chances of having a long and healthy life.

Having taken responsibility for your lifestyle in general, what are the more specific things that you can do for your heart through movement and relaxation? The suggestions above, and those which follow, are not just for people who know or suspect that they have heart trouble: they are for everyone who wants to be healthy. As a person without known heart problems, what should *you* do for your heart? The answer is: be sensible. Avoid things which strain and stress your heart without benefiting it. You may try to counteract a sedentary lifestyle with occasional bouts of vigorous exercise, but this is a mistake. Your system benefits much more from regulation and balance than from swinging back and forth from one extreme to another, which simply combats one stress with another. Milder daily exercise – done smoothly and rhythmically while breathing deeply – long walks and stretching will benefit your heart most. More demanding exercise can be done when your body is already relaxed, stretched and toned. It is, though, very important to exercise every day.

When should you start working on your cardiovascular system? You could begin in your mid-eighties, if you like, but why not begin now. The earlier you start, the more healthy years you can add to your life. The first thing you must learn is to relax – not just while lying down, not just while meditating, but during all phases of your daily life. Relaxing is something that happens to body and mind simultaneously. When you relax, the flow of blood throughout your blood vessels, down to the smallest capillary, is automatically increased *without* any extra work by the heart. The increased flow into the capillaries relieves pressure on the larger blood vessels.

We recommend that you begin with three months of daily practice of the exercises in the Circulation chapter. Take your time with each exercise, doing it slowly and thoroughly, and you will find that, along with your circulation, your body awareness and general health will gradually improve. You can start with only a few repetitions of each exercise, increasing your activity gradually at a pace that is comfortable for your body. Practice the movements while visualizing that you are expanding your blood vessels, allowing more blood flow, with less resistance. Take daily walks. Always remember to breathe deeply. Notice when you become tense or upset, and try to relax your mind. Make the needed changes in your diet. After these first critical three months, decide that you will devote a minimum of forty-five minutes, three times weekly, to working for the health of your cardiovascular system.

If you do have heart problems, you should work only with the consent and approval of your physician. If your physician is not helpful and supportive, you might try to find one who is more open-minded toward the goals of natural medicine. Use your physician's knowledge to your own benefit: to monitor your health and progress closely, to encourage you when the program works for you, to consult with if it does not help you.

Our purpose here is to give you some idea as to how to work with your heart; to suggest that you try a variety of ways to help it, experimenting until you know what works for you; and to remind you never to give up on yourself – no case is hopeless. As you learn and practice these exercises, you will notice that, as a fringe benefit, they will benefit the rest of your body as well.

Hypertrophy

One of the most common symptoms of heart trouble is called hypertrophy. This refers to an enlargement of part of your heart, mostly the left ventricle. This increased muscle mass usually results from the heart having to work too hard to pump blood; just as any other muscle will gain mass when vigorously exercised, so will the heart. At first, this increases the ability of the heart to work; eventually, however, the added work exhausts the heart. Hypertrophy is usually caused by increased resistance in the blood vessels or by heart failure, during which some of the heart tissues die from lack of oxygen. The living tissues which remain have to work harder to make up for the dead tissues. In time, the blood vessels supplying the heart cannot nourish the increased muscle mass, so the heart becomes even more vulnerable to infarction – death of tissue due to a sudden insufficiency of blood supply. If this is your condition, you must realize that your heart is injured and, on top of its injury, is being required to do more than its normal load of work. Your goal is to find ways to make the work of your heart easier for it to do, and to help your vascular system to decrease its resistance to the heart's work.

Your blood vessels run through every part of your body, so contraction and blockage anywhere in the body can interfere with circulation. The more you relax, the more you can release tension and open blockages. Tension can happen, and can cause trouble, anywhere in the body. Some of our most obvious tensions, however, are also the most relevant to the heart. The areas nearest the heart – including the shoulders, chest, neck and upper back – are extremely prone to tense muscles. You will be helping your circulation immeasurably by relaxing these areas. This is best done by a combination of massage and exercise.

Along with the exercises suggested in the Circulation chapter, you should consult the Spine, Joints and Muscles chapters for exercises relating to the areas you want to work on. Each of these chapters has shoulder exercises; some also have exercises for the neck, chest and upper back. You should receive upper-body massage as often as possible – it is not a self-indulgence but an important and very effective therapy. You may consider whether deep-tissue massage would benefit you, but be sure to consult with your doctor about this, as well as with an experienced massage therapist. The following are some suggestions which may be useful to your massage practitioner.

14–1　Your clavicle, or collarbone, runs from the base of your throat out to your shoulders. The entire area surrounding the clavicle, both above and below, should be massaged until it relaxes completely. You may find that this has a dramatic effect in deepening and easing your breathing. This is one area which you can easily massage by yourself, so do so frequently and thoroughly, especially when you feel yourself becoming tense or your breathing becoming shallow.

14–2　Continue by massaging around the sternum, or breastbone, which runs down the middle of your chest and to which many of your ribs are attached in front. Since it is composed of cartilage, rather than bone, you should never let anyone press down hard on the sternum itself. Also, many of the muscles

which surround it and the ribs are extremely tense and sensitive, so you or your therapist must adjust your touch accordingly. A gentle, steady pressure and slow movement of the hands seem to get the best results. You should be lying on your back. One good technique is to place the fingertips on the muscles between the ribs, near the back, press down lightly, and rake the fingers along the muscles toward the center of the chest. Then do the same while shaking the hands (without lifting the fingers off the chest). Next, you or the therapist can press gently, with the palms, against the side of the chest as you inhale – expanding your chest against the pressure – and then quickly let go, near the end of the inhale. Remember to breathe slowly, deeply and continuously while your chest is being massaged. Tapping on the chest, with loose fingers and wrist, is also beneficial as long as it is pleasant, and it is another thing you can easily do for yourself.

14–3　Ask your therapist, or someone in your support group, to hold your arm as you lie on your back, and to gently stretch it – upward, straight out to the side, diagonally upward and diagonally downward from the shoulder. Shaking it while pulling it will further stretch and loosen the chest and shoulder muscles. Your partner can instruct you to visualize your arm stretching farther and farther – across the room, across the street, into infinity. Imagine that your chest is stretching and expanding along with the arm, and that your ribs are lifting and separating, creating a bigger breathing space for you.

14–4　Now imagine your chest expanding from within. When the muscles of your chest and the rest of your upper body relax, they allow freer movement for the heart and the lungs. Deep, chronic tension creates a restricting posture – shoulders rounded forward, neck shortened, head sunk on chest, chest cavity cramped and crowded. Relaxing your muscles will open this whole area, allowing the constant, easy expansion and contraction upon which deep breathing – and circulation – depends.

14–5   When you have become comfortable visualizing your chest expanding from within, try the following visualization. Picture the inner walls of your chest massaging the lungs as you breathe in and out, and the lungs simultaneously massaging your heart. Imagine the lungs and heart as warm and very moist and soft. Breathe deeply and visualize the air sacs in the lungs – all five million of them – swelling with air. Then picture the same expansion in your heart, swelling as you breathe in, shrinking as you exhale.

These visualizations are, in fact, meditations. They are important. You may not realize how deeply negative thoughts have influenced, and continue to influence, the health of your heart. From your first visit to the doctor or the hospital, you have probably carried a deep anxiety about your heart, knowing how many people die of heart trouble. And this anxiety penetrates deeper with every pill you take, with every exertion or excitement that you experience or seek to avoid. This is natural, but it doesn't help you. What can help to heal you is a new thought: the image of your heart as healthy, functional and strong. This image becomes your meditation. If you have never meditated, don't let the word put you off. Meditation is not just for mystics. All it means is directing your mind the way *you* want it to go – in this case, toward thoughts of health.

How you approach the meditation should depend on your own style. You may want to sit and listen to relaxing music; close your eyes or do palming (see exercise 8–5 in the Vision chapter for this); drink a cup of herbal tea or hot water with lemon; or listen to a calming meditation tape. Say to yourself, 'My heart is allowing me to enjoy this beautiful moment; I'll send it good thoughts.'

When the music or the tea or the meditation tape is finished, take five minutes or so to simply think of your heart as strong and healthy. You may even want to have a picture of a heart to look at as you meditate, as this helps some people to focus their thoughts. There are many ways to meditate, and all of them are good. See what works for you.

14–6   No matter what you know intellectually, no matter how serious your condition really is, visualize that, though there may be some damage to your heart, most of the heart is still healthy, and working to compensate for the injured part.

14–7   When you are comfortable with that image, you may want to try a visualization of recovery. Imagine that even the damaged part is functioning, along with the rest of the heart which works perfectly. Think of healthy new tissue growing within the scar tissue, beginning to replace it. Miracles do sometimes happen, and the mind has to allow for this. Perhaps positive thinking cannot replace damaged tissues, but it creates a kind of grace that promotes greater health throughout your body.

14–8   The next visualization is of your entire heart as whole and perfect – a heart that never fails you and never will. If an accident has befallen it, no destruction has resulted. With positive thoughts, deep breathing, relaxation and healing meditation, it may be that you can change your condition completely for the better.

Promoting Circulation

The following exercises focus on reducing your tension, easing blood flow, and increasing the level of oxygenation in the blood.

If your heart is working against too much resistance, it is almost as though it is arm-wrestling with the rest of the vascular system. It is accepted that the size of the blood vessels influences the blood pressure via the autonomic nervous system, which can cause the blood vessels to dilate or constrict. In our opinion, the contraction of the muscles around the blood vessels also has a very strong influence on blood pressure. Even people with no known heart trouble benefit from getting as much blood flow as possible into the smallest vessels, the capillaries, and thus taking the load off the larger ones. This balanced flow eases the need of the heart to pump more. Warm hands and feet are a sign that the blood is flowing in the smallest vessels, those near the skin and in the body's periphery, farthest from the heart.

14–9 Sit in a comfortable chair or couch with arms, resting your elbows and forearms. Let your shoulders drop, and let go of tension in your neck and arms and chest. Breathe slowly and deeply through your nose, and visualize calm spreading through your body, releasing the blocks that hamper your circulation. Now visualize that you breathe not only through your nose but through your hands and feet as well.

14–10 Inhale until you cannot inhale any further, and then insist on inhaling a little more, and a little more still. When you at last exhale, do so slowly, letting your breath out a little at a time. Repeat this ten times. Feel how the energy rushes to your hands and feet as the blood flow to them increases.

After those three months, you won't need that exercise any more. Just sit and visualize your hands and feet growing warmer, instructing the blood to flow toward them. Feel their weight, feel the blood pulsing in them. Massage your hands (see exercises 7–1 to 7–7 in the Massage chapter), and then your feet (see exercise 5–2 in the Muscles chapter). In a few minutes you will feel the increased circulation, and your whole body will feel relaxed and energized as well. Your thoughts can help to control many of the internal, 'involuntary', functions of your body, including the action of your heart – as long as you do not become anxious or self-judging about your results.

Along with your breathing and visualizations, self-massage will help to promote circulation to your body surface and periphery – that is, to the areas farthest from your heart. Just as a person carrying a heavy burden is most tired and strained at the end of a long journey, the heart must work hardest to reach these farthest areas. The work you do now relieves it of that burden. Massage your hands and feet, legs, neck, scalp, shoulders – any place on your body that you can comfortably reach. Use all four fingers and your thumb, on both hands, palpating in a rotating motion, stroking, squeezing and tapping. Refer to the Massage chapter for ideas for self-massage. We recommend that you spend about twenty-five minutes daily on self-massage, meanwhile receiving as much massage from others as you can arrange. If you have heart problems, you should try for a minimum of two sessions weekly, but do massage yourself daily. You may want to use a massage oil or cream, or a herbal salve.

Breathing, visualization and self-massage all require concentration, focus, and some degree of stillness. This may present a problem at first, since many people with heart problems tend to be restless, impatient and driven to ceaseless activity, focused outward rather than inward. It is important to curb these tendencies when massaging yourself, to let your touch be warm, loving and penetrating, taking whatever time is needed to achieve relaxation, circulation or whatever change you are aiming for. Make the experience as pleasant for yourself as possible – and give yourself and your attention to it totally, instead of thinking ahead to the next thing you 'have' to do. There is nothing as important as what you are doing now, which is healing your heart.

14–11 After your initial three-month period, you can add alternating hot and cold showers to your regimen, if your doctor approves. This is not something you should do when you have just begun to work on your heart: it should only be done at a stage when your circulation has already improved and your body responds noticeably to your exercises, visualizations and so on. For two minutes, stand under water as hot as you can bear, then stand for one minute under the coldest bearable water, exposing all of your body to it. Switch to hot for one minute, then to cold again. Finish the shower with three minutes of cool or lukewarm water, massaging and tapping your chest under the shower spray. Repeat this procedure daily, or even more often if possible. Warm water brings blood to the

surface of the body; cold drives it into the deeper tissues: between the two, your circulation gets a real boost.

Everything we have done so far has been aimed at 'reprogramming' your vascular system, helping it to learn how to function efficiently without straining your heart. As we mentioned earlier, one of the surest signs that this has happened is increased warmth in your hands and feet after a little massage, breathing or visualization. When you can regularly achieve this, you are ready for more vigorous exercise.

14–12 Stand and 'walk' in place, moving only your heels up and down alternately – the front half of the foot should not leave the floor. Breathe slowly in and out through your nose as you do this, and keep your posture erect, with your back straight and your head up. Look forward at a point in the distance, an inch or so above the level of your eyes. Rub your hands together briskly as you move your heels. Do this thirty times at first, taking about a week to work up to 100 repetitions. Do this three times daily, always on an empty stomach. You may want to do it during a break from work, or before meals, or at any other time when you can establish it as a routine.

Take about three months to work up to 500 repetitions per day.

At this point, you should also begin to take long walks, preferably spending an hour a day walking. You can break this up into fifteen-minute periods, if you wish. If you live near a sandy beach or a park, take the opportunity to walk barefoot whenever possible. Walk sideways and backward as well as forward. As you walk, massage your arms, hands and chest, visualizing the blood running through them, warming your whole body. From time to time, place your hands over your heart and tell it to beat slowly and evenly.

Lying on your back with a pillow under your head and another under your ankles, rotate your ankles, 100 times in each direction. Massage and squeeze the muscles of your calves, then rotate the ankles another fifty times.

At this point, you have completed a series of exercises with a dual purpose: (1) to assist the heart in carrying more blood to the surface and the periphery of your body, thus restoring a balanced circulation and easing stress throughout your vascular system; (2) to slow down the action of your heart. These two things will help to preserve your heart for a longer life.

Stenosis

Along with hypertrophy, valve stenosis is one of the most common factors in heart disease. One or more of the valves which open and shut to let blood pass through the heart becomes narrowed and stiffened, impeding blood flow. Most of the exercises we have described for heart disease and for blood-pressure regulation (see Chapter 13 – High and Low Blood Pressure) are very helpful for a person with stenosis – with a few important additions and subtractions. Please read the following carefully.

Massage is particularly important for a person with stenosis, especially in the early stage of self-treatment, since too much vigorous activity may be dangerous, yet increased blood flow is essential. The techniques described

earlier are all useful; however, the best kind of self-massage for this condition is tapping on the chest. With a loose wrist, let your relaxed fingers flop against the chest, making a firm impact, but not hard enough to hurt. Tap from your armpit area to your sternum, and from your collarbone down to the bottom of the ribcage, and all along the muscles between your ribs. Stenosis is often accompanied by a rapid heartbeat. Take your pulse before the tapping (see exercise 2–5 in the Circulation chapter), tap all over the chest for five minutes while breathing slowly and deeply, and take your pulse again afterwards; you may find a difference of as much as five to eight beats in your pulse rate.

As in other circulatory disorders, increasing blood flow to the body's surface and periphery and reducing the pressure on the heart and major blood vessels are essential concerns. With your doctor's approval, you can do the exercises listed in the Breathing chapter *except* 1–11, 1–14, 1–16 and 1–18. You can do all the exercises in the Circulation chapter *except* 2–6 to 2–9. However, we strongly recommend that you do the exercises slowly and carefully, paying total attention to how they make you feel, how your body reacts to them, and when it is time to stop and rest, or to stop and move on to another exercise.

While you do your breathing exercises, visualize your heart, in particular the area where the valve is blocked. It may be useful to get an illustration of a heart from an anatomy book and study it to find where the blockage is. As you visualize the valve, imagine that you can see it slowly expanding, becoming more flexible and soft with every movement of your chest as you breathe in and out.

All movement exercises should be done at about one-quarter of the speed at which you would normally do them – unless this slowness itself causes you to strain, in which case just move slowly and with awareness. Exercise 2–16 from the Circulation chapter is particularly recommended. Practice your visualization of expansion and softening of your valve as you do your movement exercises.

After about four months of daily massage and movement combined with visualization, consult with your doctor to find out whether you have obtained any noticeable results. If you have not, do not progress to the next exercises in this chapter. If possible, consult with a Self-Healing practitioner/educator. You may choose to continue with the exercises you've been doing thus far, if you feel that they've been helpful. If your doctor reports that you have obtained noticeable results then you can begin to include walking in your daily regimen.

If you can walk barefoot, in sand or grass, this is preferable, as it brings more circulation to the feet and legs than does walking with shoes. As with all of your movement exercises, begin slowly and build up gradually. At first it may be best to walk no more than 200 yards. After two weeks, you might do this twice daily; after another week, two daily walks of 300 yards; and so on. Within six months you may be able to increase your distance to two miles, twice daily. Read the Walking section in the Muscles chapter, and pay close attention to how you walk. Walk backward and sideways, as well as forward, to bring new muscles into play; this creates a better overall circulation. Always remain sensitive to your condition; try to stop and rest *before* you become short of breath. Both walking and resting will increase circulation, but walking while under a sense of strain will hamper it.

You may also now add the exercises from the Breathing and Circulation chapters that you skipped earlier, but only with your physician's approval. Exercises 1–16 and 1–18 from the Breathing chapter are especially helpful. Continue your augmented program for another three months. At that time, you can choose your favorite exercises and continue with them. Explore the other chapters in this book for exercises you may enjoy. While doing whatever you can to improve your health, remember to be conscious of your limits – one of Meir's clients became so elated with his progress that he took a skiing trip to the Alps long before he was ready for it, and a heart attack resulted. Be in constant touch with your physician – and with your heart.

Congestion of the Lungs

When its action is impaired, the heart sometimes becomes congested, being unable to pump out blood adequately. When this happens, the blood which is coming into the heart from the lungs may back up, causing fluids to remain trapped in the lungs. This is a very serious problem and requires a physician's care, but – with your physician's approval – you may want to try several Self Healing exercises in addition to your medical treatment. You need to improve your circulation while being very careful not to overwork your heart. What will help most in this case are breathing exercises. Please refer to the Breathing chapter, and practice all of the exercises as described there. An important breathing exercise is 6–2 of the Nervous System chapter. Chest massage, especially tapping on the chest, is also very helpful (you can refer to exercise 2–10 in the Circulation chapter);

you can do this yourself, but it will be best to arrange for someone else to do it, at least four times weekly.

Edema

Edema, or fluid retention, is another common side effect of poor circulation. Baths are very helpful for this, as is swimming, since being in water helps to distribute the body's fluids evenly. After being in water, remain naked for as long as possible, allowing your skin to breathe.

Fluids often collect in the ankles and hands. You can help to disperse them by breathing deeply, visualizing your breath entering the bloated area, expanding it as you inhale and shrinking it as you exhale.

Massaging your legs will be very helpful for swollen ankles, and may help to prevent varicose veins if your doctor thinks it is advisable. Vigorously massage your ankles, calves, knees and thighs, pressing deeply with your thumbs and fingers in a rotating motion. (If you already have varicose veins, naturally you will need to be much more gentle in these areas.)

Lastly, the regimen of hot and cold showers, as described in exercise 14–11 in this chapter, may help reduce edema. And as you probably know, salt should be avoided completely, as it promotes fluid retention.

CHAPTER 15

Headaches

Headaches in some cases may result from brain tumors, from aneurysms of blood vessels, or from several other physical conditions which can and should be treated by physicians without delay. Before reading the rest of this chapter, check with a physician to find the physical state of your head and neck and whether you have a problem that demands immediate attention. In such cases our exercises can have an added benefit to medical treatment, but in no way can they replace it.

There are several other types of headache, and all of them hurt. Their causes vary, but all of them are related to stress in one way or another. Most of us have to cope daily with difficulties that cause physical tension, and for many the result is chronic headaches. General body tension, sinus congestion, neck and shoulder muscle spasm, circulation problems, constipation, eyestrain, insomnia and reactions to various foods are a few causes of headaches.

Some headaches are easily alleviated by aspirin, while others refuse to respond to any medication. Swallowing a couple of aspirins, however, is only a temporary measure which does not deal with the underlying cause of the headache. If you have headaches more than once a month, you are not doing yourself a favor by simply masking the pain with aspirin. You need to find out what is causing your headaches, and work on that rather than on the pain, which is only a symptom. By taking painkillers, you are sending a message to your body that the real source of pain is something you just can't change – and therefore the headaches will continue to recur.

This chapter will give you some ideas on how to identify the causes of your headaches and what to do for them. First, let's start with some ideas for dealing with headaches in general. Many headaches don't arise from specific health problems like bad vision or poor digestion; they develop from a combination of overall tension, tiredness, stress and overwork, with some eyestrain and bad eating habits thrown in. This type of headache is often referred to as a 'tension' headache (even though, in a broader sense, *all* headaches are tension headaches).

If you have a chronic tension headache, the first thing you must do is notice the location of the pain. This varies from person to person: it may be sharpest in the center of the forehead, the base of the skull or the sides of the face. Very often, there may be a part of the body which also seems tense and painful during a headache. If there are places that always seem to hurt worst when your head aches, you need to take care of these vulnerable spots, even when your head is not aching. If you find that your shoulders, your abdomen or your lower back are usually tense during a headache, then work with the relevant exercises in the Joints, Breathing, Muscles or Spine chapters.

Get massage as often as possible, whether from a professional, from someone in your support group, or from a friend who is willing to take the time to give you a real treatment, and focus on these problem areas. Since stress, body tension and poor circulation are the causes of so many headaches, massage is one of the most natural preventatives, and can also be a wonderful remedy.

The eye-relaxation technique known as palming is another very effective remedy. This technique is described in the Vision chapter, exercise 8–5. Palming rests the eyes and so relaxes all of the facial muscles, often making it easier for you to breathe more deeply, and thereby helping to relax the rest of the body as well. If eyestrain is a factor in your headaches, this exercise will be especially helpful; even if it is not, we recommend palming for any tension headache. While you palm, imagine that each of the areas that hurt becomes black, or invisible. Breathe deeply, and imagine these areas expanding as you inhale, shrinking as you exhale. Without lifting your hands off your face, move them in a circular motion around your eye sockets, or rub your forehead with your fingers, or massage your jaw and cheekbones with your thumbs.

After palming for at least an hour, massage the painful areas, first lightly, then more deeply. Roll the skin of your scalp between your fingers, and pull it gently away from the skull – loosening the scalp muscles in this way will allow normal blood flow to the head. Now touch the base of the skull with one finger and rotate your head, imagining that the finger is the center of the circle your head is making. Do this ten times in each direction, then move the finger down to the next vertebra, and repeat the rotation and visualization. Do this until you reach the base of the neck, where it joins the shoulders.

Exercise is another headache-preventer. We recommend long walks as a general prescription for anyone with chronic headaches. They are relaxing, aerobic and good for circulation, respiration and digestion – a combination that is hard to beat. We also recommend that you do relaxation exercises daily for chronically tense places in your body, and suggest that you read the Muscles, Joints and Spine chapters to find which exercises best suit your needs.

Exercise *during* a headache is more problematic. When you are in pain, you may not feel like doing anything but lying down and resting, and that may indeed be the best idea. But while you are lying down you can speed your recovery by doing some non-challenging body-relaxation techniques.

15–1   The first is simply to breathe deeply, in and out through your nose. Make the inhalations and exhalations as long as possible, with the exhalations longer than the inhalations. Try to do this ten times, and see whether you can make your breaths a little longer each time.

Next, visualize each separate part of your body in turn, asking it to relax. Then feel or imagine it completely relaxed and comfortable.

Now combine these two: breathe deeply in and out and imagine that you are sending your breath to each separate part of your body in turn, causing that part to expand as you inhale, to shrink as you exhale.

As you begin to relax and perhaps feel a little better, you may find it relaxing to do some limited movements, such as hand or ankle rotations, moving the head very slowly from side to side or in circles, or opening and closing the jaws or the fists.

15–2 Massage your abdomen (refer to the Massage chapter, exercise 7–23). Inhale and, while it is expanded with your breath, move the abdomen in and out and, if you can, in rotation, before exhaling.

Massage your shoulders (refer to the Massage chapter, exercises 7–13 and 7–15) and practice shoulder rotations (refer to the Spine chapter, exercise 4–30). If possible, have someone massage your shoulders as you rotate them.

Headaches and Food

Many people suffer headaches in reaction to food. Some of the most common problem foods are cheese, wheat, chocolate, wine and coffee. Foods containing yeast, mold or fungus – and this can include all breads, pickles, mushrooms, tofu, yogurt and a host of other foods – give some people headaches, particularly those suffering from a yeast infection caused by *Candida albicans*. Sugary foods can cause terrible headaches by causing your blood-sugar level first to soar and then to plummet. This leaves you feeling weak, shaky, tired and often with a headache and other muscle aches. If you have chronic headaches, you should begin to pay close attention to how you feel after eating, both immediately following a meal and during the next hour or so. If you don't feel well, make a mental note of what you ate, and see whether any of these foods causes the same problem in the future. By monitoring her food reactions in this way, one of Maureen's clients discovered that her 'killer' headaches, which no amount of aspirin could help, only happened when she ate sourdough bread. We have since learned that sensitivity to sourdough culture is not unusual.

Some people use coffee and/or sugar to alleviate their headaches. These are usually people who are addicted to these two substances, both of which are very potent drugs. Coffee causes some blood vessels to dilate, and sugar raises blood-sugar levels, so these may indeed temporarily help a headache, if it has been caused by constriction of blood vessels, as in migraines, or by low blood sugar. However, using them in this way increases your body's chemical dependency upon them. The more coffee and sugar you ingest, the more you will need in order to maintain a 'normal' feeling. And since both of these drugs have extremely bad side effects, we can't help feeling that dosing yourself with them is the worst of all possible ways to get rid of a headache. Sugar, for example, has been considered by many to be the cause of symptoms ranging from yeast infections to diabetes to fear of heights to lack of sexual drive to eczema to psychosis. Coffee can cause fatigue, shakiness, nervousness, insomnia, ulcers and other stomach diseases, kidney trouble, high blood pressure and ultimately nerve damage. If you are taking either of these drugs more than once or twice a day, be very careful – it is extremely easy to become addicted. If sugar or coffee is causing your headaches, you will need to eliminate it or to cut down drastically, and you will probably experience several days of headaches while the drug is cleaned out of your system. You can help yourself during this time by getting massage, by doing deep breathing (see the Breathing chapter) and mild exercise, and by eating healthy food. Protein is especially helpful in counteracting the effects of sugar, while liquids like water, herbal teas and vegetable juices help to flush out caffeine.

Constipation can cause severe headaches. It is important to understand that there are two basic types of constipation. One type is caused by the stools themselves. If you don't drink sufficient liquid or eat sufficient bulk and fiber, you may produce hard, dry, heavy stools which don't travel easily through your intestines. Obviously, in this case you need more liquids and more fiber. The other type of constipation is even more likely to cause headaches. It occurs when the stool itself is fine but is basically trapped inside the body by tension and spasm in the intestinal tract or the muscles surrounding the lower colon and the rectum. In this case, the pressure of the unexpelled waste can result in headaches. For this type of constipation, eating fiber is not the answer — all that will do is add to the weight already pressing on your lower tract. What does help is relaxation and exercise. Massage of the aching head itself will not be as helpful as massage of the lower abdomen, lower back and hips. Exercises which relieve constipation are found in the following chapters: Breathing (1–16), Muscles (5–34 and 5–35), Nervous System (6–5 and 6–6) and Massage (7–23).

Headaches and Eyestrain

This type of headache may be felt as a deep ache in the forehead and around the eyes, but can also manifest in the jaw area or in the muscles of the top and back of the skull. It is often accompanied by aching or burning eyes. It is best relieved by palming, referred to earlier in this chapter and described in the Vision chapter (exercise 8–5). Palming is nothing short of miraculous for refreshing overworked eyes and relieving the facial and body tensions that accompany eyestrain. Please read the entire section on palming carefully and follow the suggestions there, especially those regarding visualization. Imagining a deep, restful darkness helps to relax your brain as well as your eyes. Overworking your eyes causes the muscles around them to tense; palming will help them to relax. Palming also restores moisture to eyes dried out by staring.

Next to palming, facial massage as described in exercise 8–1 of the Vision chapter is the best way to relax the area surrounding your eyes. You can always do this for yourself, but it is even more relaxing if someone else does it for you. Even a couple of minutes of massage can sometimes make the pain vanish.

You can also make a compress of cotton or a washcloth soaked in black tea or eyebright tea. Place this over your closed eyes for several minutes while you lie down, breathe and relax. The compress can be either warm or cool, as you prefer, but should not be either hot or cold, as this could make your eyes tense up again.

Prevention is the best cure. If you know that you are going to spend more than an hour working hard with your eyes — reading, writing, drawing, sewing, working with a computer or at any skill that requires intensive eye use – then the best thing to do is take ten minutes to palm and five minutes to massage *before* you begin to work. This is comparable to the warm-up exercise that dancers or athletes do before their hard work. When you are finished, take the same amount of time to palm and to massage, just as athletes always cool down with slow exercise after a workout. In this way you can prevent eyestrain and its attendant headaches from ever developing. If you have to work for many consecutive hours with your eyes, take frequent palming breaks. The Computers and Office Work chapter may offer you some useful ideas.

Sinus Headaches

The sinuses are a very common source of headaches. Sinuses are cavities found in certain facial bones, with mucous linings that connect with the mucous linings in the nose and throat. When these cavities become congested with mucus the facial areas that contain them may ache fiercely. If you have pain in your forehead, cheekbones, bridge of the nose or eye sockets, there is a good chance it is caused by sinus congestion.

There are several ways to relieve this congestion; try them and see what works for you – a combination of methods will probably work best. The first and easiest is facial massage. You will find a complete description of facial massage in the Vision chapter (exercise 8–1). Consult an anatomy book or your doctor to find exactly where your sinuses are and concentrate your massage on these areas. In addition, massage your forehead with rotating motions using your fingertips; massage along both sides of your nose while inhaling and exhaling deeply and fully; massage between your eyes just above the nose; hold the bridge of the nose and move it from side to side, as though trying to loosen it from the skull. Massage helps to drain fluid buildup, which makes it effective for relieving congestion. If you have chronic sinus congestion you should do this facial massage daily, whether or not you have a headache, because it will ultimately help to eliminate the condition.

15–3 Inhaling aromatic steam can also help relieve congestion. Boil a cup of water. While it is still steaming you can add one of the following: lemon juice and salt; bark or oil of eucalyptus; comfrey leaves; oil of menthol; or oil or extract of one of the aromatic herbs such as sage, rosemary or peppermint. Hold the cup an inch below your nose. Inhale and exhale deeply, through the nose. If one nostril is completely clogged, close the other with your finger and try to inhale some steam through the clogged nostril. After several repetitions you may find the nostril starting to open up.

By far the most important approach is to improve your breathing. Find out whether you have any allergies that may be causing the congestion, and see whether you can eliminate their source from your life. (These can often include food allergies.) Congestion does not have to come from allergy or illness, however – it can be the eventual result of improper breathing. If you breathe shallowly or through your mouth instead of your nose, your nasal passages – which connect with your sinuses – don't get the volume of air they need to clean them. Just as wind sweeps debris away, deep breathing clears the breathing passages. Please read the Breathing chapter and practice all of the exercises there. Remind yourself as often as possible to breathe deeply through your nose, whether you are active or at rest. Remembering to take deep breaths when you are feeling stressed will be especially helpful. Mild exercise such as walking does wonders for breathing, as does more vigorous exercise *if* you remember to breathe through your nose.

Cervical Syndrome

A common reason for headaches is severe cervical tension or cervical damage. The headaches could result from referred pain from the cervical spine. To relieve the cervical tension, you will need to elongate the spine and fully mobilize it through balanced movement of all the neck muscles. Do not be tempted to start with neck movements, as you most likely tend to move the neck through tension. You need to loosen the rest of your body first, to give your neck better support.

During the first two weeks, work mostly with exercise 5–23 of the Muscles chapter. You can benefit much from receiving massage. Have someone massage your scalp, pulling the skin away from the head, and use exercise 7–31 of the Massage chapter.

Later you may try exercise 5–40 of the Muscles chapter, as shown in fig 5–40C, but only if that does not cause a headache or increase it. Work with exercise 4–30 of the Spine chapter. Alternate between hot towels and ice on the back of your neck. Massage the scalene and sternocleidomastoid muscles at your throat, but do not squeeze your throat. Walk backward and sideways daily, for a distance which feels comfortable.

Only after working for two months with these techniques can you start working with neck rotations, as described in exercises 4–26 and 4–27 of the Spine chapter. Emphasize moving the head from side to side, 200 to 300 times, twice a day, while massaging your neck muscles through tapping and gentle squeezing.

Insomnia

You may find that you develop a headache if you do not get enough sleep. If the insomnia persists, the headaches too may become chronic. There are as many causes of insomnia as there are insomniacs. It may be that your insomnia is caused by a very serious emotional problem that is demanding your immediate attention, but insomnia may also be caused by simple muscle tension brought on by lesser irritations. Often sleep will come easily if you can relax your mind and body a little.

Breathing deeply is a good way to start. Maureen's favorite home remedy for insomnia is to start on thirty long, slow, deep, full, extended breaths – making the exhale longer than the inhale. She has never yet reached thirty. Several clients of ours practice palming while lying in bed, with their arms supported by pillows, and say that this helps them to sleep.

Meditating before going to bed is an almost certain cure for insomnia. The problem with this, however, is that if you are too tense to sleep you may also be too nervy to meditate. Relaxation, hypnosis or meditation tapes can be a good substitute for meditation itself. If you are being kept awake by disturbing thoughts, it may relax you to hear someone else's voice soothing you to sleep with words and thoughts that are more uplifting than those running around in your own mind. With enough practice, you may eventually be able to summon relaxing images and ideas of your own when you need them.

If nothing else works, the best thing to do is to get out of bed, lie down on the floor, and do a series of very slow, gentle body movements. These can include:

- rolling the head from side to side;
- rolling the head in circles;
- pulling the knees up to the chest and moving them in rotation;
- holding the knees to the chest and rolling from side to side;
- stretching the arms out to each side and (i) opening and closing the hands slowly, (ii) moving the forearm in rotation, from the elbow, and (iii) slowly swinging the whole arm in rotation;
- bending the knees and lowering them, together, to either side;
- or any other exercise which is relaxing rather than challenging to your body. Too-vigorous exercise will only stimulate you further.

If you know that a particular part of your body is chronically tense, then select exercises from this book which are designed to relax that part. Neck tension is one of the most common culprits, so, if you don't know where you are tense, the neck might be a good place to start. See the Muscles and Spine chapters for exercises to relax your neck.

Migraines

Whether you have a migraine once a year or once a week, it is always an unforgettable experience. The pain can reach such extreme levels of intensity as to cause vomiting, vertigo and temporary blindness. On a less spectacular level, sufferers report nausea, blurred vision, sensitivity to light and smells, and weakness in addition to the migraine's sharp persistent pain. Migraines are typically localized on one side of the head, often above one eye. A bodyworker can often trace a very distinct path of muscle spasm from the pain site, along the side of the skull, into the neck and often into the shoulders and back, sometimes reaching all the way down into the lower back and abdomen.

Migraines are known to be caused by narrowing of the blood vessels leading into the head, with subsequent overdilation of the blood vessels *in* the head. We have found that, by finding and releasing the path of muscle tension, migraines can be relieved – perhaps because circulation is normalized.

Maureen suffered from moderately lethal migraines about twice monthly for four years. For more than a year, no medication or massage would stop the pain. Two hours of massage would do no more than relax her enough to allow her to sleep – and the migraine would be waiting when she woke up. After several months of this treatment she gradually relaxed enough during the massage to be able to fall asleep and wake up without the pain. About two years down the line, Meir was able – after four straight hours of massage – to work out 95 percent of the pain, and a bowl of chicken soup finished off the rest. This was an important turning-point for Maureen, because she had learned that the pain – which had seemed insurmountable – could be overcome. It took another two years for her to eventually learn which movements, massage techniques, breathing exercises and other tools she could use to cut short the migraines, and even sometimes to feel them coming on and stop them before they started.

Some migraine specialists believe there is a 'migraine personality', which they describe primarily as perfectionistic, relentlessly demanding upon the self and anxiety-ridden. We don't know whether this is generally true as a description of the migraine sufferers themselves, but it does seem to be true that the corresponding emotional state – which can occur in anyone, even if he or she is usually relaxed and easy-going – does create the kind of tensions which can lead to migraine. Maureen found that migraines often struck at times when she felt overwhelmed by work and other obligations. In fact, sometimes they seemed like the one indisputable way of getting out of doing something that just seemed too hard. (During the final editing of Meir's first book, she felt one creeping up on her and said to it, 'I know what you're trying to do, and thanks a lot, but there's no way out of it – this has to be done by tomorrow.' The pain left in seconds. Needless to say, this doesn't always work, but when it does it gives you a wonderful feeling of self-mastery.)

Even more than for other types of headache, curing migraines consists largely in preventing them. This means making some changes in your daily life (if your lifestyle and health regimen are already perfect, please skip this section). The best way to prevent a migraine is to create balanced circulation throughout your body. We have mentioned our belief that muscle tightness in the neck and shoulders can cause the simultaneous constriction of blood vessels *to* the head and overdilation of blood vessels *in* the head that leads to migraine. Muscle spasm in other areas can also contribute to migraine; relieving these chronic knots can

help in preventing migraine. Some of the most common areas are the abdomen, lower back, buttocks and outer thighs. Migraines also seem very often to be accompanied by spasm in the lower colon. Many of our migraine-afflicted clients experience belching and flatulence in the process of recovering from the migraine; the passing of this trapped gas seems to contribute greatly to the relief of the head pain.

All of the above is to explain why we recommend the following precautions as migraine preventatives.

Walk for an hour a day if possible. It is best if you can walk barefoot on some yielding surface. If you can, spend a little time walking backward and sideways as well as forward, in order to use a few different walking muscles. Walking is one of the best digestive aids known, gently promoting the action of the colon. It stretches and strengthens the lower-body muscles. It deepens your breathing, which automatically improves your blood circulation.

Strengthen your abdominal area. This does not mean harden your abdominal muscles: it means stretch, stimulate and mobilize an area that, in many migraine sufferers, is virtually paralyzed with tension. Exercises for the abdomen are in the Abdomen and Back section in the Muscles chapter, exercise 1–16 in the Breathing chapter, and exercise 7–23 in the Massage chapter. For the same purpose, strengthen your ring-shaped sphincter muscles with exercises 6–5 and 6–6 in the Nervous System chapter.

For you especially, a healthy diet is crucial. Liquids and fiber are very important to have. Sugar and coffee are just plain deadly. Other foods, such as fried foods, foods with various additives, or mold-containing foods, may also be affecting you. Pay close attention to your diet and see if any food regularly causes you to react. (Hint: pay close attention to your favorite foods, because we often crave the very thing to which we are allergic.)

Get massage regularly. We recommend once a week. Because many people who suffer migraines tend to be under pressure, this is essential. If you have a support group, exchange massages with the other members as often as possible.

When You Get a Migraine

First of all, get someone to massage your abdomen. This will help you to breathe deeply and relax your lower tract.

Visualize. Either while being massaged or while lying on your back in a dimly lit room (migraine often makes your eyes more sensitive to light), imagine that your body expands each time you inhale and shrinks each time you exhale. Then concentrate on each separate section of your head – forehead, top of skull, back of skull, base of neck, jaws, eye sockets – and imagine them expanding as you inhale, shrinking as you exhale. Do the same with your neck, your shoulders and each separate part of your body.

Try to get a full body massage. Find a position that is comfortable for you, since you may find it more painful to lie on your stomach or back at first. We have found it most helpful to work first on the abdomen and back, then work up the back to the shoulders and neck, and to work for about forty minutes on the body before touching the head. Shifting the position every few minutes also seems to help, as it helps balance circulation. The person being massaged can lie on the side in a fetal position, or facedown with pillows under the abdomen or chest, or even sit cross-legged on the bed or floor. He or she can do slow movements while being massaged if this feels good. Palpating or shaking motions using all of the fingertips usually feel much better than deep pressure – a person with a migraine is under enough pressure. Deep breathing will make the touch much more helpful, especially when combined with visualizing the breath expanding the part being massaged.

Several exercises for the spine are incredibly effective in both preventing and relieving migraine – refer to the Spine chapter, exercises 4–8, 4–12, 4–18, 4–27, 4–28 and 4–30; to the Breathing chapter, exercise 1–10; and to the Circulation chapter, exercise 2–25.

Massage seems to increase in helpfulness from one migraine to the next, so don't be discouraged if it doesn't help greatly the first time. Experience any measure of relief or relaxation it brings; this will increase over time.

If your migraines are severe and persistent and have required medication, we do not recommend giving up your medication without your doctor's full approval. Combine the suggestions in this section – especially those regarding prevention – with your medication, and you will find your migraines becoming less regular and less intense. That will be the time to discuss discontinuing the medication.

We suggest that you follow this program for at least six months, keeping a journal to record your experiences and progress. We would like very much to hear about them.

CHAPTER 16

Diabetes Mellitus

In this chapter we will discuss both juvenile and adult diabetes.

People with juvenile diabetes will always remain dependent on insulin treatment, though we have found that the amount of insulin needed can be reduced. In cases of adult diabetes, the need for insulin can often be eliminated through correct diet, massage, exercises and avoidance of unhealthy substances.

If you manage to reduce the amount of insulin intake, do it very carefully and conservatively. Test yourself at home, and have your physician supervise you.

There are no shortcuts. You cannot improve from diabetes if you smoke, drink alcohol or eat a lot of unhealthy food. Many diabetics stop having diabetic attacks once they cut down on junk food. We strongly suggest that you try to eat healthy food with no preservatives or pesticides.

Our focus in this chapter is on several of the secondary problems which may result from diabetes, rather than on the diabetic condition or attacks. For example, lack of circulation to the feet can result in gangrene. Retinal myopathy, a result of poor circulation to the retina, may cause partial or complete blindness – sometimes overnight. Both of these can be prevented.

We would like to start by sharing with you the story of one of our students, and then suggest a program for you to work with. The vision exercises we mention are described in the Vision chapter unless noted otherwise, and will be referred to in detail later in this chapter.

Rachel, a very beautiful young woman, had suffered from diabetes since childhood. At the age of twenty-two, after her retinas had been damaged by recurring lesions and growth of blood vessels, she was left with practically no vision. Laser therapy, which is often helpful in these cases, could not help her. She still had some indistinct, blurred vision in her left eye, but she no longer even tried to see out of her right eye. That was when she decided to try our vision exercises.

It was important for her to not give up on the right eye. When the brain has decided that a part of your body cannot work, it assigns much more responsibility to another part that can work. If you have become mostly dependent upon one stronger eye, the brain works hard to suppress the vision in the overall weaker eye and keep it from doing anything. This effort leads to overall fatigue and strain that eventually translate into even less vision.

In order to activate the right eye, Rachel would lie down in the dark with her better eye covered. A red light-bulb blinked on her right side, near the blind eye. She could not identify the light's color as red, but she could see the light going on and off. At first, the only light her eye could see was the red light. Gradually she became able also to see the blinking of other colors — yellow, blue and green.

Rachel spent many hours on vision exercises, concentrating on palming, sunning and shifting. Within three sessions she was able to read printed letters, one inch in size. Shortly after that, she was able to read, from the distance of five feet, the first three lines on an eye chart. When she directed a small flashlight toward her weak, right eye, the vision in her better eye improved immediately: she could read the fifth and sixth lines on the chart, and even see some letters from ten feet.

We worked mainly from five feet, and very slowly her vision improved. Rachel chose to join Meir's Self-Healing practitioner training class as an opportunity to work intensively on herself. The class was a very supportive environment. When the class was over, Rachel was able to see much better. A year later, she was back in college, doing her own reading and working part-time as a bookkeeper. In another two years, she regained her driver's license.

Due to diabetes, Rachel had originally lost much of the peripheral vision in her left eye (her stronger eye), and many of the cells in the center of the macula were also damaged. Through exercises, she was able to train herself to use those parts of the macula which were not afflicted by the retinal myopathy. The vision in her left eye is 20/40 with correction, even though she cannot use the center of her macula, where the clearest vision is found. Her vision in this eye has improved from non-functional to normal vision.

Rachel's overall health also improved during the time we worked with her. The special massage technique we have been using for diabetes helped her circulation, and allowed her to cut her insulin intake in half within a year. Her doctor gave her the cleanest bill of health she has had since she was diagnosed with diabetes.

Dealing with Diabetic Problems

It is important for you to improve your circulation. This is what will prevent gangrene, help wounds heal faster, and even help prevent damage to your retina. Better circulation will mobilize insulin faster. We have found that tapping on the bones helps circulation greatly, especially in cases of diabetes. Bones are where blood cells are produced. It is known that diabetic patients are not necessarily anemic; however, we feel that in some way the vibrating of the bones does the diabetic a lot of good for the circulation.

Spend a month studying and working with the Massage chapter, and then focus on bone-tapping. Tap on the bones you can reach, and get at least three sessions a week from a therapist or friend. Bone-tapping is the most effective technique we have found for diabetes.

Refer to the chapter on Osteoporosis, exercise 18–1, for a description of bone-tapping. Favorites for tapping are the tibia, all the way from the knee to the foot, and the bones of the skull (excluding the temples). You would enjoy all of this best if someone taps on you while you relax in a dark room. Close your eyes and breathe deeply. WARNING: WHEN YOU RECEIVE A MASSAGE, YOUR SUGAR LEVEL MAY DROP AS IT DOES DURING OTHER PHYSICAL ACTIVITIES, EVEN THOUGH YOU ARE PASSIVE. HAVE JUICE OR A FRUIT HANDY IN YOUR MASSAGE SESSIONS.

Besides bone-tapping, we recommend sitting in jacuzzis, which have a somewhat similar effect.

The most important chapter for you to work with is the one on Circulation, but you should also refer to the Breathing chapter, exercise 1–16, and to the Massage chapter, exercise 7–26, for important techniques to improve your circulation.

Retinal Myopathy

If you have had laser treatment for retinal myopathy, you may find that some parts of the retina are non-functional, while others were saved. If you are lucky and your central vision remains intact, or if the damage was minimal, then you may sense some loss of vision in some areas, but functionally your vision may not be impaired; your brain may be able to allow good vision in spite of the damage. In this case, palming (refer to the Vision chapter, exercise 8–5) will allow relaxation and recovery of the eye, and will help the brain while it relearns how to use the healthier parts of the retina. In addition to palming, sun your eyes frequently (refer to the Vision chapter, exercise 8–6) and then work through the Vision chapter step by step.

If the center of your retina is damaged and you can only see well in your periphery or parts of it, then we definitely recommend working with vision exercises. For two weeks, practice palming and sunning as described in the Vision chapter. After that, follow your palming sessions with peripheral stimulation by candlelight, as described in exercises 8–13 and 8–14 in the Vision chapter.

Sit in a dark room, and move a lit candle back and forth exactly in the areas where your eye cannot see. For a split second move it to where your eye can see and then back to where it cannot see. Don't move your eyes – they should be looking straight ahead – only the candle is moving. Now close your eyes and imagine you are seeing the candle right where you know it is.

Move the candle from an area where you can see it to an area where you can hardly see it. Move the flame back and forth, again and again, until the border between the seeing area and the blind area is less distinct. Close your eyes from time to time to imagine again that you can see the candle. Gradually expand your visual area, by moving further away from the originally clear area. Sooner or later you may find that you can use more of your retina.

If one of your eyes is badly damaged and your other eye sees much better, don't neglect to stimulate the damaged eye. In the case of damage to a large area of the retina, or to the central vision, you may find it difficult to adjust to the great loss of clarity. In this case, it is up to you to teach your brain about all that is available, to stimulate it and to use it well – through palming, sunning and fusion exercises (exercise 24–10 in the Vision Problems chapter).

If one of your eyes is partially damaged and the other is almost completely damaged, start working with your vision by activating the weaker eye. Work with exercise 24–11 in the Vision Problems chapter.

16–1 After several weeks, try shining a light from a small flashlight directly into the weak eye, while you read or practice shifting in the sunlight with your better eye. Wiggle the flashlight quickly, and you may find that your reading is better. Make sure that the strong eye does not see the flashlight. If necessary, put a piece of black paper between your eyes to separate the visual field of one from the other.

Close both your eyes from time to time and visualize that each letter is very black, and that its background is very white.

If both eyes are badly damaged, one more than the other, but you can still read from both, your exercises will be different. Choose a distance and an angle from which you can work with the eye chart comfortably, and work with the eye chart with all the exercises described in the Myopia section of the Vision Problems chapter. You may need to work from a particular angle, and familiarize yourself with that angle. Don't let letters fade away – keep moving until you find the exact angle that allows you to use the healthy parts of your retina. Always return to that angle to read, and gradually your brain will develop the ability to see better from there.

Refer to exercise 24–7 in the Vision Problems chapter, and work mostly with the third paragraph (see fig 24–7).

If you need to get closer to the chart to read with your weaker eye, then do that. Even if your weak eye can read only from two feet and your better eye from ten, you will find that, after practicing from two feet, reading

with your better eye from ten feet will be easier, because the stimulation of your weaker eye will have eased the tension caused by the brain's suppression of that eye. What you can also do, besides walking back and forth, is cut large letters from black paper and post them near the chart, so that you can practice reading with your weaker eye from a larger distance. Make the letters as large as you need them to be – even if that is one or two feet high.

George, a diabetic client who used this exercise, came to see us when his vision was 20/600 in his better eye and insignificant in his weaker eye. He claimed he could not read at all. An active eighty-seven-year-old, he worked joyously and energetically with the eye exercises, and soon the vision in his better eye was measured at 20/200. His weaker eye improved to 20/600. He was then able to read large signs and catch the bus by himself – achievements that made his life much more independent. We also found that one of the reasons that George was not able to read was that he had been trying to read from the same distance he had been reading from before the diabetic attack. By experimenting with a much shorter reading distance, George was able to use his newly developed vision for reading. After several months George was able to read regular-size print for half an hour at a time, without glasses. No matter what your degree of improvement, it is worth your time to try to improve your vision.

If you have lost your vision altogether, you may still be able to see blinking lights – perhaps only after bodywork sessions. Even if your vision does not improve any further than that, the stimulation of your visual cells by the lights is healthy for you, because all the cells in your body should be stimulated.

CHAPTER 17

Arthritis

What a joint does is to permit movement. When it stiffens and begins instead to *hamper* movement, it is absolutely crucial to encourage it to keep moving. As long as the joint has some mobility, you can not only prevent its permanent loss, you can also regain all or most of the mobility that was lost previously. For a person with any form of arthritis, this may seem next to impossible, because of the pain involved. For the person embarking on the task of recovering from arthritis or injury, it is important to remember two things. First, every movement can be done by degrees, and even the smallest amount of movement in a joint helps to preserve its movement capacity and prevent further damage to it. If you have an arthritic ankle, no one expects you to perform ballet exercises, and indeed these could be extremely damaging. What will help you is to find the range of motion that your ankle will enjoy, no matter how small, to perform that range of motion regularly, and very gradually to expand it.

The second important point to keep in mind is that not all of your pain is directly caused by the condition of your tissues. Some portion of it depends upon other factors, such as fatigue, the general condition of your body,

and most especially your state of mind. Research has shown that pain is often partly due to perception. People with chronic conditions such as arthritis often suffer more pain than they need to, because their emotions cause them additional tension and stress. They may be fearful because of the memory of past pain, angry and resentful at having to deal with constant discomfort, frustrated because their illness limits them in what they can do. Does this sound like you? If so, your feelings are absolutely justified. However, they will hurt you almost as much as the disease itself if they come to dominate your outlook. You must be willing to have the feelings and then let them go – at least during the time which you spend working on yourself. Try to come to your exercise periods with an open mind, and suspend – at least temporarily – the difficult thoughts and feelings which can increase your perception of pain. Emotions have an immediate, tangible, measurable and provable physical effect on your body: they can contract your muscles, slow or speed up your circulation, alter your digestive processes, and suppress your breathing as well as all other functions of your autonomic nervous system. Tightened muscles and slowed circulation of body fluids will only make your condition worse. So remember that your frame of mind, both when you work on yourself and at other times, is very important. You may not be able to avoid having negative feelings, but try at least not to encourage them, to dwell on them or to add to them.

View your exercise sessions as a time to treat yourself gently, to take things easy. If you are in the habit of doing things strenuously, forcibly or mechanically, you will have to learn new habits, since these are the ones which have been contributing to your problem. You will have to develop patience with your body, but your patience will be rewarded by lessening of pain and return of better, and in some cases of full, function. Many arthritic patients who have learned to work on themselves in this way have found flexibility and ease of movement far beyond what they had had before their illness.

You will find your best results through working on your entire body, rather than just on your problem areas. Each movement of a joint affects many other joints. Arthritis in your hip may be worsened by the way you move your ankle; chronic tension in a shoulder may be contributing to the development of arthritis in your fingers. Also, if you know that you have the tendency to develop arthritis, it makes sense to take preventive measures so that no further joints will be affected.

Water Exercises

All of our clients with arthritis have used water exercise at one time or another. Moving in water – especially warm water – without having to fight the pull of gravity dramatically reduces stress on your joints. Try to get access to a warm pool; most cities have such a facility – at a community center or YMCA, for example. Many of the exercises described in this chapter and in the Joints chapter can be done while sitting or standing in warm water, preferably with the part of the body you are working on fully immersed. Find the ones that you can do easily. Doing these movements under water will double their effectiveness and, as an added bonus, will help to regulate the fluid balance in your body.

There are numerous conditions which have been identified and loosely grouped under the term 'arthritis'. We shall describe programs for a few of these conditions. If your condition is different, you may still find suggestions which are applicable to you.

Osteoarthritis, or Degenerative Joint Disease

In osteoarthritis, the cartilage facings of the bones within a joint first lose their glossy surface, becoming rough and pitted so that the bones no longer glide smoothly but instead create friction, with the surfaces 'catching' on each other, making movement slower and more difficult. The cartilage eventually will fray and shred, gradually wearing down so that finally the bone surfaces are exposed to each other. This can make movement not only difficult but also very painful. Sometimes little spurs, called osteophytes, will develop on the bone surfaces where the cartilage has worn away, and these too may or may not cause pain. This condition is especially noticeable in the finger joints, where these knobby growths replace damaged cartilage, eventually swelling and deforming the knuckles. These knobs are known as Heberden's nodes and are one of the most common signs of osteoarthritis. Bony spurs can also develop on vertebrae where a disk (one of the tough elastic cushions found between spinal bones) has worn away, and this condition may also be classed as osteoarthritis.

Everyone is predicted to develop some degree of osteoarthritis at some stage of life. Obviously, this prediction includes you.

It is oversimplified to consider osteoarthritis a 'wear-and-tear' process, but weight-bearing joints and those which are under repetitive stress over long periods of time are more prone to it.

During the second half of this century, more than in any earlier time, osteoarthritis has become increasingly related to life management. In other words, this is a stress-related illness. This is where we believe that you have a choice. There is much you can do to prevent osteoarthritis.

First of all, you need to reduce your stress. This whole book is devoted to just that. By working with the first part of the book, chapter by chapter, and focusing mainly on the Joints chapter, you can prevent osteoarthritis. Work with all the exercises for the joints which are easy for you to do, to increase the range and smoothness of your motion. Do not be vain, assuming that you are flexible enough already, and do not be humble, assuming you cannot do anything. Work with your body, teaching yourself new ways of operating. Moving constantly will keep you moving indefinitely.

The second important thing to do is to reduce the salt and sugar in your diet and to not smoke or consume alcohol and caffeine. Your diet should be as healthy and as sensible as possible, including the freshest fruit and vegetables. We suggest that you also fast from time to time, to cleanse your system.

Your body needs daily work – not weekly or occasional. Checkups with your physician are important, but not nearly as much as maintaining your body daily.

Be vigilant with your body. Recognize a problem joint and stop the process of its deterioration as soon as you can. Change your lifestyle with the first signs of osteoarthritis; do not wait for it to escalate.

Many people are not satisfied with what conventional medicine offers for joint damage, and therefore search for alternatives. We suggest that you *start* with alternatives. If you believe in your body's natural capacity to be strong, firm and loose at the age of forty-five, fifty and even eighty, then you may have the motivation to change your body for the better. If you do not believe in your body's capacity, then we hope that with time we will manage to convince you. Your body's healing mechanisms do have the capacity to prevent deterioration and stiffening.

17–1   One method you may enjoy working with is hydrotherapy. Alternating between hot and cold water can increase the flexibility of the joints. If possible, try to spend some time at hot springs, and remember to jump into a cold pool once in a while. If you can, and if your physician approves, go swimming in a cold pool or lake or ocean on a hot summer day (we know some people think that this is torture), and you may find yourself more flexible after the swim.

If your hip joint is arthritic, you will sometimes feel pain in the hip joint itself; at other times you will suffer pain in your knee, resulting from the stress produced by the lack of mobility of the hip. Because we usually walk in shoes, on concrete, we tend to stiffen our ankles. When the ankles do not move to their full range, the movement of the knees is limited, in order not to stress the stiff ankles. In the same manner, the hip joints will not move fully, so as not to put stress on the knees. To reverse the process which led to an arthritic hip joint, you would focus your work on developing mobility in the ankles and strength in the calves and shins. This mobility and strength will support the knees and hips better, allow better mobility in the knees and hips, and place some of the pressure on the calves rather than on the hips. The pain will then decrease from step to step. When the impact of movement is repeated on the same part of the joint, it causes deterioration of the joint. We suggest, therefore, that you walk and run on an uneven surface, on a soft substance such as grass or sand, and alternate between going forward, backward and sideways – refer to the Muscles chapter, the section on Learning to Walk.

Your program should consist of walking barefoot, to increase the mobility of your ankle; walking in water, in a pool or in the sea, which creates a pleasant, massaging resistance; walking backward to activate groups of muscles which tend not to be in use; and loosening the hip through massage. Whether you massage your hip joint or someone else helps you with that, you may find that tapotement is most effective – gentle, quick tapping which will promote circulation to the area which needs to heal. Work also with the Muscles chapter. Start with exercises 5–1 and 5–2 for the feet, and continue with all the exercises you feel comfortable with in the section on The Lower Body.

If your shoulders are arthritic, before working on your shoulders you will want to work very much on your fingers. Refer to the Massage chapter, exercises 7–1 to 7–7 and 7–24; refer to the Musicians chapter, which has many exercises and stretches for the fingers, some of which are 10–6 and 10–11 to 10–15. Becoming more aware of the fingers and activating them will ease the work of your shoulders.

If your problem is in your elbow, focus your work on your forearm and your wrist. Refer to the Joints chapter, the section on Wrists, and to the Musicians chapter, exercises 10–3, 10–4, 10–8, 10–9, 10–10, 10–18 and 10–21.

Whenever you have a problem joint, your work with your body should be toward increasing the balance of your working muscles. By building up muscles in the periphery of the problem joint, you can ease the load of the arthritic joint, which was the cause of the deterioration in the first place.

When you work on increasing the flexibility of a joint, remember to make sure that all parts of the joint are moving. For example, if you are working to increase the extension of your elbow (straightening the arm), remember also to work on increasing the flexion, or bending. Move each one of your joints thoroughly.

17–2   Imagine that your head goes all the way up to the sky, and that one shoulder goes all the way to the east and the other all the way to the west. Visualize that there is a large space between each one of your vertebrae. Imagine each one of your joints elongating. With every movement you make, think of the joint as long and flexible. For example, as you bend forward, think of your back as elongating from behind. As you straighten your back, imagine it elongating from its front.

If you are very afflicted with osteoarthritis — to the point that you are confined to a wheel-chair — we urge you to use the joints that you can to the extent that you can. Your support group can help you mobilize each joint to its full range, in a balanced way. Perhaps a few people can work on you simultaneously. You will need four or five sessions a week to increase your mobility substantially, but there is also much that you can do for yourself.

If you find it difficult to open and close your hand, work with exercise 17–6 in this chapter.

Lie on your back, put your head on a pillow, and move your head from side to side. Visualize that the muscles of your neck are long, and that the joints of the neck are soft. Imagine your head rolling from side to side with ease, and you may find that it is indeed rolling more easily.

In the same manner, imagine that each part of your body moves with ease, and work toward that. Read the rest of this book, to find the visualizations and stretches that work right for your specific condition. Once you are more familiar with the principles, you may find yourself inventing the movements that are best for *you*.

17–3 One good way to increase mobility is to try different postures from the ones you are used to. For example, lie on your back and rest your bent legs on a high mound of pillows. This may give your hips a stretch. In this position, have someone pull your buttocks from the sides to give your lower back a stretch. You may be able to do this pulling yourself as you breathe slowly and deeply.

We suggest that, after working with this chapter, you continue with the Breathing chapter before you go on to other chapters.

Return to the Breathing chapter from time to time, because it can always help you work better with your body.

TMJ — Temporomandibular Joint Syndrome

TMJ is a very common form of osteoarthritis. The medial pterygoid muscle, which composes the inner cheeks and takes part in elevating the jaw and moving it from side to side, tends to be very tight, limiting the mobility of the jaw. In the case of TMJ, this tightness is extremely excessive. There are dentists who work on changing the shape of some of the teeth in order to change the alignment of the jaws when one bites, and in many cases that does help release some tension in the muscles of the jaws. We find that working directly with the tight muscles is very effective, and we recommend that you try releasing the jaw muscles first, before considering having dental work done.

We suggest that your dentist, or physical therapist, or other therapist whose knowledge of anatomy is good, massages your inner cheeks (using gloves) to release the spasm of these muscles. This area can take deep-tissue massage, as the muscles are very strong and powerful. Massaging the outer muscles of the cheeks, and the whole area of the joint, is also very helpful. After eight to ten sessions of such massage, you may find that your jaw is loose enough to allow wide opening of the jaw and much sideways movement.

17–4 Open your mouth as wide as you can, several times, tapping on your cheeks to loosen them. Rotate your head as you palpate your cheeks with one hand over the other. Open

through your nose. You may want to record for yourself a tape which you can then follow, something like: 'My right ankle expands as I inhale, and shrinks as I exhale ... My right knee expands as I inhale, and shrinks as I exhale...' and so on. Go through all the joints, one by one, and focus mainly on those which are sore and swollen. This visualization has been helpful in reducing the swelling for many of our patients. Spend at least thirty minutes a day with this visualization, either in one stretch or in shorter segments, even five minutes at a time.

After you complete your breathing meditation, move each one of the joints separately to get a feeling of the mobility you do have in them.

We recommend that you read the first section of this *Handbook*, whether or not you can practice its exercises. Have a sense of the movement you desire to have in your joints, but do not try to force it upon yourself. Judge for yourself, with the help of your support group and perhaps professional therapists, which of the exercises we offer work best for your body.

17–6   If you find it difficult to open and close your hand, try to imagine your hand opening and closing with ease. If you can instill that sense in your mind, you may find opening and closing the hand easier. Visualize that your fingertips are leading the motion of opening and closing the hand twice, and then actually move your fingers once. Whenever you start to alternate between visualizing and moving, visualize twice as many movements as you actually make. With time you can change the ratio – visualizing two movements, and then moving thirty or forty times.

It is most important to have a sense of increased mobility. For example, if your fingers do not move well, imagine them getting longer. Then take each finger with the other hand and actually stretch it, as if lengthening it physically. Now open and close your hand and you may find yourself doing it with more ease.

You can do the same exercise with your hands in warm water with dissolved mineral salts, such as Epsom salts, English salts or others.

Finish the exercise by washing your hands in cold water for a minute or two, to stimulate blood circulation.

We recommend that you receive massage every single day for a period of four months in order to reduce the swelling in your joints. Swelling can be reduced by passive motion. Your therapist can move each needy joint in circles, at the range that your joint allows – even if it is minimal – being careful not to cause any pain. The rotations will help drain the joint. The swelling can be reduced effectively by pinching the skin near the joint and squeezing it between the fingers, while tapping on the area with the other hand. (Refer also to the Massage chapter, exercise 7–21.)

Sometimes this type of massage may be as effective in reducing the swelling as drugs can be. In most cases it is less effective, and we prefer it that way. We believe that the swelling is needed to a certain extent as a protective mechanism against excess movement in the problem joint. If you move without the confinement that the swelling imposes on you, you may create more destruction in the joint by increasing the friction. (By using painkillers you make yourself unable to feel how you destroy the joint even further.) On the other hand, by decreasing the swelling gradually you will be increasing your mobility more gradually, at a pace that your body can handle safely. With time, through movement, massage and visualization, you can remove the swelling altogether.

17–7　Pain is a very subjective feeling: it may be minimal in areas where there is a good reason for pain, and may be excruciating in other areas with very little reason. Meditation always seems to be helpful in reducing it. Return to exercise 17–2, and now visualize that the pain in your joints leaves through your periphery. If you suffer neck pain, visualize that it leaves through your shoulders, arms and fingers to the open air. If your hips hurt, imagine the pain traveling down through the thighs, calves and ankles to the feet and then leaving through your toes.

We found working with the autonomic nervous system very effective for rheumatoid arthritis. Work for at least six weeks with the exercises for the sphincter muscles, exercises 6–5 and 6–6 in the Nervous System chapter; later add to these exercises 2–6 to 2–9 from the Circulation chapter and 6–1 to 6–4 from the Nervous System chapter, 1–14 from the Breathing chapter and 5–34 from the Muscles chapter.

　After working with these exercises for three to four months, you may find that the balancing of your autonomic nervous system will lead to a general improvement in metabolism.

Exercises in a Pool

For the next six weeks, spend an hour to an hour and a half every day at a warm pool. The water should be no less than 85 degrees Fahrenheit (29 degrees Celsius), and best is 94–95 degrees Fahrenheit (35 degrees Celsius). In the pool, do many easy movements in the most relaxed way.

17–8　Supporting yourself by holding the wall or leaning against it, rotate each foot, slowly, in both directions. Rotate each calf, from the knee, in front of you, to your side and behind you. Do the same with your leg straight, rotating it from the hip. Stand on both legs and rotate your hips as described in exercise 4–5 in the Spine chapter.

Refer to exercises 5–9, 5–10 (if not painful or too difficult) and 5–44 of the Muscles chapter for more exercises in the pool.

　We also suggest that you swim a lot. When you swim, imagine that your toes are pushing you, that your fingers are leading you, and that no effort needs to be made by the arms, legs, shoulders, back or abdomen.

　You will find that these exercises will make a very big difference in your capacity to move. Be aware that for the first few times when you become much more mobile in the water you will be much less mobile outside of the water. In this case you need to take a rest immediately after the exercises in the pool, because your muscles will have difficulties dealing with gravity after moving with less gravitational resistance in the water.

　In addition to the exercises mentioned above, refer to all the exercises described in the Osteoarthritis section or referred to from there.

　If after six months of working with the program we suggested you feel that you have had a substantial improvement, you may want to visit your specialist for a new series of X-rays and tests. You may find your improvement greater than ever expected – if so, please write us about that.

Ankylosing Spondylitis

This condition is called 'attachment arthritis', because it involves inflammation of the area where a ligament attaches to a bone. Ankylosing spondylitis affects the spine almost exclusively. Until recently, the disease had been found only in men, beginning between the ages of twenty and forty. Over the past ten years, however, the disease has been found increasingly among women, which may be connected with women's increased participation in the stressful and sedentary aspects of business.

Initially, people with ankylosing spondylitis will experience pain when they try to move the affected areas, since the tendons and ligaments are inflamed. Eventually, however, the inflamed areas will harden into bony ridges, making movement no longer painful but simply impossible, which is why people with advanced ankylosing spondylitis will complain of stiffness much more than they will of pain. The ultimate result of severe ankylosing spondylitis will be a spine consisting of one giant bone connecting the pelvis, vertebrae, ribs and skull, with bone connected to bone by ligaments which have themselves become bony. However, such an extensive reaction is extremely rare: only one in 100 patients diagnosed with ankylosing spondylitis will progress to great limitation or deformity. There is some danger of lung infections such as pneumonia in people whose ribcage has become too stiff to permit full expansion of the lungs.

Not surprisingly, the best known antidote to this condition is movement and posture correction. Since the tendency of the joint attachments is to harden and contract, they must be constantly encouraged in the other direction by movements which stretch and separate them. Perhaps one of the reasons men suffer more frequently from this condition is that their spinal muscles and connective tissue tend to be stronger and tougher, and thus much more chronically contracted, than most women's. For social as well as practical reasons, men end up doing more heavy lifting and hauling type of work than do women. They tend to prefer exercises which increase muscle strength, while what is needed to prevent this disease is muscle flexibility.

If you suffer from ankylosing spondylitis, you probably find it difficult to lie on your abdomen. An important exercise for you is to lie down on your back in various positions, gradually developing the ability to lie on your abdomen again. This will not be easy, because the structure of your back will create pressure and discomfort in that position, and because your abdominal muscles are probably tense.

Start by massaging your abdomen gently as you lie on your back (refer to the Massage chapter, exercise 7–23), or have someone else massage your abdomen to release its tension (Massage chapter, exercise 7–33).

After reducing the tension in your abdomen, work on reducing the tension in your legs, which may be extremely stiff. Refer to exercise 4–13 of the Spine chapter, and have someone massage your legs as you lower each knee toward the floor. You can also tap on the outer side of your thigh as you lower your knee.

To loosen the muscles of the pelvis, refer to the Spine chapter, the section on Loosening the Hips and Pelvis; exercises 3–7, 3–8 and 3–11 of the Joints chapter; and exercises 2–25 and 2–28 of the Circulation chapter. You may find that working with these exercises can make lying on your abdomen possible. You can put a pillow under your abdomen or chest if that helps you feel more comfortable. However, lying on your abdomen without a pillow will give your back a good stretch, and will help you breathe deeply without much resistance.

Breathing deeply can be a very relaxing and effective part of your therapy. We recommend working with all the exercises in the Breathing chapter that you feel comfortable with.

Be aware that, because your connective tissues have a tendency to harden, changing postures is not an easy task — and the earlier you start working on your mobility the better. A good practice would be to stretch sideways and then stay in that position for a while. Stand with your back to the wall and try to extend your back until much of its area touches the wall. Go through this whole book to find the stretches which are good for you now — we cannot suggest any specific ones because the condition varies a lot from one person to another. Find the postures which are not impossible or even hard for you to move into, massage yourself while in those positions,

and stay there for a while, breathing deeply. Use the help of your support group to invent exercises which would lead to the posture you have in mind. If lying on your side is difficult for you, then support yourself with pillows on both sides and move a little from side to side to avoid staying too long in an uncomfortable position.

17–9 Lie on your back, bend your knees, keeping your feet on the floor, breathe, and move both knees to your right. Breathe deeply, massage your buttocks, and tap on the outer side of your left leg — or have someone else do that for you. You may want to use a bonger — a ball connected to a flexible handle — to reach leg muscles which you cannot otherwise reach. Now move both knees to the other side.

Flexibility is a result of good circulation and mobility. We would like to emphasize that, as you create more movement in your body, you should try to make your movements as fluid as you can, rather than rigid.

CHAPTER 18

Osteoporosis

When bones lose a large percentage of their calcium content, they become porous and fragile. This is usually a problem of the elderly, of women past the menopause and of people whose diet is rich in fats. It is more common among women than men.

Changing one's diet to one which is lower in fat and richer in calcium is easy. In addition, conventional medicine often offers hormones to women past the menopause. We prefer not to promote the use of hormones, but leave you to consult with your physician about that option. Your program to counteract osteoporosis may, however, include our bone-tapping massage – a technique we have found very effective.

Meir's mother was diagnosed, at the age of sixty, as having 60 percent calcium loss in the bones of her lower spine, and therefore being at high risk for fractures in her spine. She was asked by her physician to come in for an observation every three weeks. It took Meir quite a bit of labor to convince her to visit him twice a week for massage. (Parents are not always the first ones to accept your unconventional methods of treatment.)

Her treatment started with deep-tissue massage, to release the hardening of connective tissue which surrounded the muscles of her lower back. Then Meir added extensive tapping on the bones.

18–1 Bone-tapping Bone-tapping should be done on any bone which is close enough to the surface to be felt: the vertebrae, the ribs, the fingers, knuckles, wrists, forearms, elbows, shoulders, skull – but *not* the temples, which are too sensitive for tapping – jaw, feet, ankles, shins, knees and pelvic crest. In short, wherever you can feel your bones. Do familiarize yourself with the shape of your skeleton and the location of the bones, though – your throat may feel hard, and some very tight muscles may feel like bones, but they are not what you want to tap on. For example, you do not have bones running down the sides of your neck, even though it may feel like you do.

This type of massage is a light, constant, quick (about three per second, just to give you an idea) tapping with the fingertips of all five fingers, with a very loose wrist and a sense of fluidity. Tap for long periods of time – a steady, rapid, drumming tap – alternating your hands. This tapping on the bones increases blood circulation and aids in bone construction. If you do not have any special weakness in your thigh muscles, you can tap with an open fist on your thigh, and the vibration of this tapping will reach the femur bone, while relaxing the thigh muscles. You can do the same with your arm. If you can feel parts of your humerus (the upper-arm bone), tap on it with your fingertips; otherwise, tap with an open fist on the strong arm muscles.

Do not tap too hard, because that would be traumatic for the fragile bones; but do not tap much too lightly, as this will have no effect: the tapping should be pleasant to your fingers as well as to the person who is receiving the treatment. You may find it amazing how relaxed a person can become when his or her bones are tapped.

Before you tap on your bones or on someone else's, do spend some time working on loosening your wrists. You can refer to the Joints chapter, the section on the Wrists, and to the Musicians chapter, exercises 10–4, 10–8 to 10–10 and 10–18.

We owe you the end of the story. During Meir's six-week visit in Israel, he worked on his mother ten times. She wouldn't do the exercises he showed her (we do recommend that you do yours). Mom's physician checked her again, reported that bone brittleness was no longer a problem, and suggested that she come in for a regular checkup a year later.

We have seen similar success stories. Ruth, a very kind, energetic and active ninety-two-year-old, used to come to the Center for Self-Healing for regular sessions with Darlene, and worked on improving her joints and muscles. One thing she did not improve was her posture; her back was stooped, and seemed to be getting worse. Meir dropped by her session one day, and spent half an hour tapping on her vertebrae. Not only did her back straighten remarkably, it stayed that way for at least two more years.

The bone-tapping technique may sound too simple to be true, but it indeed works like magic.

Often people who have osteoporosis tend to believe that their health will deteriorate no matter what they do, but the truth is that you can stop that degeneration or slow it down, and even reverse it. You must apply your intuition and kinesthetic awareness to choosing the exercises which will help you and avoiding those which are too difficult and may harm you.

18–2 One exercise to start with, if you are comfortable with it, is lying on your back and alternately bending and straightening your legs as your feet glide on the floor. Imagine that your feet are leading the motion with ease, and try not to involve the muscles of your abdomen and back in the motion. Move your legs quickly and lightly.

Another exercise which you can do at the early stages of your work is the following:

18–3 Stand up, and shake each one of your limbs. Imagine that each one of your hands is wet and that you are trying to shake off the water. You can shake your legs with both feet on the floor – mostly moving the knees quickly. If you feel stable enough, lift one foot off the floor and shake the leg. Now shake the other one.

When your bones become less fragile, we recommend that you work with the rest of this book, starting with the Joints chapter – always being careful to choose exercises that you are ready for.

CHAPTER 19

Back Pain

Low-Back Pain – General

We offer this program for people who suffer
spasm of their lower backs, or people suffering
from structural problems such as ruptured
disks.

Learn from your physician about your situation. If surgery is not recommended immediately, it will be worth your while to experiment
with various techniques which may help your
back.

If you suffer severe low-back pain, the very
first remedy you need is gentle massage of the
painful area. Have a member of your support
group or a massage therapist help you with
that (refer to the Massage chapter, exercises
7–29 to 7–31, and to the Nervous System
chapter, exercise 6–3), and massage your lower
back by yourself (refer to exercise 7–17 in the
Massage chapter). Be sure not to forget to
breathe deeply and to relax as fully as possible.

19–1 Your lower back may be inflamed. We
have found that one solution for that is sitting
in a hot tub with ice against your lower back
(the ice will be immersed). This may sound
funny, but in fact it combines relaxation of the
muscles with reducing the local inflammation.

If you do this repeatedly, you will find your
pain decreasing.

Avoid movements which will increase your
pain. Trying to flex or extend your back
beyond its present limited capacity will hurt
it even more. It is important, however, to
promote movement in painful areas and areas
near them. Gentle, non-vigorous movement
increases circulation, muscle-fiber flexibility
and strength, and is essential for healing. We
suggest the following movements:

19–2 Lie on your back, bend your knees
(keeping your feet on the floor), and move the
knees together from side to side, while rolling
your head to the opposite direction. Put a hot
towel under your back to increase the circulation to that area immediately. That will
help you stretch the back muscles as you
mobilize the rest of your body. Breathe deeply.

After five days of using the exercises above,
try these: exercise 2–29 of the Circulation
chapter, and exercises 4–4, 4–9, 4–10, 4–11
and 4–13 of the Spine chapter.

In order to ease tension in your back, you
need to strengthen your calves and balance

the use of the muscles of your legs. When you achieve that, you will not use your back muscles to support you with your walking. Start by giving your feet a good massage, as described in exercise 5–2 of the Muscles chapter. Then continue with the following exercises for the feet: Circulation 2–30, 2–31 and 2–34; Muscles 5–1 and 5–11 to 5–15; Joints 3–33.

19–3   Standing, lift one foot forward and rest it on a chair or a low table. Rake your hamstrings with your fingers, pulling from behind the knee toward your buttocks.

19–4   Lie on your back, breathe deeply and slowly, and feel whether breathing causes pain in your back. If it does, slow down your breathing. The slower you breathe, the less you will feel pain. Lying on a hot towel will help you breathe with less tension. Lying on your side, massage your back with round, warming strokes.

When you reach a stage where breathing is not painful any more, try the next exercises.

Refer to exercise 12–1 in the Asthma chapter and to exercise 3–15 in the Joints chapter. This latter exercise will help you ease the tension in your upper body and use the correct muscles to do the work. As you rotate your foot around the chair, tap with your free hand on your buttocks and your lower back to loosen them.

By loosening the leg muscles, your legs will be able to carry the torso more easily. To loosen your legs, work with exercises in the bathtub: refer to the Muscles chapter, exercises 5–3 to 5–5 and 5–7. Use a tennis ball to loosen the thigh muscles, as described in exercise 5–25 and in the following exercise.

19–5   Sit on the floor with your legs stretched forward but without locking your knees. Place a tennis ball under your hamstrings, press on your thigh with your hands, and bend forward. Repeat this exercise with the tennis ball under different areas of your hamstrings. You can use your fist, rather than a tennis ball under your thigh, if this does not create pain in your hand.

To summarize, your work on your lower back should be focused on increasing circulation and mobility in the lower back, and preventing movements which are painful to it.

A hurting, injured back will normally take three to six months to get to the stage where the pain is manageable. If you find that every week your pain is somewhat decreased, then you will probably benefit from continuing the same exercises that have helped you. To relieve the pain permanently, first the injury must be allowed to heal. When it has healed, you will need to continue with a program of movements which will help you maintain muscle strength and flexibility, as well as a healthy, balanced posture – refer to the Spine and Posture Problems chapters for ideas.

Sciatica

Sciatica is a pain that radiates along the course of the sciatic nerve, which is the longest nerve in the body, running from the lower back all the way down the leg and into the foot. The pain resulting from compression of the nerve may be experienced along the entire neural pathway or only along a part of it. A mild sciatica is one where there is a sensation of aching in the buttocks or lower back. A severe sciatica may be painful from the lower back all the way along the leg and into the foot. The path of the pain is characteristic: beginning in the lumbar area, it goes through the buttock, down the outside of the thigh, across and into the inside of the calf and into the arch of the foot.

Sciatica is very common and very unpleasant. It can flatten its victims like a migraine. It often results from a nerve-root compression between the fourth and fifth lumbar vertebrae, but it can occur from a variety of other causes, such as pressure on the nerve by overly tight buttock muscles. One of our clients, a flute player, developed agonizing sciatic pain as a result of sitting crosslegged, twisted to the right and holding a flute several hours a day for twenty years. No degeneration of the disks showed in his X-rays, but the unbalanced position of his muscles, held for extended periods of time, had, in our opinion, produced muscle stiffness that led to the nerve irritation.

People suffering from sciatica often have trouble sleeping because of the pain. Some find it difficult to sit, stand or lie down for more than a few minutes. If you have sciatica, treat your body with respect – don't ignore the pain, but use it to learn what is best for your body.

19–6 You may find that lying down on the side that doesn't hurt is most comfortable. Bend both knees, and place the upper foot near the lower knee. Your first exercise should be done in this position. Tap rapidly and gently with your fist on your buttocks, to release the tension in them, and along the side of your thigh, to relax your leg. You might ask a friend in your support group to relax your

thigh and calf by massaging them as you lie on your side, starting with gentle strokes, and later very lightly squeezing the muscles. Refer your partner to the Massage chapter for more techniques. While receiving massage, practice subtle hip movements, such as rocking the hip slightly back and forth, moving it in a very small circle, or tightening and releasing the buttock.

If you don't have any problem with your upper back, you may benefit from deep pressure there: deep massage strokes, rotating pressure with the thumb, or lying on tennis balls as described in exercise 4–33 in the Spine chapter (use the balls only in areas that are not sore and not extremely tight). In contrast, your sensitive lower back should be 'babied'; it should be massaged gently, using a cream or oil, and so should your buttocks and the painful sides of your legs. Self-massage can be very helpful. Breathe slowly and deeply, and try not to tense your upper body while working on yourself. As you lie on your side, visualize that your hip joint expands as you inhale, and shrinks as you exhale. Do that for several deep breaths and then massage the side of your leg gently. Only after two or three sessions of this gentle treatment, and only if your pain level decreases considerably, can you become a little firmer with your massage. Always be sensitive to your painful areas.

We have found that taking short walks, barefoot, on sand or grass has helped to increase the strength of the calves and ankles and to relieve much of the sciatic pain. This kind of walking eases the stress of the hips by distributing the weight more equally throughout your feet and legs. Practice walking backward and sideways, to involve muscles that usually do not take part in walking. Please read the section on Learning to Walk in the Muscles chapter for more ideas.

Practice foot rotations. When your foot does not have enough mobility, your ankle will stiffen, then your knee, and ultimately so will your hip and lower back. Learn to feel each part of the foot as you step or stand on it. Familiarize yourself with the ability of each one of its muscles by following the instructions for foot massage – exercise 5–2 in the Muscles chapter. You may find it difficult to bend your toes upward, or to rotate your whole foot outward, because of constant spasm in the muscles of the instep and arch of the foot. You may also find that it is easier to bend your toes down after pulling them up. Massage your foot, ankles and calves as described in the Massage chapter, and with time and patience your mobility will increase.

For a period of time your sciatic pain may come and go no matter what you do about it. But, if you continue to work on your body, it will eventually decrease. Please read the section on Muscular Atrophy in chapter 21, Muscular Dystrophy and Atrophy.

Your next exercise is exercise 4–5 in the Spine chapter. Do this very gradually: start with very small rotations, and then larger and larger ones. Stay within a radius that is pain-free; if it begins to hurt, make the circle smaller. Follow with the other exercises in the Loosening the Hips and Pelvis section of the Spine chapter. Then practice the Spinal Flexion exercises, alternating between them and lying on tennis balls as mentioned above.

Work with exercise 19–5; massage all sore areas of your legs with your palms, then squeeze, stroke and shake them.

When you get to a stage where your pain subsides almost completely, and not before ten weeks of this kind of therapy, you can benefit from deep-tissue massage: squeeze the sides of your legs strongly, breathe deeply, and visualize your legs expanding as you inhale and shrinking as you exhale.

After you recover from sciatica, you can prevent its recurrence by continuing with self-massage and Self-Healing exercises, taking long walks, swimming and learning how to avoid straining your back.

In order to avoid back-strain, you need to apply several principles of movement: isolation, centering and visualization.

The first principle you need to learn is isolation. Each of your body's muscles should do its own work. More specifically, you need to isolate your back from your limbs. By loosening your hips you will prevent tightening of the lumbar spine, which is the cause of sciatica. By strengthening and balancing your calves and shins you can prevent your hips from tightening. This chain of tension starts with walking stiffly and with a need for the thighs to compensate for weak legs. Refer to the section on Learning to Walk in the Muscles chapter.

To demonstrate to yourself the involvement of your back in the work of the legs, pay attention to how you climb stairs. Try to use only your leg muscles and to relax your back completely. The chances are you will find that difficult. Another example of an unnecessary involvement of the back in a movement which is none of its business is sitting down on a chair and standing up again. Do you bend forward to do either of these movements? If so, you are unnecessarily involving your back. This is where we come to the next principle of correct movement, which is centering.

'Centering' is a conscious awareness of the exact physical center of your body, combined with a sense of moving as though every move-ment began in and flowed from, your center. Having an awareness of your center will give you better posture and more balanced move-ment. It will help you to align your body evenly, so that gravity can work *for* you – to keep you well-balanced – rather than against you – to distort your posture and movement. Since people with sciatica have a tendency to stand, lean, walk and even sit more heavily on one side of the body than on the other, centering is especially important. For some people, centering is experienced as a feeling of connection with the center of the earth, result-ing in a sense of stability. You may find it helpful to imagine that the area just below your navel is connected to the center of the earth through a flow of energy. When your body is tense and its energy flows are restric-ted, you may begin to move as though some other part of your body, such as your chest or your neck, is your gravitational center. This throws you completely off-balance, desta-bilizing and tensing the entire body.

The following exercise will demonstrate to you how centering can relax your back. It will also help you get in and out of a chair with less strain on your back muscles.

19–7   Sit on a chair, without leaning against its back, with your feet apart. Imagine that your navel is connected to the center of the earth. Tap with your feet, alternately, on the floor, in a quick rhythm, and tap with your hands on your navel. It helps if you say aloud 'Center–center–center' as you tap. A little com-plicated? Well – we gave you the easy version. (Besides, remember that you are helping your central nervous system whenever you practice coordination exercises.) Now go on with this tapping for about a minute, and then stand up quickly. Continue the tapping while stand-ing, and then sit down quickly (make sure that the chair is still behind you!). After you have done this a few times, place one hand on your chest and one on your lower back as you sit down or stand, and you may find that you are sitting and standing without bending your back.

Notice that the exercise you used for centering actually resulted in a more active, 'isolated' use of your body's periphery. Your legs, rather than your back, were doing all the work of lifting you and putting you back in your seat. It is crucial for you to develop this ability to isolate your muscle use, to let your back work for itself and your legs work for themselves. Without it, your spine will continue to hurt. Centering, therefore, is another method of achieving isolation.

19–8   Another important technique in keeping the back uninvolved in motions that are not its concern is using visualization. The best visualization is of using your body's periphery: when you walk, visualize that your feet are lifting your legs – this will help you to give up the tendency to lift your legs by tensing the hip and back muscles. Looser hips and lighter walking will ease the sciatic pain. When you use your arms, visualize that your hands or fingers are leading the motion – and then, perhaps, you can stop using your back muscles for writing, drawing, driving and so on. By visualizing that you are using the periphery, you give the body a feeling of lengthening beyond the muscles which are involved in the motion. This allows release of the central – mostly back – muscles.

19–9 You need to learn to lift objects without tensing your back. If you are going to lift a heavy object, first of all bend your knees. Take hold of the object, and hold it close to your body (fig 19–9A). Now use the strength of your knees to lift your whole body up (fig 19–9B), bending your arms to keep the object close to your body. If you can get help lifting the object, please do. Every time Maureen's mother has another sciatic attack, it happens as a result of lifting. Whenever she isn't trying to carry grandfather clocks, however, she keeps her sciatica well under control with our exercises.

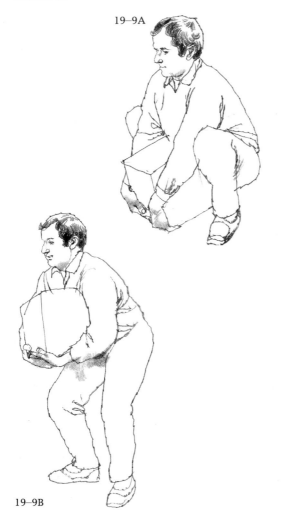

19–9A

19–9B

Stenosis of the Lumbar Spine

Lumbar spinal stenosis is an uncommon form of sciatica. The spinal canal at the lumbar area narrows and compresses the roots of the nerves leading out from the spine to the legs. In many cases surgery is effective in reducing the pressure, and if you suffer much pain it may be worth trying. The effects of surgery are often temporary, however, and to reduce the chances of recurring stenosis you would need to work on reducing the muscle tension which contributed to it in the first place. If your physician approves of delaying surgery, you might try to help your back and perhaps prevent the need for surgery altogether.

One feature commonly seen in lumbar spinal stenosis is great tension in the abductors (the muscles of the outer thigh). If you feel stiffness and rigidity along the outsides of your thighs, you probably have this problem. Massage the sides of your thighs by raking and pinching the muscles and rolling the skin between thumb and fingers. You can press your thigh on a tennis ball, as described in exercise 5–25 in the Muscles chapter. Work with the following exercises for the legs.

19–10 Lie on your back and put the soles of your feet together, keeping your knees apart. Lift your right knee and bring it over to your left, and then back to its original position. Now bring your left knee to your right, and back to its place.

19–11 Raise both arms to shoulder level, and kick sideways, as high as you can, alternating your legs. Keep your toes pointing forward and not toward the side you are kicking to. If you can reach your hands with your kick, raise your arms further. If you tend to lose your balance with this exercise, hold onto a table, counter-top, ballet bar or any other stable object.

For more exercises, refer to the Joints chapter, exercises 3–11, 3–31 and 3–32, and to exercise 2–31 in the Circulation chapter.

Neck Pain

Lack of sufficient space between the cervical vertebrae can often result in pressure on the nerves which extend from the neck down throughout the arm. This pressure can cause pain and loss of function anywhere along the nerve pathway, from the base of the skull all the way to the fingertips – and that is a real 'pain in the neck'.

If your condition has become uncomfortable to that degree, or even if your neck is just tense, painful or limited in mobility, there are a few things you can do about it.

You will benefit from massage of the scalp and the back. Refer to the Nervous System chapter, exercise 6–3, and to the Massage chapter, exercises 7–29 and 7–30, for ideas. If your pain is very severe, or if you are very sensitive, the massage should be very gentle.

We recommend stretching the back rather than using traction, because traction may be too stressful for the tight neck muscles.

19–12   Refer to exercise 4–30 for shoulder rotations. Now, in the same position, rotate your whole arm several times. Rest your arm and visualize that you are rotating it smoothly and without effort, and then rotate it again.

Repeat this several times before rotating the other arm.

19–13   Lie on your back with your head supported by a pillow. Move your head from side to side. Let your head rest lightly on the pillow, and try to make the motions as effortless as possible. Breathe deeply as you roll your head.

The main goal of the exercises for the neck is to lead to isolation – that is, separation of movement – between the arms, the shoulders and the neck. We tend to use the entire upper torso as though it were one rigid piece, contracting *every* part of it whenever we use *any* part of it, and the result is chronic tightness and pain throughout the area. Exercises which can help develop isolation between these parts are exercises 2–20 to 2–23 in the Circulation chapter. Repeating these exercises will create a feeling in your fingers that they can do their own work without the involvement of the neck, which is just doing *its* own work. The exercises will also strengthen your fingers, and allow them to do such things as writing, typing or playing music without tightening the muscles of the shoulders and neck.

For isolation of the shoulder muscles, refer to the Joints chapter, exercises 3–16 to 3–28, and to the Spine chapter, exercise 4–29.

19–14   Sit cross legged or, if you can, on your calves. Pull your head upward with your hands, your thumbs pressing on the base of your skull, and move your lower back forward and back, and in rotating motion. The motion of the lower back can relax the neck.

19–15   Sit in front of a table, place your hands palms-down on the table, and move both hands on the table in circles, making sure both move equally. Next, rest your arms on the table, lift the forearms but leave the elbows on the table, and rotate the forearms. Let your shoulders and chest relax completely as you move the arms. You will find that this loosens your neck. Imagine that your forearms are heavy, while your head is floating up to the sky. A variation of this exercise can be done by moving your head in rotation while circling with the hands.

19–16 Hold your head with both hands (see fig 5–43B in the Muscles chapter). Let your hands carry your head in rotating motion with no resistance or help from the neck muscles. This exercise may make a great difference to how your neck feels.

You may want to return to exercise 19–3 in this chapter. Refer also to exercise 6–17 in the Nervous System chapter.

Shoulder Pain

We have found that shoulder pain always involves deep tension in the middle-back and chest muscles. It may also be connected with tightness in the abdomen and diaphragm. So, in order to relieve shoulder pain, you need to loosen up these areas.

Deep breathing is what you need most, in order to stretch, expand and loosen your chest, middle back and abdomen. Please read the Breathing chapter carefully. Practice any of the exercises that appeal to you, and pay special attention to exercises 1–5, 1–7 to 1–10, 1–13, 1–15, 1–16, 1–19 and 1–20.

Massage your abdomen, and the muscles underneath your ribs. Exercises 2–2, 2–3 and 2–10 in the Circulation chapter will give you directions for massage of these areas. You will probably need help for massage of your middle back: not only is it hard to reach, it is often rigid. Your massage partner can release it by gentle pinching, upward pulling of the skin and rolling the skin between thumb and fingers. He or she can also refer to the Massage chapter (exercises 7–29 and 7–30) and the Nervous System chapter (exercise 6–3) for further back-massage techniques.

To release the chest and upper back through movement, we highly recommend exercise 2–15 in the Circulation chapter.

After working with these, you will probably benefit from practicing exercises from the entire Spine chapter, with special emphasis on shoulder rotations (exercise 4–30). Massage your shoulders (Massage chapter, exercise 7–15), or have them massaged by someone else, and work with the section on Shoulders in the Joints chapter.

To summarize, we would like to stress again that back pain will not disappear permanently before the body, and in particular the spine, is in proper alignment. The muscles should be working in a balanced way; there should be isolation of movement between separate parts of the body, and free, relaxed motion. We would like to refer you again to the chapters on the Joints, the Spine, the Nervous System and the Muscles. Working with these chapters one by one will help your pain decrease or subside.

Be careful, but not fearful. Avoid motions which may be wrong for you, but do not avoid those which may help you. Ease slowly into stretches and gentle movements. A solution to your situation will take time, so don't rush. Be patient with your body – it's the only one you've got.

CHAPTER 20

Posture Problems

Lordosis, Kyphosis, Scoliosis

All of these names refer to changes in the normal shape of the spine.

Lordosis is another name for swayback or an abnormally deep inward curving of the lower spine, in the lower lumbar and sacral areas. Many people develop this condition as a result of everyday habits such as slouching at a desk, wearing high heels or carrying around a heavy belly (pregnant women have to be careful to avoid this condition).

Kyphosis describes an abnormal outward or convex curve of the upper back and shoulders. People with this condition used to be called hunchbacks, and it is still sometimes called 'widows' hump' since it is often found in older women, though by no means limited to them. Kyphosis tends to depress the upper ribs and press the head toward the shoulders, so it affects the posture of the entire upper torso.

Scoliosis is a lateral, or sideways, curvature of the spine, which may also cause individual vertebrae to rotate sideways. This condition is often the most dangerous of the three. It can distort back posture, sometimes radically. It can also change the positioning of the ribs, which may lead to smaller lung capacity. Scoli-

osis usually develops in childhood or the early teens from a variety of causes. These may include:

- illness (for example, polio, which may weaken muscles around the spine);
- accidents;
- poor posture;
- a pattern of inactivity, leading to weakness and consequent muscular imbalance;
- unknown causes.

Lordosis

Some people may have lordosis but suffer no pain, while others have pain varying from mild to excruciating. If you suffer severe pain, work first with the chapter on back pain. If pain is not a major problem, start by spending one to three months with the Spine chapter. Then work a few weeks with the Joints chapter, and later a month practicing the exercises in the Muscles chapter. After practicing the general exercises for a total of four to five months, start working specifically with your lordosis.

You can reduce your lordosis by activating your lower back, thus increasing its flexibility and mobility, and by releasing tension in your abdomen.

20–1 Read the following exercise and dictate it slowly and in detail onto a tape, so that you can listen to it and use it as a meditation while you do the exercise.

Lie on your back, with your feet together and your knees apart. Breathe deeply, press your lower back to the floor, relax and exhale. Now inhale again, press with the lower part of your lower back onto the floor, relax and exhale. Continue to feel the different parts of your lower back – its middle, its upper part, its right and left sides. You will be activating many muscles that you normally do not use. Do the same with your middle back and upper back.

Do this exercise slowly, so that you will have time to really distinguish between the different areas in your back. Work with this exercise for a month, and then turn to the next variation.

This time, pull your right knee to your chest, and press the upper-right, middle-right and lower-right parts of your lower back to the floor. Now bring your left knee to your chest, and press to the floor the three parts of your lower back on your left side. Pregnant women should consult their therapists and feel for themselves whether this exercise suits them. Your therapist may suggest that you pull your knee more to the side. After two weeks of work with this variation, work one week with exercise 4–3 in the Spine chapter.

Refer to the following exercises: Circulation 2–26, Musicians 10–1, and Spine 4–12 and 4–13, which will help you flatten your lower back. Two very important exercises for you are 9–7 and 9–8 in the Running chapter.

20–2 You can benefit from having your back massaged as you kneel and bend forward, giving your back a good stretch. A recommended massage technique is rotation of the palm over the muscles of the lower back, starting from the center and moving toward the periphery, to stretch the muscles and straighten the curvature. The person massaging you can guide you in visualizing that your muscles are stretching outward laterally.

Whenever you develop more sensory awareness of an area in your body, you help that area heal. Increasing your ability to feel your lower back will help it straighten.

20–3 Kneel on all fours, and place a book on your lower back (fig 20–3). The book will help you sense the muscles of your lower back. Move your lower back up and down, without straining your abdominal muscles.

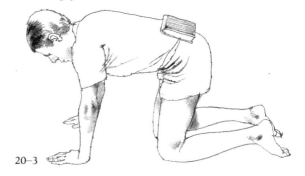

20–3

Two exercises from the Massage chapter will help you balance your muscles and loosen them. Work with exercise 7–19, pressing your lower back to the wall, and with exercise 7–20.

Spinal-flexion exercises 4–9 to 4–11 from the Spine chapter will be helpful, and so will bending the spine in the opposite direction, as in exercises 4–15 to 4–17 and 4–35 to 4–37. Alternating these will limber the lower back considerably.

You will also benefit from massage of the abdomen (Massage exercises 7–23 and 7–33), and from strengthening your legs as a means of support for the lower back – refer to exercise 5–23 of the Muscles chapter to strengthen your legs. To relax your legs, turn to exercise 18–2 of the chapter on Osteoporosis.

Your middle back is probably tense, and may welcome deep-tissue massage. Another area which tends to be tense and is partially responsible for the lordosis is the buttocks. Loosening the buttocks will also be helpful in straightening the spine. Refer to exercises 3–1 to 3–6 in the Joints chapter.

Kyphosis

If you have kyphosis but are free from pain, begin your exercise regimen by working for three months with the Joints chapter, emphasizing the work with the shoulders. The exaggerated backward curvature of the spine affects the posture and motion of your chest, shoulders and arms. By loosening your shoulders you will expand and free your chest.

For a period of one month, devote as much time as you can – up to twenty minutes a day – to the isolation of your arms from your shoulders. Refer to exercise 2–23 in the Circulation chapter and exercise 3–42 in the Joints chapter.

Next work for one month with the Spine chapter and then for two weeks with the exercises described above for lordosis – all but exercise 5–23 from the Muscles chapter. Add

to your list exercise 4–2 from the Spine chapter and, an exercise that we recommend you emphasize, Circulation exercise 2–15. During periods that you work intensively on yourself, try to receive frequent massage sessions.

The stretching exercises described below can be very helpful, but they are difficult and could be dangerous if they are done before you increase the flexibility of your back. Kyphosis often results from extreme muscle stiffness; the stiffness should be relieved gradually, to avoid damage to muscles or other tissues.

Practice exercise 2–14 from the Circulation chapter, but do not strain your middle back. When you feel ready for a greater stretch, ask a friend to help you by pulling your arms backward while you hold them in the position shown in fig 2–14B. Breathe slowly and deeply as your arms are stretched.

20–4   Lie on your abdomen and place your hands, palms-down, underneath your forehead, fingers interlaced. Lift your head and upper back up and rotate your whole upper body (fig 20–4).

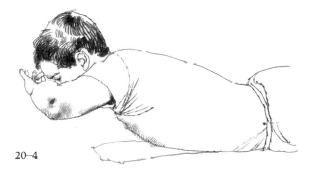

20–4

Practice the following exercises: Breathing 1–11, Spine 4–17 and 4–25, Muscles 5–39 and this next one.

20–5 Plow Lie on your back, lift your legs and lower back from the floor, and bring your legs above your head as you support your back with your hands. Now bring your feet to the floor behind your head, bend your knees, and try to bring your knees to the floor on both sides of your ears. Stretch your arms to the sides and rest them on the floor. Breathe deeply and feel your back expanding as you inhale. The third stage of this exercise – the rotating plow – is one of the most effective exercises for straightening your spine: lift your stretched legs from the floor, keep them together, and move your whole body in rotating motion.

Another very effective exercise for straightening your back is exercise 4–23 of the Spine chapter.

Scoliosis

Most doctors believe that only braces or surgery can correct scoliosis. Our experience with cases of scoliosis, however, has disproved this 'rule' many times over. In cases which are not severe, the spine may be straightened fully through massage and exercise. In cases of severe scoliosis, the progression of the lateral movement can be stopped, and the posture can be improved to a great extent.

You will need to invest a lot of time in correcting your scoliosis, as will your massage therapist or support-group partners. Try to arrange to have three or four massage sessions a week, and plan to spend three hours daily in exercises by yourself. Get your doctor's approval for the program, especially if you are elderly or weak. The results will almost certainly amaze you.

The displacement of the vertebrae which creates the sideways curve of scoliosis may be due to an inequality in the strength of the muscles on the two sides of the spine, which are called the erector spinae. The stronger muscles on one side will become overly contracted and rigid, exerting a strong pull on the weaker muscles of the opposite side. Since muscles and their surrounding connective tissue are part of what hold the bones in place, the bones themselves will eventually be pulled, along with the weaker muscles, toward the stronger side, and thus the curvature is created. The weaker side of the back will be flatter. Nor is the back alone affected: the uneven pull of the muscles will, in time, also change the position of the ribs, usually bringing them somewhat closer together and tightening the intercostal muscles between the ribs. You may be able to see this even in the chest: the ribs will be closer to each other on the weaker side. The imbalance and rigidity may extend to the muscles of the upper and lower back, causing changes in the position of the hips or shoulders. A scoliosis condition may result in one calf becoming thinner and weaker, usually on the weaker side. Often one side of the abdomen will be contracted.

We recommend the following exercises for scoliosis. All of the exercises in the Spine chapter will be helpful for you. They are designed to relax tense muscles and strengthen weak ones, and to promote equal use of all parts of your back. Begin with the section on Spinal Flexion, and add other spine exercises gradually, as you become comfortable with those you have already learned. Spine exercise 4–33 should be done only after warming up the back with stretches. You cannot use the tennis balls in the same manner as described there, because excessive pressure on the weaker areas of your back may cause you harm. If the curvature of your spine is in the middle back, you can press the tennis balls under the lower back, but, when you get to the middle back, put the tennis balls only under the stronger, tighter side, while on the weaker side you bring the ball all the way up to the shoulder.

After working with tennis balls, work with exercise 20-1, but do it very slowly.

Every scoliosis is different. It may be in the lower back or the upper back; it may benefit from different exercises. The one thing in common is that the back is very tight and its muscles are surrounded by hard connective tissue.

20–6   Lie on your back, with a pillow under your knees so that they are slightly bent, and rotate your feet slowly. Start with twenty rotations in each direction, and build up daily until you can do at least 100 in each direction. This helps to strengthen your ankles and calves, which will give a stronger basis of support to your back, so that the muscles there will not have to 'work for' your legs.

Toward the same end, exercise 5–23 in the Muscles chapter will help to strengthen your thighs.

20–7   This exercise will help you loosen your hamstring muscles and your back. Sit on the floor with your legs stretched in front of you, the feet as far apart as possible. Bend forward with your arms stretched ahead, and then stretch to the left and to the right of each one of the legs.

Now stretch with a twist: try to bring the back of your right shoulder toward your left knee, and then do the same on the other side. You may find that you are much more flexible on one side than on the other. Often people with scoliosis are flexible but not in a balanced way. The more even your flexibility, the less curved your back will be.

Another good stretch for the thigh muscles is exercise 3–8 in the Joints chapter. Work mostly with the bend shown in fig 3–8A. Remember to breathe deeply.

20–8   Refer to exercise 4–30 for shoulder rotations, and do them while lying on your tighter side and rotating your weaker shoulder. This is an important exercise for strengthening the muscles of the shoulder. We also recommend repeating the exercise while receiving massage. Now, in the same position, rotate your whole arm several times. Rest your arm and visualize that you are rotating it smoothly and without effort, and that the fingertips are leading the motion. Now rotate it again.

Massage Techniques for Scoliosis

Massage is every bit as important as movement in the treatment of scoliosis. If the muscles of the back are too tight to allow movement, exercise will not be very effective. Initially, massage will be the best way to loosen the muscles.

If you are going to be working on someone with scoliosis, please read the Massage chapter thoroughly first. When working with scoliosis, it is especially important to be able to distinguish strong from weak muscles, as different techniques are required for the different conditions – and you will be encountering both of them on the same back.

Do not begin directly on the muscles around the curvature. Start with the thighs, work up to the hips and buttocks, then to areas of the back which are less affected, and last to the region of the scoliosis itself. In most scoliosis cases, the massage therapist will find that the muscles and connective tissue which surround the curvature are extremely hard and tight. This may make it difficult to tell the weak muscles from the strong ones. You will need to soften the muscles first without using deep-tissue massage, because deep-tissue work on the weak muscles may be both painful and harmful. A good technique to start with is to pinch the muscles upward, rolling them between the fingers and pulling them away from the spine, as far as can be done comfortably. You can pull both horizontally, along the width of the back, and vertically, along its length. This both loosens the muscles and begins the breakdown of accumulated connective tissue. Deep-tissue massage may follow, but only in those areas where the strong muscles have become rigid.

Where strong pressure is appropriate, be sure that you begin with a lighter pressure and build up gradually to deeper pressure. You can then concentrate for an extended time on the rigid area. You can move your hands in a slow rotating motion over the area, moving the pressure from thumbs to palms to fingertips. Tapping with the fingertips and shaking the muscles while pressing down with your hands will also help to loosen the muscles. When the back begins to feel warmer and the muscles less rigid, you can use the same pulling and pinching technique on the flesh directly over the vertebrae.

On the weaker areas, use a much more gentle touch. Avoid deep pressure. Instead, use a warming and stimulating oil or cream and rub gently in wide circles with the entire palm, as though you were simply spreading the oil on the skin. Placing the palms flat and shaking them lightly against the muscles is another good technique. Passive movement is also good: have your partner lie on the tighter side while you move the shoulder of the weaker side slowly in rotation, lift the arm and move it in rotation, and very gently rock the hip back and forth.

Massage the intercostal muscles, between the ribs, by exerting a light pressure with your fingertips and moving them along the length of the muscles. If this tickles, deep breathing will help. Do this both on the back and on the chest, and encourage your partner to do this himself.

CHAPTER 21

Muscular Dystrophy and Atrophy

Muscular Atrophy

We will first discuss those muscles which atrophy, or become thin and weak, as a result of prolonged lack of use. This may happen after an illness which has kept one in bed for about four months or longer. It may happen as a result of wearing a cast on a broken limb. It can happen to older people who tend to be less mobile.

If this is the situation you find yourself in, you should practice caution with your movement as you work to regain strength in your muscles. If your legs have weakened because of prolonged bed rest, be careful to move out of bed slowly; if you don't, your stiff joints may become even stiffer or dislocated, and your weak muscles may be destroyed even further. Have a massage therapist or a friend massage your legs gently and move your legs while you are passive and relaxed, neither helping nor resisting the motion. (Refer especially to the Massage chapter, exercise 7–26, rotations from the hip as shown in fig 7–26A.) In areas where resistance is felt, tapping and massage will help. Gradually increase the range of passive movement.

It is important not to massage the muscles deeply, and that the movement of the muscles is gentle, without tension. After massage and passive movement have made you stronger, you can begin to strengthen the legs by taking walks. Gradually increase the duration of your walks.

The same applies for work with an atrophied hand. Working with the hands – writing, rubbing them together, cutting with scissors, squeezing a ball – can strengthen a hand further after the initial strengthening with massage and passive movement.

If you work with this condition slowly, results will occur quickly. If you rush, you can destroy the muscles even further, to the point where damage is permanent. Slow movements done in a sensitive, aware and thoughtful way can build up your muscles.

Study the Joints chapter, and work with each one of the joints gently and slowly at a pace at which the joint feels comfortable or almost comfortable with the motion.

Muscle cells do not divide, but that does not mean that lost muscle mass cannot be regained. Regeneration occurs in skeletal muscle fibers when satellite cells, found just outside the outer boundary of the muscle fiber, become new muscle cells. There are many muscles in your body, some of which you have not used and developed to their maximum capacity, and there may be fibers within a damaged muscle that were not damaged that can carry on with the function of that muscle and be strengthened to compensate for those fibers which cannot recover. So, even if some fibers are lost, the healthier ones can take their place.

Please read the Nervous System chapter to better understand the following concepts.

Much of the recovery involves changing the brain's concept of how the weak area functions. As a result of the prolonged lack of use of certain muscles, the brain accepts the lack of movement as the normal state of the tissue. In order to bring more life to the area, you need to demonstrate to the brain that a different state is possible, and you can do that only by bringing more mobility to the area that needs to heal. When you break the old patterns of limited motion, when you vary the stimulation to the area by increasing your variety of movements, your brain responds to the change by reorganizing its motor control of that area. It can then stimulate the tissues and make them work better.

The same is true in cases of muscular atrophy where nerve damage is involved, such as sciatica and spinal injury. The damaged nerve does not send the muscles connected to it enough neurological stimulation, and that causes their deterioration. On top of that, the pain involved in many cases results in less movement. By demonstrating to the brain which possibilities of function still exist in spite of the atrophy, you can increase the stimulation of the tissues by the brain. (For sciatica, see also the Sciatica section in the Back Pain chapter.)

We would like to tell you at this point about one of our students, Irene, who suffered from post-sciatica atrophy. She was referred to Meir by her doctor, a homeopath with a background in surgery. Irene was hesitant about working with Meir until she met him personally at a health fair, but the personal meeting changed her feeling about his capacity to help her. (It is often the case that the person who helps you is the one you trust and feel most comfortable with.)

Irene suffered back pain, and her right calf was very thin, with very little muscle mass. We worked with massage and a variety of exercises. The best one was the broomstick exercise: Irene would lie on the floor, a broomstick under the length of her spine, and bend her knees. The broomstick gave her no choice but to relax her back and straighten her spine: as long as she didn't, her back hurt. (See the description of this exercise in the Muscles chapter, exercise 5–39.)

Gradually her spine straightened, and a result of that was that her breathing became deeper. She also became more mobile, and the feeling all over her spine was that of release. A bit tired of life but looking forward still, she had all the energy she needed to help herself, and that is really what it took to improve her.

Irene's body was foreign to her, and to some extent she was afraid of it. We worked with massage three hours a week, spending an hour using mainly the 'buildup' motion (described below in the Muscular Dystrophies section) on the calf. She took long walks on the beach and climbed hills, to strengthen her weak and immobile leg. And then one day, at the beginning of a session, Irene's face looked as if something awful had happened. 'I have a tumor in my right calf,' she said. Low and behold, new muscles had started to work, and her calf had become thicker. Meir congratulated her for her success, but it took her five more minutes to understand that this unfamiliar expansion of her thin and deteriorated muscle was not an inflammation or a tumor.

Muscles can be rebuilt. It took Irene three months to rebuild hers, and this was a beautiful example of what can be done for destroyed muscles. Function can be restored by waking up the fibers that were just sitting there waiting to take over.

Muscular Dystrophies

The diagnostic tools to distinguish between the various types of muscular dystrophy are becoming more and more sophisticated. Geneticists are identifying the genes involved, which leads to genetic counseling. We have been working in a very different direction: helping those who have it already to regenerate.

We have worked with a variety of muscular dystrophies, mostly with the Duchenne, Becker, limb-girdle and facioscapulohumeral types. In general, our work with muscular dystrophies involves a few basic concepts:

- Dystrophic muscles should never be worked to a degree of exhaustion, as that would cause further deterioration.
- Strengthening of dystrophic muscles should start with very gentle and supportive massage, and continue with passive movements: only when a muscle gets stronger can it be exercised actively.
- Typical exercises for muscular dystrophy would be easy movements, repeated very many times – building up to hundreds or even thousands of times. Rotational motion

is of course a very balanced and therefore preferred method: it activates each of the muscles around a joint, and allows the smaller ones, as well as the large ones, to develop.

We do not have statistics to demonstrate our success in rehabilitating sufferers of these illnesses, but we have documented a few of them during the course of their treatment.

Unlike Duchenne muscular dystrophy, which affects young children, facioscapulohumeral muscular dystrophy usually begins in early adolescence. Life expectancy is normal, and typically the muscles of the face and shoulder girdle weaken. Most of the people we have seen so far with this condition also suffered weakness in the pelvic girdle, thighs or shins.

Michael had facioscapulohumeral muscular dystrophy. A pharmacist with a strong preference for homeopathy and alternative pharmacology, Michael was a lively young man with a kind, bearded, smiling face and a sense of humor. He said that Meir's book *Self-Healing: My Life and Vision* happened to fall on his head in a bookstore, so he just had to open it – and then he realized that there was quite a bit that he could do to help himself.

Fortunately, Meir was teaching a practitioner-training class when Michael came for his first sessions. The students helped not just by joining the therapy but by documenting it on videotape, and for the first time we were able to show what progress can be achieved with muscular dystrophy. (The documentation is available at the Center for Self-Healing.)

Michael, whose body was slender, had lost a great deal of muscle mass from the muscles in his arms, shoulders and chest. The hamstrings of his left leg were so weak he could not bend his knee against gravity (for example, lift his foot from the ground backward). His facial muscles were thin, but not especially so when compared to other people with the same muscular dystrophy; the movements of his mouth were not impaired in any way.

Michael was ambivalent about his ability to recover. With one part of his mind he believed that he could overcome the disease, that he could struggle his way out of it, but another part was haunted by it. It is easy to feel powerless physically and mentally when facing an illness which weakens you progressively – sometimes even daily – but to recover from it you need to use all your mental power and to have a sense of your inner strength. You need to give yourself credit for every improvement, as it is a physical manifestation of your strength of mind. Each improvement is a sign of your potential for long-lasting progress.

Massage Techniques for Muscular Dystrophy

We started by working on Michael's upper arms, using massage and exercises. The first form of massage was what we call 'support': a very light, though penetrating, rotating, gentle massage, with the fingertips of all ten fingers, warming the muscle while hardly touching it. When the area being worked on is very small, only one hand works there, and the other touches the body elsewhere. What do we mean by 'support'? The muscle tissue is weak, perhaps even dead or dying in places. Regeneration is taking place but may be outstripped by cellular death. The healthier muscles near it have not been much used, because their mobility has been limited. The first thing we

want to do is to give the area a feeling of being supported. With that feeling, and with better circulation, it will then become stronger. The massage creates a feeling of warmth and of penetration. Remember, this is not a deep-tissue massage – it is extremely light – but it will be effective if both the person giving massage and the one receiving it imagine that the fingers of the massage therapist are penetrating the tissue, caressing it from inside.

The 'support' massage goes on and on – for anywhere from thirty to ninety minutes. One of the results is that the muscle starts to puff: the tissues will enlarge, and their tone will improve. This enlargement will remain for about six to eight hours, but it will take several months of work to make it permanent. When the muscle is puffed, you can feel inside it those fibers which are tight. If you feel fibrous, rough or tight areas surrounded by the soft tissue, you need to try to loosen them.

This is where the 'release' technique is used. 'Release' is done by touching the limb with the fingertips, fingers spread apart, and shaking delicately, ever-so-lightly, to release the tension in the muscles. YOU SHOULD NEVER USE ANY VIGOROUS MASSAGE ON DYSTROPHIC MUSCLES.

Use these two techniques for about two months, before you attempt to start building up the muscle. If you feel that your hands are sensitive enough to feel the change in the muscles, you may want to start this earlier, at about two to three weeks. When it is obvious that the muscle you worked with has puffed, it is time for the third technique, which is just slightly less gentle than 'support': the 'buildup'.

Like the 'support' technique the 'buildup' is a light stroke. Gently rotate both thumbs, gradually moving them toward the heart. The more concentrated pressure of the thumbs effectively builds up the weak muscle that they are touching. Never forget that the muscle you are working with is not healthy. Alternate between the 'buildup' and the 'support' and 'release' until the muscle is ready for the next step – passive movement.

As Michael lay on his back, he rotated his forearms from the elbows, slowly, helping to strengthen the muscles of his upper arms. He did this both during massage and also independently of the massage. He exercised his breathing, by inhaling and moving his abdomen up and down before exhaling (exercise 1–16 of the Breathing chapter). Later he relaxed while kneeling and bending forward as we massaged him to build up his upper back. The improvement in his breathing had a great effect on his ability to move. Better oxygenation of his body helped to increase muscle mass in the undamaged cells.

When we built up Michael's upper back, we were not able to build up his trapezius, which spans over the whole upper back, but we were successful in strengthening the smaller rhomboids, which could compensate for the weakness of the trapezius because of their similar role in pulling the shoulder blades toward the spine. However, after a year of treatment and exercise, Michael developed muscles that we hadn't believed would ever recover. Michael's conclusion was that even destroyed muscles can heal, and not just be compensated for by strengthening of fibers which were not used much. Medical science supports this conclusion in part. Regeneration is known to take place in dystrophic muscles but does not match the pace of destruction. Apparently regeneration did overtake the degenerative process in Michael's case.

There are surprises of both kinds with muscular dystrophy. You may find that you lose mobility in muscles that generally don't 'belong' under the category of your disease, but you can also strengthen muscles that were 'doomed' to deteriorate, or find that they never do degenerate in the first place.

Michael eventually developed enough strength in his arms to lift them above and beyond his head – a motion he was lacking when we first met him. The most effective tool was massage – first of all the 'support' massage, then the 'buildup', and last the 'release'. We could watch Michael's muscles puff as we worked on them, and those supposedly weak and immobile muscles gained strength as they puffed up.

In spite of the massage, Michael was not able to bend his left knee, because of the weakness of his hamstrings. We had to develop a new method for that, and we did – the result of which seemed like a miracle to us. As he lay on his abdomen, we massaged his hamstrings and then asked him to bend his left leg by lifting his left foot with the help of his right foot. Michael would breathe slowly and deeply, and then bend both legs together, supporting his left leg with his stronger right one. Once he had his left knee bent, he was able to move the calf of that leg from side to side and in rotating motion. These were motions he was not familiar with, but once he started practicing them he was able to strengthen his hamstrings by working mostly on the muscles adjacent to them.

It was essential to alert his brain, along with his muscles, to the partial control that was still available in the weak areas. Because certain key muscles were paralyzed, others which were able to function had not been given the opportunity to do so. The left leg had not received enough circulation, and therefore it became stiff. As a pharmacist, Michael's work caused him to stand for many hours, and that created a tremendous strain on his muscles and ligaments.

Michael's improvement was interesting to follow. As he built some muscles, others began to hurt. In fact, his shoulder hurt for months. That is typical of about 40 percent of the patients with facioscapulohumeral muscular dystrophy we have worked with: as some muscles build up while others don't, a lot of pressure develops in the shoulder girdle, and eventually one of the cervical nerves may be pinched.

We had to stretch Michael's shoulder to correct that, but we were very careful with the stretching – he was not yet strong enough to withstand a stretch without risking dislocation of his bones. We had to stroke him, using oils to reduce the friction, and warm his muscles to loosen them. We also used a technique that for people with muscular dystrophy is considered rough, and which we therefore usually avoid in such cases: Meir placed the palms of his own hands on both sides of Michael's shoulder and shook it, thus releasing a few tight fibers of the levator scapulae (a muscle that shrugs the shoulders), which had pinched the nerve. Later he taught him an exercise in which he would shake his hands, shake his wrists freely, and then shake his shoulders.

Hot towels were used to relax and loosen some of the newly built muscles. Within three months the shoulder pain was gone and has never returned. As more and more muscles were built up in Michael's shoulders and upper arms, his musculature became more balanced.

Michael had improved to such an extent that he regained most of his lost mobility within a period of one year. The problem that took longest to help was his inability to bend his left leg at the knee by itself.

One day we decided to work in the bathtub. Because we wanted the hamstrings to work, we had Michael lie on his abdomen, with his arms hanging over the side of the bath. At first he couldn't bend his left leg even in the water, where gravitational pull is less. But when Michael received shoulder massage in that position, his whole upper torso relaxed, and he was able to bend his knee and reach his foot all the way to his buttocks. All the students of the training class were crowded around him, excited and cheering. Michael's first success in bending his knee was video-taped, and we find it exciting to watch again and again. The combination of a supportive massage to his thigh along with the loving massage of his shoulders allowed him to start strengthening his weak muscles.

Many people do not understand the importance of relaxation in movement. The habit of tensing-up in order to move is deeply ingrained, and harmful. Michael realized that, the more effort he put into tightening muscles that are not needed for the movement in question, the more he had actually blocked the movement he was capable of. Giving up the tension was his next step – and will hopefully be yours. An important part of healing is reorganization, which means using only the correct muscles for a specific action without compensating with others, and not tensing muscles other than the ones you need to move.

Several weeks after bending his knee for the first time in the bathtub, Michael was able to bend and straighten his knee outside the water. During the year after that, he gradually developed stronger and stronger muscles.

When we met him again, a year after he had

learned to bend his knee, we learned that his fingers had withered, and that was a new task to work on. It is important to remember, that even when its symptoms are overcome, the disease is there. Perhaps in the future a cure will be found – either in the shape of medicine or genetic engineering – but in the meantime don't just sit and wait for it. There is a way to prolong the life of muscular dystrophy sufferers, and to relieve their paralysis. Your body has all the resources it needs to heal itself with. Use them to heal yourself. Take charge of your health – because the means are available.

Meir met Beatriz in Brazil. Suffering from facioscapulohumeral muscular dystrophy, she had been helped by a physical therapist who had learned from Meir how to work with muscular dystrophy for the benefit of her own son.

Beatriz had a slight limp, because her tibialis anterior (shin muscle) in her right leg was dystrophic, and it was difficult for her to lift her right foot. This definitely made dancing difficult for her, and, being a Brazilian, she hated to give that up. She was unable to lift her arms higher than her shoulders. Her neck was tight, with one tendon too short, but her main problem was her weakened facial muscles. She had already lost over twenty pounds; her weak muscles did not allow her to eat enough. She was too weak to chew, and by the middle of a meal she was not able to close her mouth. She was very upset with her deterioration. Her mother, who suffered from the same disease, was her model of what to expect: wheelchair-bound, her mother suffered chronic back pain, as her tight abdominal muscles and weak back created a painfully arched back.

Beatriz found herself in tears every day, but she came to see Meir full of hope. Something in her told her that life must be different, that she must be able to lift her arms higher, to walk better, to have stronger muscles. She realized how painful her condition was, and that was her first step toward changing her condition for the better.

When people become comfortable with their handicap, they may not make the effort to overcome it. People don't hurt the same: one will suffer when his vision is less than perfect, while another wouldn't mind using powerful glasses; one may hurt when she has to give up running, but another wouldn't mind walking with a cane. In short, some people hurt when their body is not at its top capacity, while others accept their body's deterioration. It is not healthy to fight a condition which is irreversible, as that could lead to very negative feelings. On the other hand, it isn't healthy to accept limitations. Sadness is often the emotional tool that brings change.

Beatriz saw Meir for only two sessions in Brazil, after which she felt lighter and found walking easier. She managed to arrange a grant through the University of San Carlos to come to San Francisco and research the application of the Self-Healing method to muscular dystrophy. Six months later, she managed to get through the red tape and arrive in San Francisco, her condition quite the same as it was when she had met Meir in Brazil. In spite of having to adjust to a new country and locate hard-to-find housing, she was so energized by her quest to be healed that she devoted all her attention, heart and soul to the therapy. Beatriz worked hard on her research. She trained with Meir as a student, came for therapy sessions, and designed a detailed questionnaire for all the current and former patients with muscular dystrophy that Meir and his students worked with.

Meir and his trainees used the same massage techniques with Beatriz as they did with Michael. They used 'support' massage for her shoulders, and asked her to rotate her forearms repetitively. Repetition – without strain – not only builds up the muscles involved, it also informs the brain again and again of the new situation: that the body demands more movement, more strength. The brain, in turn, takes charge of strengthening the muscles next to the destroyed ones. It teaches the body how to adjust to the disease while still functioning well, how to compensate in a way that will not harm the compensating parts.

The reason Beatriz worked so much with forearm rotations was that the muscles around her elbows were much stronger than those around her shoulders, and forearm rotations did not cause her strain. By rotating her forearms she was able to increase the circulation and get the message to the brain that more movement was needed in the arms. Her ability to rotate her forearms increased quickly, and with the new strength she was able to work on the muscles which were much weaker.

With massage, she developed muscle mass and strength in her pectoralis (upper-chest) and trapezius muscles. At that stage a new passive exercise was developed for her: Meir would swing her arm back and forth while she was standing. Her arms, which were at first very limited in their upward motion, were gradually able to move with more and more ease.

Beatriz worked on herself four hours a day. Some of her exercises were designed specifically for the weak muscles, like rotating her forearms, or lying on her back and lifting her arms alternately above her head. Other exercises worked muscles that were close to the afflicted ones, allowing better circulation and

nutrition to the areas which needed to heal. She learned to isolate between her abdominal muscles and her leg muscles, and to mobilize her chest and abdomen with ease. With the movement exercises she combined resting and just visualizing that she was doing the motion. We find visualization to be an important technique for muscular dystrophy, because it increases circulation to the part of the body being visualized, it is not tiring, and it helps the brain find the muscle fibers which are not too weak to do the motion.

Beatriz developed the ability to lift her arms up all the way above and behind her back – after not being able to lift them more than ninety degrees. Most important was the work on her facial muscles, which was our main focus. Beatriz became able to close her mouth easily, blow out her cheeks, smile better – and eat.

Program for Muscular Dystrophy

People suffering from muscular dystrophy need a great deal of support in their therapy. They will participate at all stages of their therapy, and when they are strong enough they can continue by themselves. We have dedicated a great deal of this chapter to the therapist, who may be a friend, a family member or any supportive person who will be working with you.

If you suffer from muscular dystrophy, it is important that you receive frequent massage sessions. For people with Duchenne we recommend five sessions a week; others can make do with four.

Only the School for Self-Healing teaches the

touch and other methods that we describe here and which have been so effective with muscular dystrophy. We cannot recommend working with muscular dystrophy without this training, but, if you do not have an opportunity to do that, we recommend learning at least some massage and anatomy, and then spending two months studying and working with the Massage chapter. A professional person would need to relearn massage, in a way, using the chapter on Massage in this book. We also recommend that your therapist(s) read the rest of this book to become familiar with our approach. Another recommendation to the therapist is to strengthen his or her fingers and fingertips, and to develop their touch-sensitivity. Developing the correct touch is very important. Refer to the Massage chapter, the section on the hands, and mainly exercise 7–1. (There are more exercises for the hands in the Musicians chapter.)

Beginning to Work

How can you recognize which are the dystrophic muscles you should concentrate on? First of all, note where mobility is lacking. Is it difficult to lift the arm? to bend the knee? to move the foot? Ask a professional person which muscles are dystrophic; use the help of a muscle chart to learn where there is thinning of the muscle belly, and perhaps also of the origin and insertion – the ends where the muscle is attached. When the thin areas are massaged, are any gaps felt within the muscle mass?

When massaging dystrophic muscles, use a massage cream or oil – preferably a herbal salve or vegetable oil, but not one with a petroleum base. We often use cold-pressed olive oil with herbs such as lavender. When you are inexperienced, massage the weak areas very slowly and gradually massage faster.

Whether your therapist is massaging you or you are massaging yourself, the 'support' touch should be very smooth and light. Both the therapist and the recipient should visualize that the massaging fingers are penetrating deeply into the tissue – soothing it, warming it and building it up. You will find that, in spite of the fact that the touch is light, it feels as though it penetrates deeply. The same kind of touch is effective even with healthy limbs. Try this: massage a friend's forearm for a moment, using the 'support' method described above, then let him or her rotate both arms at the elbow. The massaged arm will usually feel lighter and more vibrant.

It will take your therapist about two to three weeks, or eight to ten sessions, to develop the sensitivity for the 'support' touch.

You will love the massage, and you will find that the more you are massaged, the more those muscle gaps will 'patch' and puff. The therapist can very gently squeeze the muscle which is touched, between the thumb and four fingers, to release it, and can use the vibrating 'release' motion – with the fingers or with the whole hand, emphasizing the vibration of the thumb. You may find that, as that is done, the puffing increases. When that happens, your therapist can start working with the 'buildup' motion, rotating the thumbs gently. This technique should also be done slowly by beginners, who will gradually develop the ability to do it fast correctly.

If worked on early enough, the deterioration due to muscular dystrophies can in most cases be stopped. If you are already confined to a wheelchair, you may not be able to develop enough strength to stop using it, but you can develop more mobility in your limbs, which will ease your situation.

You will have to find what movements you can do with ease, and work with them. If, for example, you find it difficult to bend your arm, but you can move it from side to side once it is bent, then bend it with the help of your other hand and practice moving it from side to side. In this way, your increasing strength and improved circulation to your arm will allow strengthening of the weaker areas adjacent to those which are moving. If most of your body is dystrophic, you can still find the areas which are stronger, the movements which are easy, and do them repetitively.

People with muscular dystrophy need a lot of support, but they can use that support to become more independent.

Fascioscapulohumeral Muscular Dystrophy

This type of muscular dystrophy involves a variety of areas, which can include the face, the neck, the shoulders, the upper back and upper arms, the back or front of the thighs, and the shins. Our strategy with facio-scapulohumeral muscular dystrophy is to work on all the needy areas from the start. If necessary, greater focus is given to areas of greater difficulty. For example, if you have a problem chewing, concentrate a lot of work in the facial muscles.

Massage should be combined with a lot of movement. Typically there is a weakness in the face which is apparent when you try to blow out your cheeks or pucker your lips, or whistle. Facial work would concentrate on massaging the cheeks, at first with 'support'

massage, and later with 'buildup'. The following exercises can help to strengthen the muscles of the face.

21–1   Blow out your cheeks, let go, and blow out again. Repeat this ten to twenty times if you can do so without effort.

21–2   Open your mouth widely and move the lower jaw to the right, left, front and back, and then rotate it.

With fascioscapulohumeral muscular dystrophy, there is a pretty good chance that you are partially paralyzed in the shoulders, and cannot lift your arms beyond shoulder level. You will need to have your therapist massage the front and back of your shoulders for many hours. We recommend combining this massage with movement of muscles that move well and easily, as follows.

21–3   Lie on your back, rest your elbows on the floor, and rotate your forearm from the elbow, visualizing that your fingertips are leading the motion. Now close your eyes, visualize the motion, and return to the rotations. We suggest practicing with one arm at a time, for half an hour a day each, and then both together for ten minutes a day.

Refer to exercise 2–21 in the Circulation chapter for rotations of the wrists. Work with each wrist separately for ten minutes a day, and then with both wrists together for five minutes.

If your quadriceps are not damaged, refer to exercise 18–2 in the Osteoporosis chapter. At first bend and straighten your legs fifty times a day, and gradually build up to 500 times a day. This exercise improves the circulation and the posture, and indirectly affects the shoulders.

Refer to exercise 4–30 in the Spine chapter for shoulder rotations.

21–4   Lie on your back. Try to bring one hand up and then to the floor behind your head, keeping your arm straight. Now, with your hand on the floor behind your head, try to lift your arm again and bring it back to your side. If you find this difficult, practice the 'snake' first: bend your arm at the elbow, bringing your palm close to your shoulder, and then climb up with the hand to the air, straightening your arm and extending it all the way until it touches the floor behind your head. Bending the arm and using the 'snake' motion on the way back may again be easier than moving a straight arm. Many repetitions of this exercise may be very beneficial, provided you take care to stay below fatigue level. Gradually building it up to hundreds of times per day may make flexing and extending a straight arm possible within a few weeks.

After you have repeated many hundreds of times those movements which are easy to do, you will be able to challenge the strengthened body with new passive motions which are still too difficult to be done actively.

21–5   After practicing the shoulder exercises described above, you can challenge the shoulder by trying abduction: lie on your side and vertically lift your arm. If you are not able to do that, have your therapist there to complete the missing motions through passive movement – to abduct and adduct (bring the arm down straight) the arm hundreds of times in each session.

Once you are able to develop a new motion actively – that is, by yourself – your therapist's goal will be to find easier ways for you to do it. A difficult new movement should not be repeated in a position that requires more effort. For example, if you develop the ability to move your arms up and down – to flex and extend them – when you are sitting or standing, it may be easier to do that while leaning or standing with the back to a wall. Another way to make this easier is to swing the arms up (above and behind the head, if possible) and down, behind the back. Swinging will give the motion the momentum to go on with greater ease. Don't ever strain to lift your arm.

21–6   After developing the ability to lift the arms all the way up, exercise your shoulders in an unfamiliar position. With both arms stretched, hold onto a bar which is as high as you can reach, and then rotate your shoulders in that position. This will allow passive contraction of your deltoid muscles, and will strengthen muscles that had not had the opportunity to move before.

One of the more common problems with facio-scapulohumeral muscular dystrophy is an arched back. The lower back is usually extremely tight, but the upper back is extremely weak because of the dystrophic trapezius muscles. The middle back is not dystrophic, but is simply too weak to support the upper back. The strategy to deal with this is first of all to build up strength in the trapezius, mostly through massage and the exercises described above for the shoulders.

The next step is to work with hip rotations to strengthen the whole hip area and relax the tight, strong buttock muscles. Refer your therapist to exercise 7–26 in the Massage chapter (specifically the rotations demonstrated in fig 7–26A). If your thigh muscles are not damaged, practice similar hip rotations actively, as long as the exercise does not create fatigue.

By stretching the middle and lower back, releasing their tension and balancing the work of the back, you can allow the back to strengthen further. Refer to exercise 12–1 in the Asthma chapter; practice the Cow–Cat stretch, described in exercise 5–40 of the Muscles chapter. Also search for exercises in the Spine, Joints, Muscles and Nervous System chapters which work best for you.

If your hamstrings are not damaged, work with the first part of exercise 5–16 of the Muscles chapter, rotating each calf separately. Alternate between actual rotations and visualizing that you are rotating the calf with no effort. Build up gradually to hundreds of rotations. If you do have dystrophic hamstrings, they need to be built up and strengthened before practicing this exercise.

How will you build up the hamstrings? Your therapist should start working on your hamstrings with massage, using the 'support', 'release' and 'buildup' methods. After about six weeks, use passive motion: when you lie on your back, your therapist can bend and straighten your leg quickly, tossing your foot from one hand to the other – from near your buttocks to further down on the massage table. You can try bending and straightening your leg by yourself a few times.

Now work in the bathtub with exercise 5–7 of the Muscles chapter. If one of your legs is stronger than the other, you may be able to work with the second part of exercise 5–16 of the Muscles chapter – passively rotating the weaker leg by leaning it on the stronger one.

It is important to realize that you may sometimes feel pain as muscles develop. To ease the pain, you can use hot towels or have someone warm your muscles by massaging you with round motions, using the whole palms. Refer to the Massage chapter for more helpful massage techniques.

If your shin muscle – the tibialis anterior – is dystrophic, this will be apparent in its lack of tone, in the gaps felt when massaging the muscle. You will find it difficult to flex the foot (to point the toes toward the knee). Perhaps you will have a tendency to drag the foot while walking. Strengthening the tibialis anterior will make walking much easier.

Strengthening the tibialis anterior is somewhat similar to strengthening the shoulders – starting, as before, with a lot of massage. If the tibialis anterior has survived the strain of walking for so long, it means it may be strong enough to take passive movement sooner than the shoulder muscles.

A passive movement that we have found very helpful is stretching the calf by bending the foot toward the shin. This is easy to do if your therapist leans your foot against his or her own chest. That will allow use of all of his or her bodyweight for the stretch. The stretch will relax the tight gastrocnemius (calf muscle), the Achilles tendon (at the ankle) and the soleus muscles (at the bottom of the foot), and it will also passively contract the dystrophic tibialis anterior. As the tibialis anterior is contracted, it should also be massaged gently.

How much passive contraction can the tibialis anterior take? That depends on the degree of its weakness. It may be too weak to take passive movement; in that case don't practice the movement described above, or do it only very lightly. You can tell that the muscle is too weak when it hardly bulges at the middle, at its 'belly', and when there is a sense of a very weak tone even when the foot is stretched as described above.

To massage the tibialis anterior, you or your therapist should use the same 'support' and 'release' strokes we described earlier, and then rotate your foot passively.

Another exercise you can do to help strengthen the tibialis anterior (if your peroneal muscles – the muscles on the outside of the calf which, among other things, help move the foot so that the sole faces outward – are not damaged) is to move the foot so that the sole faces alternately inward and outward. That will bring more circulation to the area.

There are, of course, many more exercises and pointers that we could describe, but we believe that, with the help of this chapter and through familiarizing yourself with the rest of this book, you can develop your own program. We believe you can handle muscular dystrophy with great success.

Your program will vary with time, according to the needs and abilities you have at each stage. It will include a variety of rotation exercises. An example of one that you probably should not attempt until you have completed about a year and a half of prior work is lying on your back, intertwining your fingers, and moving both arms in large circles together. It will take a long while and an incredible amount of patience until you develop enough strength to do this.

With time, when your muscles are stronger, you may want to exercise with weights. Start with half-pound weights, and never use weights heavier than five pounds – do not forget that your muscles are dystrophic. You can rotate your forearm from your elbow, or rotate your wrist while carrying a weight in your hand. You may want to use a light weight when you swing your arms up and down. Never use weights with muscles which are paralyzed. When you start practicing with weights, work first with the same motions that were always easy for you, and only about six months later exercise the muscles that you had to rebuild. Never practice to a degree of fatigue: it is always better to repeat a motion many times easily than to prove to yourself that you can lift something heavy and then tire after a few motions.

Limb-Girdle Muscular Dystrophy

Because people suffering from this disease often have a very weak back and find it difficult to straighten from a bending position, it is important to do a lot of work on the back. Distinguish between the stronger areas, which tend to be tight and need release, and the areas which are weak and need support. Improving the state of the back will improve both your total posture and your circulation, and allow the regeneration of your dystrophic muscles.

The back tends to get weak because of the incredible burden it has to carry. It compensates for the limb girdles that became dystrophic.

You may have a very narrow region in the lower part of your middle back which is strong and tight and needs mostly releasing. In that case, we advise that your therapist use the vibration technique and not deep-tissue massage to release that area. This is just as a precaution: although that area of your back may not be dystrophic, it is adjacent to dystrophic muscles that can be harmed by deep-tissue massage.

The rest of your back will need much 'support' massage and, with time, 'buildup'.

The program we suggest for limb-girdle muscular dystrophy is similar to that for facio-scapulohumeral muscular dystrophy, but with an emphasis on the back muscles. Even though the degeneration is different, the work is much the same. Once the posture improves and the back gains mobility, the deterioration can be stopped or reversed.

Don't work just by the book, however: find the muscles that need more work and focus on them.

Duchenne Muscular Dystrophy

We are dedicating this section to parents of children with Duchenne. If this is not the group you belong to, we apologize – this chapter is for you too. We hope to help you realize the extent to which light massage and correct exercises can create an impact. Even if the effect is temporary, it is worth working for. In many cases, though, it is long-lasting and even permanent.

Children with Duchenne are usually diagnosed between the ages of seven or eight, though sometimes earlier or later. They often have difficulties standing on their heels, because their gastrocnemius muscles are tight; they may find it hard to lift their arms all the way up; or they may just suffer general weakness that makes any motion a little more difficult. Blood tests will indicate that muscle tissue is being destroyed.

The earlier you start working with Duchenne, the better your results will be. It will take four to six hours of Self-Healing massage and exercise per day, for at least two years, to help your child recover. This is the time to decide whether you are willing and able to put in the time and energy needed. Physically you

don't need to be strong, but you need to be sensitive. This is a very demanding task mentally.

In order to develop the sensitivity in your hands, we urge you to work with the Massage chapter and do a lot of massage on your hands. Work with the first part of this book to make your body stronger and more agile. Only a body that has created a change in itself can create a change in another.

Any muscle may be vulnerable with this type of illness, therefore all muscles should be massaged with a 'support' touch.

At the early stages of the dystrophy it is possible to mobilize each one of the joints. You can use the Joints chapter for ideas, or simply rotate each joint in all directions. You can do this slowly or fast – let your fingers lead you – but always do it very gently.

Take, for example, routines for the ankles and toes: rotate the ankle fifteen times in each direction, mostly slowly, sometimes fast. Now stretch the foot – pointing the toes toward the knee. Massage the upper shins (the tibialis anterior, whose job it is to lift the foot). Now stretch the foot in the opposite direction, pointing the toes down, and massage the calf (the gastrocnemius, whose job it is to pull the foot down). Repeat the whole process ten times. We suggest that you start with this regimen and, if needed, vary it later.

Now rotate each one of the toes ten to fifteen times. They may have a tendency to point upward because the muscles at the ball of the foot are dystrophic. Massage the foot above and under the toes very gently. Now hold the toes with one hand, stretch them upward a little, and massage the foot underneath them. Pull the toes down, and massage the foot above them.

Part of the recovery and prevention of

further deterioration has to do with the life-style of your child. Make sure he avoids strenuous movements. (We refer to the child as male as that is so in the majority of cases.) Don't send him to a school where he has to climb too many stairs to get to his class – either have the class relocated, or move him to another school. How many stairs are too many? If your child is making an observable effort to climb them, even if there are only one or two steps, there are too many. You may have to let him stay away from school for a day or a few days every once in a while, to prevent excessive effort. Prohibit rough play and riding bicycles, as these can hasten his deterioration.

Repeat very frequently movements that he can do with ease, especially rotating movements.

Emphasize exercises in the bathtub or pool. Working with less gravitational resistance is much easier for the muscles and helps them get stronger. Refer to exercises 5–3 to 5–5, 5–7, 5–9 and 5–44 in the Muscles chapter, and also the following.

21–7 Standing in the pool, with the back to the wall, rotate the leg from the hip; facing the wall, rotate the leg backward. Always rotate both clockwise and counterclockwise.

Some of these exercises may be easier to do in a small tub, so get one that suits the size of the child. The exercises in the pool and tub should not last more than half an hour at a time, whether or not the child feels fatigue. The activity may diminish the sense of fatigue which does exist in the muscle. The water should be pleasantly warm, so that the muscles can relax as they move.

It is important to massage the child using the three strokes – 'support', 'release' and 'buildup' – before and after the water exercises.

Find out what motions are possible, and practice them. Even if your child is very disabled perhaps he can move his head from side to side as he sits or lies down. If so, practicing this will improve his circulation and strengthen his muscles. This is true for other possible motions as well.

Becker Muscular Dystrophy

Becker muscular dystrophy is similar to Duchenne but milder. The work needed is quite similar to that with Duchenne. Work with all the muscles, but focus on those which are deteriorating fastest.

The muscles you would want to work with the most are the back muscles.

You may have an arched back for years before becoming confined to a wheelchair. The arch results from weakness in parts of the back while other parts are incredibly contracted. To help the distorted posture, have your therapist massage the weak muscles with the 'support', 'release' and 'buildup' motions, and release the tense, stronger muscles. You may find that improving your posture improves your overall physical condition.

As in Duchenne, you may find that some of the muscles become thicker even though they are not stronger; the tissue becomes hard and immobile. We suggest that you have these muscles stretched and shaken to loosen them.

We refer you to Meir's book *Self-Healing: My Life and Vision*, where you can read about the program that Danny worked with on his muscular dystrophy.

CHAPTER 22

Polio

This chapter is dedicated to Vered Vanounou, our friend and colleague, who has had remarkable success in rehabilitating herself and improving from paralysis inflicted by polio and surgery. We thank her for her input to this chapter.

The polio vaccines have been extremely effective in stopping the spread of polio throughout the world, so new cases of polio are relatively rare. Recent outbreaks of the disease, however, indicate that its threat is by no means extinct. Some recent cases have been attributed to the vaccine itself, rather than to random occurrence of the disease. If your child contracts polio, you should, in addition to getting the best medical care available, make sure that your child receives daily massage, in the manner described in this chapter, and a program of exercise to encourage regeneration of the weakened tissues. With some exceptions, we recommend being hesitant about surgery.

Many people who contracted the polio virus as children now suffer from a condition known as post-polio syndrome. This condition affects particularly individuals who demand much of themselves and have worked hard to improve their lives and achieve their goals, and it reflects the stress of such efforts on bodies weakened by disease. The symptoms can include strokes, heart disease, lung disease, severe back pain and other muscle pains, and intensification of already existing polio symptoms. It has been estimated that about 40 percent of all polio victims develop some degree of post-polio syndrome.

To some extent, all polio sufferers will experience residual physical problems, even if these are not diagnosable. Polio strikes non-symmetrically. This lack of balance will result in a number of pathological difficulties. If these patients receive medical treatment such as physical therapy, in most cases the treatment will tend only to *increase* this imbalance. Patients will typically be encouraged to build up and strengthen only the muscles on the unafflicted side, the idea being to make that side strong enough to compensate for the weak one. The weak side is regarded as useless, and little or no attempt is made to improve it. It is generally believed that the polio virus leaves some motor parts of the nervous system permanently unable to function – that once these parts have been afflicted by the disease they will never be useful again. In our practice, however, we have had the wonderful experience of seeing lost movement regained and lost function restored, permanently.

Some of Meir's earliest work was done with polio patients, and his success with them was part of what motivated him to become a therapist. We have had wonderful results in our work with polio victims – partly because they themselves have brought so much creativity and inspiration to their own Self-Healing. Before we describe polio exercises, we would like to tell you about some of these people.

You may have read about Vered in Meir's book *Self-Healing: My Life and Vision*. Vered was stricken with polio at the age of three, and left with a weak, wasted left leg and hip. Until the age of twenty-four, she was able to lift her left foot only a couple of millimeters off the ground, and usually would not do even this, finding it easier simply to drag the foot behind her. When Vered met Meir, her doctors were suggesting an operation in which they would break and fuse the knee joint, locking it permanently and making it easier for her to drag the leg. In two and a half years of intensive work, Meir and Vered succeeded in making it possible for her to lift the foot three inches off the ground, and to raise it regularly during walking.

This in itself was a major accomplishment, and one which helped to strengthen every muscle on the left side of the body used in walking. Vered, however, carried her progress to amazing lengths. For several years after Meir left Israel, he and Vered were unable to work together, so she continued to work on herself alone. On a visit to San Francisco, she attended one of Meir's practitioner training classes. The class discussion revolved around paralysis – not total paralysis, but partial paralysis such as that caused by polio – emphasizing what an extreme shock it brings to the mind and

body of the victim. The traumatic experience of paralysis may in fact convince the brain and nerves that movement is impossible, where in fact some movement may still be possible. Using Vered as an example, Meir asked Vered to raise her foot and put it on a stool, six inches off the ground, which was twice as high as she had ever been able to lift it. She said, 'You're crazy.' Meir answered, 'OK, that's true, so why don't you lift your leg onto the massage table.' This was about three feet off the floor. She laughed and demanded, 'How do you expect me to do that?' but even as she spoke, she tried to comply. She did not succeed, but, as she lowered the leg, Meir quickly asked her again to lift her foot onto the stool – and she did. Somehow, the effort to go way beyond her limitations, to visualize doing something so seemingly impossible, had enabled her to succeed in a task that had seemed only slightly less impossible. Her effort, of course, was both mental and physical, but it showed how much a thought can influence the body.

Meir massaged her thigh, then asked her, 'Try again to lift it up to the table.' She shook her head, repeating, 'You're crazy.' One of the students asked Vered, 'What would *you* like to accomplish here?' She replied, 'I don't care about accomplishing anything; I'm just doing what feels right for my body.' But, at Meir's insistence, she did try, and kept trying. Several attempts failed. Each time Meir would massage her thigh and tell her to try again. And at last she actually succeeded in lifting her leg onto the table, to the amazement of everyone – but especially herself. She covered her face with her hands and literally fell over backward, overcome. She had lived thirty-four years not knowing what potential power her leg really had.

Something in Vered, and in her leg, was ready for this new development or it would not have happened, though the potential was there all along. There are many more people suffering from paralysis who are also ready for such a change, but have not had the opportunity to find out how to accomplish it. Both their own – and often their physician's – lack of belief in their ability to improve and their lack of knowledge and training in how to produce such an improvement are responsible. No one expects paralyzed parts to move, so no one tries to get them to move, so they don't move. But, as Vered and others have proved, when you give your body the proper encouragement it often will give you back more than you could ever have hoped for.

Vered's new movement capacity gave her a new body image, and changed her entire self-image. She is still adjusting to the change. There are movements she cannot do, and there is a lack of balance in her use of her body, but every year this imbalance is reduced and new movements are acquired. Many of the exercises described here are the results of her experience.

Vered could have opted for the knee-fusing operation (it would have been her sixth experience of surgery), which would have left her dependent on an orthopedic boot or brace for the rest of her life. She could have resigned herself never to use her left leg or hip. The imbalance in her body would have gradually, continually increased. As an active, self-motivated person, she would have gone through life working too hard with her strong side to support and compensate for her weak one. With time, she would have become prone to symptoms typical of post-polio syndrome. Instead, she is working toward balance and

strength for her *entire* body – and she is achieving it.

It is common knowledge that if you have a stronger eye the brain oppresses the weaker one, and if you have a weaker limb the brain overactivates the stronger one. Most eye doctors understand the implication of having one strong eye and one weak one: they know that this will lead to poor vision and damage both eyes. However, this principle is not always applied to the rest of the body. Physical therapists and physical educators work toward enforcing the unbalanced pattern rather than working toward balance.

In our work we emphasize increasing balance in the body, and offer the means to achieve that.

Meir worked with Vered for many years. Another polio client, Wilma, he saw for only a few treatments. She was forty-four years old, a respected psychotherapist and an intelligent, independent woman. She was using crutches, as one of her legs was almost completely non-functional and the other partially so. She also complained of back and neck pain. Meir showed her movements she had never tried before, such as lying on her abdomen, bending her weaker knee, and moving the calf from side to side. This strengthened her leg so that she was eventually able to lie on her back with the afflicted leg bent at the knee and the foot flat on the bed. Previously the muscles of that leg had been too weak to hold the leg in that position. This posture relieved her back pain. Wilma was surprised that, after living with her post-polio limitations for forty years, she could yet discover new movement possibilities and get relief from chronic problems.

Body self-image is enormously important in working with polio. A person convinced that a body part has become totally useless is not apt to make much effort toward nurturing it. One client, Ruth, was stricken with polio in both legs, one worse than the other. During her thirty-year lifetime she had undergone twenty-nine corrective operations on her legs – none of which increased her mobility. When she began to work with Self-Healing therapy, she was willing to work only on the (slightly) stronger left leg, and would not at first even consider 'wasting time' on the right leg. It took a lot of arguing for Meir to persuade her to try to move the right leg. In fact, it took much more time to talk her into trying than it did for her to get the leg to move. To her amazement, she found that after only several tries she was able to swing it back and forth from the hip and from the knee. Needless to say, after this she was ready to attempt other 'impossible' movements.

Thus, when starting to work on yourself, it is as important to be aware of your self-image as it is to do the exercises. Polio victims often embody or identify with a sense of weakness, of enfeeblement, which can make it hard for them, emotionally, to take charge of their situation. Developing self-confidence is a difficult but essential task. Remember that, besides the residual effects of the illness, you are a healthy individual with many strengths. While it is true that you are being challenged more than the average person, you also can find the strength to meet that challenge. Remember, too, that those individuals who did not write off their own potential for recovery often ended up regaining as much as 50 percent of their 'lost' movement capacity. In some not-too-severe cases, we have seen near-total recovery.

Exercises for the Legs and Feet

Let us visualize a polio patient, perhaps yourself, with one calf that is weak and immobile. You may have lost muscle mass. You can move your foot only partially, and the toes are probably thin and weak. The big toe may stick up, and the bones at the base of the toes may protrude downward, with only a thin layer of muscle covering them. Your arch might ache frequently as a result of the foot's weakness and deformity.

22–1   To strengthen your calf, you should first work on the areas adjacent to it – the foot and the thigh. Sit down, rest the weak calf on your opposite thigh, hold the foot in the opposite hand and rotate it 100 times in each direction. As long as your muscles are still weak, this type of passive movement is best for them; active movement may challenge them beyond their present capacity. As your muscles grow stronger, over a period of a month or two, you can gradually increase the number of rotations to 400 in each direction.

22–2   You should also massage your foot and ankle. It is important that your attitude toward your foot should be warm and loving for the massage to have its best effect. Many people, feeling that their bodies are deformed or paralyzed, relate to them with strain and hostility. You might find it helpful to first practice your massage on your stronger leg, or even on another person altogether, before you try to massage the afflicted foot. Your hands, which will enjoy working with healthier tissues, can then carry with them that positive feeling when later working on the weak foot. Perhaps you can find a nice massage cream, such as a herbal salve, which will help to relax your muscles.

First warm the muscles with a very gentle touch. Visualize that your hands are soft and warm, and that they create a fluid effect where they touch. Try to keep a sense of smooth, rhythmical movement of the hands. After thoroughly massaging each part of the foot, stand and feel that now you possess two whole legs, instead of barely one and a quarter.

By massaging the foot, you have brought more circulation to it. Now massage your calf with your thumbs, in a very gentle circular motion, working on the calf muscles one by one. To relax your calf muscles, spread your four fingers far apart from your thumbs, and position your thumbs in the middle of your calf and the fingers along the shin bone (see fig 7–22 in the Massage chapter). Moving the fingers in a rotating motion, with the thumbs anchored in place, gradually move the fingers back and around toward the thumbs. Then do the same thing with the fingers firmly in place, moving the thumbs around and in front toward the fingers. Be gentle and nurturing toward your leg. Then hold the calf with both hands, the thumbs on the opposite side from the fingers as before, and move your hands back and forth on the calf, one moving forward while the other moves backward, in a gentle circular motion. Start at the top of the calf and do ten such motions in each area, then move down to the next area until you have reached the ankle. Spend as much time as you can in massaging the calf this way: it is one of the most effective ways to build up muscles weakened by disease.

22–3 This next exercise is done in the bathtub – make sure it is all right to spill some water on the floor, since you will be splashing. Partly fill the tub with warm water, and sit down in it with your legs stretched before you. See to what extent you are able to bend your knees in the water. Fill the tub as full as you need to make this movement as easy as possible. Now bend and straighten your knees alternately – as one bends, the other straightens – and take as much time as you need to complete the movement. Slide your feet on the floor of the bathtub as your legs move. Repeat the motion several times and then stop and imagine that you are doing it. Bend and straighten your legs again.

Doing exercises without the hampering resistance of gravity is another good way to strengthen muscles without straining them, and the mobility you gain in the water will eventually be retained outside the water. When you start to develop new movement, you will find that your muscles are starting to be somewhat tight and feel tired. This is a good sign.

22–4 This next exercise should be done in a pool. Stand in the water and hold onto something for support. Standing on your stronger leg, kick the weak one forward, backward, out to its own side, and crossing over to the opposite side. Do this first with the leg held out more or less straight, swinging the leg from the hip, and then with the hip partly bent, swinging the leg from the knee. You can also pull the knee up toward the chest and kick forward; you can hold the leg out to its own side and then bend the knee, so that it slants diagonally toward your other leg; you can bend the knee so that your foot points in the direction of your buttocks; and from all of these positions you can gently kick the leg. You can also sit on the steps or lean on the wall of the pool and rotate your foot several hundred times. Stop sometimes to rest and visualize doing the movement, and then resume the rotation. You will find the foot rotation one of your most important exercises. Even if you can do very little of it, be sure to do it as much as you can.

As paralyzed limbs gain some movement in water, without the exhausting pull of gravity, they are learning that they are capable of some motion after all. Eventually, they will retain some of this knowledge out of the water as well. Much of Vered's ability to lift her foot off the ground happened as a result of many hours spent in the sea, hip-deep in the water, lifting the leg again and again. In the water, she could eventually bring the foot almost two feet off the ground. This translated to being able to lift it more than an inch off the ground on dry land. Bending and straightening her knees under water in the bathtub eventually enabled her to do the same out of the water – something she had previously been too weak to do.

To make your water exercises effective, practice them for an hour and a half every day for three months.

Here are some exercises you can do out of the water.

22–5 Sit on the floor with your knees bent, pulled up to your chest and touching each other, and your feet flat on the floor. Slide your arms under your knees and hold each elbow with the opposite hand. Lift one foot off the floor and with it draw circles in the air, clockwise and counterclockwise (fig 22–5). The movement here is from the knee rather than from the ankle as in foot rotations, but visualize that the foot itself is leading the

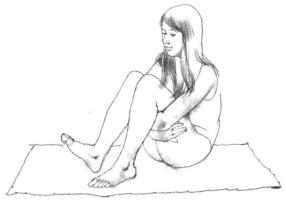

22–5

motion, as though there is a string tied around the toes and someone else is pulling it. Rest that foot, breathe deeply, and do the same thing with the other foot.

22–6 In the same position, move both feet in circles at the same time, first moving them in the same direction – that is, either both clockwise or both counterclockwise – and then, after resting them, moving one clockwise and one counterclockwise simultaneously. This might sound complicated, but it is what most people do naturally. You may need to lean against a wall to do this exercise.

22–7 Many polio patients have very stiff hips as a result of the difficulty and imbalance in their walking. Here is an exercise that will give your hips a great stretch. Lie on your back with your knees bent and your feet flat on the floor, and let your knees rub against each other, with one moving forward as the other moves back (fig 22–7). Then rub them in a circular motion, as though you are riding a tiny bicycle, without lifting your feet from the floor. Do this at first for five minutes at a time, and try to build the time up to twenty minutes.

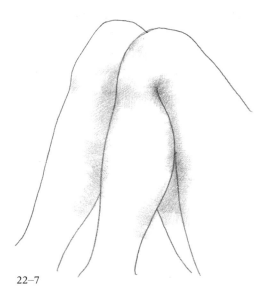

22–7

Also good for making the hips flexible are hip rotations. Refer to exercises 4–5 and 4–6 in the Spine chapter, but do them only if you don't find them too strenuous.

You should do these beginning exercises for about two months before going on to more challenging ones. After these two months have passed, you are ready to do some exercises more geared toward strengthening your muscles. A good way to begin is by taking walks on an uneven but yielding surface such as sand, dirt or grass. Perhaps you are lucky enough to have a sandy beach to walk on, and good company to go with you. These help a lot, but are not essential. If you wear a brace, see whether you can walk a little without it, as this will be helpful both for strengthening the muscles – by making them work for them-selves – and for flexibility.

If your weak muscles are in the thigh rather than the calf, your exercises will be somewhat different. Again, strengthening the adjacent areas will be very helpful, so working on the calf will ultimately make it easier for you to work on the thigh. As always when working

with very weak muscles, begin your self-work with lots of gentle massage on your thigh. Do this yourself, whenever you can, and get friends, family or members of your support group to massage you too.

The next stage should be passive movement, in which someone else holds and stretches your legs. The strong leg needs stretching to relax from the tension it builds up through working for both legs; the weak leg needs stretching for elongation, as the unused muscles tend to grow smaller. You will find this passive movement very pleasant, both in itself and because it gives your legs a sense of moving with ease that they otherwise lack.

22–8   Your partner should first hold the leg at the ankle, flexing the foot so that the toes move toward the shin, then extending the foot so that the toes point away from the shin, then rotating the foot in as large a circle as possible. Your partner can then hold the ankle and lift the leg straight up, so that it is at a right angle to your body, and let it sway from side to side; then lift it a little higher so that your hip comes off the table. With the leg stretched out flat, he can stand at the foot of the table or bed and pull the leg straight toward him, shaking it a little to loosen it.

Spend a lot of time with exercise 22–1, as this will increase the circulation to the feet and strengthen the calves. Because of the proximity of the calves to the thighs, the thighs will benefit from this strengthening.

Continue with the next exercise, in the bathtub.

22–9   Sit in the bathtub with both legs stretched forward, and now stretch them farther alternately, past each other.

The next two exercises are done on the floor.

22–10 Kneel and support your back against a wall. Now slowly raise one knee, lower it, and then raise the other one. You may need to support yourself with your hands on the floor. If the weaker thigh cannot raise the knee by itself, assist it with your hands, but visualize the thigh lifting by itself; even this semi-passive movement is good for the thigh muscles. Then, if you can, lift each knee in turn and move it in rotating motion, assisting with your hands if you need to, making the circle as small as you need to and as large as you can comfortably.

22–11 Kneel, move your legs out to either side until your knees are about two feet apart, then lower yourself so that you are sitting between your thighs. In this position, lift one knee at a time, as far off the floor as you can without straining (fig 22–11). As in the previous exercise, try also to move the lifted knee in a circular motion, assisting it with your hands if you need to.

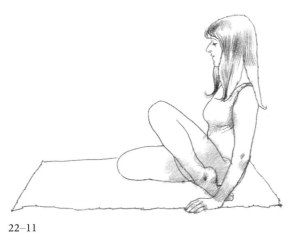

22–11

22–12 Stand on a stair, holding onto the banister or wall for support, and let your weaker leg dangle down toward the stair below the one you are standing on. (You should be standing sideways on the staircase, rather than facing up or down.) Swing the dangling leg from side to side, and move it in rotation if possible. This loosens your hip as well as strengthening your thigh. You can expect your thigh to become stronger and more supple within a few months.

Now you can start your attempts to bend your knee. This should be done mostly in water at first. Work with exercise 22–3, and when you are comfortable with it continue with the following exercise in a pool or, better yet, at a sea, lake or river.

22–13 It is best to be helped by a good supportive friend who can hold you as you do this motion. Stand in water up to your chest, and quickly bend and straighten each leg alternately, lifting the foot slightly off the floor. If the motion becomes easier, bring your knees up to hip level. A third stage of this exercise is to keep moving the legs quickly and easily but this time bringing the knees as high as you can toward your chest. This exercise is fun to do.

22–14 Now you can try to alternate bending and straightening your legs as you lie on your back, as you did in the bathtub in exercise 22–3, keeping your feet on the floor. Try not to tighten your abdomen or back muscles when you do this, and do it as slowly as you need to. You will get best results if you first return to the exercise of bending and straightening your legs under warm water in the bathtub, and then immediately proceed to this exercise when you come out of the water. Your leg muscles will retain some of the relaxation and sense of ease they experienced in the water, and carry it into this exercise.

22–15 Next, roll onto your abdomen, slide your stronger foot under the weaker, and slowly bend your knees, so that the stronger leg is lifting and carrying the weaker one. Lower the legs slowly, letting the 'passive' one relax completely. Repeat this several times. You may find that a stiff, immobile leg becomes much more flexible.

Now try it with the weaker leg supporting the stronger one. This may sound impossible, but after receiving the support of the stronger leg the weaker one can often bend in this position, even under the stronger one. If you cannot actually do this, then visualize doing it, and keep trying. Even if you can only raise the legs an inch, you have achieved something important.

You may have had damage in both legs, necessitating use of braces. If so, you may want to try all the previous exercises and see if they work for you. Your next exercises are the following.

22–16 Lying on your back on a mattress, bend your knees, keeping your feet flat on the mattress, about hip-width apart. Lean your knees toward each other, and stay in this position for as long as you can. Merely keeping your legs in this position, unsupported, will strengthen the leg muscles. Now move the knees slowly away from each other. If they tend to fall over when you do this, notice at exactly which point this happens, and try to stop before this point; even if you can move the knees only a fraction of an inch apart

without their falling, stop at that point. Your challenge here will be to very slowly, very gradually, expand this distance.

22–17 In a bathtub, bend your knees and put your feet flat on the tub floor. Let your knees rest against each other, and move them, together, from side to side.

All of these exercises, and the progression from one exercise to the next, must be undertaken by you at your own pace. Much damage has been done to polio and other neuromuscular-disease victims by forcing them to work harder than their muscles can endure. You will need to maintain a deep awareness of your body and its responses as you work on it. Don't go on to harder, more challenging, exercises until you really know you are ready for them; don't compete with yourself and don't push yourself. You may spend months on just one exercise before you are ready for the next.

Exercises for the Upper Body

Polio may also strike the upper-body muscles. Perhaps your problem is the deltoid muscle, which connects the upper arm to the shoulder. When this muscle is thin and wasted, it is very hard to lift and move the arm, and the other arm muscles may suffer from lack of use as a consequence.

As before, you may find it best to begin with the areas adjacent to the weak muscle, rather than with the afflicted muscle itself. So begin with massage of the forearm, from wrist to elbow, using the same circular palpating motion you used on the calf (exercise 22–2).

22–18 Now rotate the forearm, supporting your elbow on a table or with your free hand. This motion may be difficult at first, since the weak deltoid limits movement throughout the arm; eventually, however, the forearm rotation will help to activate the arm muscles.

Stop the forearm rotation after circling the arm at least ten times in each direction, and rotate the wrist instead, visualizing the fingertips leading the motion. Now return to the forearm rotation. Do you feel a difference now?

Tap all of your fingertips against a table or other firm surface, about twenty times, keeping your wrists loose. This focuses your attention on a peripheral area and away from the afflicted area itself. The arm experiences movement that doesn't strain the weak muscles but allows them to move with some ease, which tends to relax them. Rotate the forearm again, visualizing that the fingers, which are now warmed and perhaps tingling, are leading the motion. Make the circle of movement as large as you can. Stop and rest the arm while you visualize rotating it, imagining the motion to be smooth and easy; then repeat the rotation.

After about three months of doing these rotations, you may be ready to work on your shoulders.

There are a few phases to building up strength in your shoulders. At first, build up your capacity to move in water, where you have less gravitational resistance.

The following simple arm movements should be done daily for about three months before you proceed to some shoulder exercises.

22–19 Begin by working in water deep enough to allow you the full range of motion of the arm, preferably up to your shoulder. First let the arm float. Outside the water, you may have trouble lifting the arm to shoulder height; in the water, it can float freely at this level. This allows freer movement not only of the arm itself but of shoulder, chest, side and upper-back muscles which don't normally get much chance to move. Now move the arm in as many ways as you can think of. Let it rise from your side to the shoulder and lower it again. Swing it in front of your body and across your chest, then stretch it as far behind you as you can. Rotate it from the shoulder, the elbow and the wrist. Bend your elbow, place your hand on your chest, and raise and rotate the arm in that position. See whether you can discover any other motions.

22–20 Standing out of the water, you can have a friend or a member of your support group move the arm for you in all the ways described above, or as many as feel comfortable. While this is being done, visualize that you are moving the arm by yourself, with total ease and flexibility.

22–21 When you feel ready, try moving the arm by yourself. Begin by swinging the weaker arm, quickly, as far up as you can reach, and as far down and back as you can, visualizing that the fingertips are leading the motion. Breathe slowly and deeply, even though the actual movement should be fairly rapid. If you are simply unable to make the movement rapid, then remember to inhale before lifting the arm and exhale while lifting it. Then stop and imagine yourself raising and lowering the arm. If you cannot imagine it, then simply say to yourself, 'I am moving my arm up and down.' If you can imagine it, do so in as much detail as possible: imagine the size, the length and the weight of the arm, and the feeling of moving it through space.

Continue with this exercise, and now imagine that you raise your hands higher and higher with each lifting of the arm. Even if this is not the case, the visualization will help to make the movement easier.

22–22 Lie on your side, on a bed or massage table or the floor, and have someone massage your shoulder and move it passively. (Refer to the Massage chapter, exercise 7–32, for ideas on shoulder massage.) Then try to rotate your shoulder, with your arm lying relaxed along your side or resting in front of you. Visualize the outer edge of your shoulder leading the motion. After this, return to the previous exercise, and this time try to actually lift the hands higher each time, as well as visualizing this. If you find exercise 22–21 easier now, repeat it as often as you can.

Be sure not to neglect the massage, since weak muscles tend to tire and stiffen easily, and the massage will nourish and relieve them and keep them from becoming exhausted. At first, you will benefit most from the extremely gentle massage described in the Muscular Dystrophy and Atrophy chapter as 'support', or supportive massage. Later, when your muscles have acquired some mass, they can benefit from a rather more vigorous massage.

For the shoulder and arm, a good technique is for your partner to press the deep curve between her thumb and first finger around the curve of your muscle, and rub her hand from side to side; this moves your muscle as well as exerting pressure on it. You can also do this yourself if you have one hand which is strong.

After about two months of the arm-lifting exercise, continue to do it while holding small weights, such as an apple or an orange. You can gradually increase the weight, graduating to a grapefruit. However, do not try to progress until you know that you have gained movement and strength and are ready to go on.

22–23 The next step is first to lift the arm as high as possible, and in that position to move it from side to side, swinging it across your body and then out to its own side. When you have mastered this, do the same holding your 'weights'.

Next, with your arm raised, move it from side to side and at the same time twist back and forth from the shoulder, so that the straight arm is the axis of the small rotations. This exercise encompasses a variety and range of motion not far from normal.

Last, we recommend that, having explored and discovered where your weaknesses and strengths lie, you try exercises from other chapters, particularly the Muscles, Circulation, Spine and Joints chapters. Each of these chapters contain headings which are relevant to the parts of the body you are most likely to be working on, so please turn to these headings, read the exercises, and see whether there are any which sound right for you.

CHAPTER 23

Multiple Sclerosis

We have worked with a great many people with multiple sclerosis. Some were able to decrease the number of symptoms they had, others noticed that no new symptoms occurred after they started working with their bodies. Very few were able to eliminate their symptoms altogether. This kind of work may help you get rid of some of your symptoms and better manage the rest. What this program can do is strengthen the central nervous system thus relieving many symptoms; it cannot cure the disease.

Be aware that the program for multiple sclerosis will take about an hour and a half per day for the rest of your life. It is pleasant, it is worth your while, and it is likely to help you. You will need to work with kinesthetic awareness and not mechanically, because the same exercise that can help you recover can also cause you damage if done wrongly, or at the wrong time.

We would like to refer you to *Self-Healing: My Life and Vision* by Meir Schneider. Read the chapters on The Mind and on Multiple Sclerosis. These will give you a better sense of how to work on yourself.

Multiple sclerosis is a disorder of the central nervous system. Its symptoms result from inflammatory damage to the myelin sheath, or insulator, of nerves. This demyelination later scars to form 'plaques', but even then the conduction of the electric current through the nerves remains hampered.

There is no typical case of multiple sclerosis, because the symptoms may be quite varied. If you suffer from multiple sclerosis, you will need to develop the sense of what exercises suit your needs best, because we are not able to cover all the possibilities. We do, however, hope to help you develop your intuition.

We would like to start by telling about some of the people we have worked with.

One of the first people Meir saw after moving to the United States was Kathy. A woman in her early thirties, she was leaning on a cane and limping. And she was very frightened about her illness.

Kathy was diagnosed with multiple sclerosis at the age of eighteen. After being stable for some time, she started having frequent attacks. Kathy hesitated about seeing Meir, because he was not a medical doctor. However, in a phone conversation, she shared with Meir some of the anxieties regarding upcoming events in her life, and Meir was able to help her reduce the level of anxiety involved. Kathy realized that a sense of calm was something she needed.

We have the feeling that rigid mental patterns, such as great fear and unresolved anger, contributed to Kathy's symptoms, and definitely made them worse. She recalled her resistance to returning to college as a student and her sensation that that would actually make her ill. She did return, and did get ill.

Meir's impression of Kathy, from the very first session, was of a pleasant, kind and gentle young woman. His intuitive impression, at the same time, was that Kathy's skin and weak muscles were in a process of deterioration. The Self-Healing therapy highly supports working with one's intuition, and Meir felt he was fighting against the odds. Kathy had very little control over her bladder, and suffered weekly bladder infections in spite of the antibiotics she was taking. This condition is very common with multiple sclerosis and often means weakness of the total system. She suffered from fatigue, though not as badly as is sometimes the case with multiple sclerosis. She was numb in her arms and legs, and – most important – she was very fearful of her deteriorating condition. Kathy wanted affirmation that she had no good reason to be fearful, but Meir had to tell her that her chances of needing a wheelchair were greater than of not needing one.

Kathy didn't like hearing that and was upset, but the sessions calmed her nonetheless. Meir did cranial massage and cranial manipulations, moving the nasal bone a little. Meir massaged her to improve her breathing, and taught her several simple exercises. She gradually learned to control rotating her leg while lying on her abdomen, to massage herself, to move each part of her back in isolation, and to move her head in one direction and her feet in the opposite direction. She practiced bouncing on a trampoline and walking barefoot on sand.

Within six months her numbness disappeared, her walking improved, and she appeared to have mastered her fear as well. Within a year and a half the major process of regeneration was completed. She had gained control over her bladder, and gradually gave up using antibiotics. In the thirteen years since, Kathy's illness has been relatively stable, with a few symptoms coming and going. She has suffered a slight deterioration in her capacity to walk, but her gait is still much better than what it was when she first met Meir, and she can walk for a mile.

One of the symptoms Kathy had experienced from the very beginning was dizziness, which was a result of lack of circulation to the head. She had tried a variety of exercises to solve that. Eventually, about five years ago, what worked for her was a combination of the skying exercise with closing and opening the jaw. She had watched someone else do that as a vision exercise (exercise 8–7 in the Vision chapter), and she realized that that was the exercise she needed. The fact that it helped her demonstrates that circulation blockage can take a different form in different people. In Kathy's case she needed releasing of the muscles of her jaw and neck.

Robert had been diagnosed with multiple sclerosis at age forty-three, seventeen years before he came to see Meir. Thus far his disease had taken a moderate course. His legs were numb and he walked like a drunk – very unstable, clutching at walls and other objects to balance himself.

A very pleasant man with a great sense of humor, Robert carried deep emotional wounds from his childhood and his first marriage. He did not tend to fatigue in a pathological way, like other multiple-sclerosis patients, but he had a sense of low energy which often comes with a deep inner conflict that does not surface. He came to sessions regularly, and took many workshops with Meir. Although he quickly came to understand his body, gave up his fears, and gained systemic strength, in other ways his improvement was slow.

Because exercise did not fatigue him, he was able to exercise with a stationary bicycle (riding backward and forward with no resistance, to minimize the effort), and to take walks on the beach. He had a pattern of balancing himself which did not work well for him: he used his leg muscles very little, and relied more on his hands holding onto walls, street signs and parked cars. To change his pattern of balance, he needed to learn to isolate his upper body from his lower body. He had to learn how to stop contracting his neck and arms, in order to allow more blood and energy flow to his legs, and to not contract his whole body for every movement, because through contraction one has less control over fine movement. (We feel that in the future the importance of not using unnecessary muscles will be appreciated more by most professionals in rehabilitation.)

Robert practiced lifting his legs one by one onto a stool, without supporting himself with his hands. By changing his habits he changed his posture, and learned to depend on his legs – rather than developing the eventual need to use a cane or crutches.

One day, as Robert was practicing his exercises at home, he didn't pay careful attention to his surroundings, lost his balance, and fell and broke his collarbone. While recovering in bed, he started contemplating walking again, this time differently. Before this incident, even though he understood the concept theor-

etically, he could not imagine himself walking without tensing his neck and arms. After two weeks of lying on his back and visualizing a more efficient method of walking, his walking improved dramatically. He did not walk like a drunk any more: he just had a slight limp.

Robert's gait slightly improved every single year for the next sixteen years.

Robert did not get rid of all his symptoms, but he improved enough to cause his neurologist to suspect that the diagnosis had been wrong in the first place; according to his neurologist, no one can overcome symptoms of multiple sclerosis. Similarly, Kathy's neurologist told her she might have a lifetime remission, but that she couldn't heal from multiple sclerosis. It is important to recognize what is indeed possible in rehabilitative health care. There are some drugs that may help symptoms, but none so far has proven as effective as learning how to use the body better.

The Program for the First Eighteen Months

The most important thing for you to monitor is your fatigue level. There is healthy fatigue and unhealthy fatigue. If as a result of activity you feel tired for twenty to thirty minutes, that's fine. If as a result of practicing the exercises we are suggesting you become aware of the hidden tiredness in your body, that's very good. The exercises and the awareness will help you to gradually eliminate your fatigue. An unhealthy fatigue is when you get very tired for a long period of time, after making very little effort.

Your exercises should be restful and

refreshing – and that is the criterion by which you must judge them. If your exercises tend to cause unhealthy fatigue, change them or the way you do them.

One of the solutions for a tendency to be fatigued is to practice a great variety of exercises and not to repeat any one of them too often: you do not then overtire any one area but instead work many different areas briefly. For example, if you find it difficult to lift your legs, you can massage them, move your feet together from side to side, lift your legs one by one onto a chair, do many relevant exercises – but none of them for more than five or six times.

We have found that it takes normally six to eight months for someone's fatigue level to decrease. Once you tend to be less tired, you can repeat exercises more frequently.

Spend a week reading and practicing the Breathing chapter daily. It will help you achieve the relaxation you need to allow change in your body and brain.

Your next step would be to read the chapter about the Nervous System, and work with it for three weeks. Work with your peripheral as well as with your central nervous system. Many of the exercises are applicable to you, though some, such as crawling, may be too vigorous. This is especially true if you have gait problems or paralysis.

A favorite coordination exercise which has helped many people with MS is the following.

23–1 Sitting in a chair, move your feet in small circles without lifting them off the floor, one clockwise and one counterclockwise. Try not to tense your thighs and pelvis. Now move both hands in circles above the feet – try to make this movement parallel, as if each hand is connected by an invisible thread to the foot

below it. When you manage to coordinate these movements, challenge yourself with another one: as you move your hands and feet in circles, rotate your head.

Symptoms of multiple sclerosis may vary, so we have chosen to describe our work with a few common ones in the following sections. These all may form part of the program for the first eighteen months.

Lack of Systemic Strength

In addition to fatigue, two other main aspects of systemic weakness are poor bladder control and heat-sensitivity.

Bladder Control

Most of the people we have met who have a problem with bladder control also have weak bodies. Some of the systemic weakness may result from the bladder and kidney infections involved in urinary incontinence, or from the repeated use of antibiotics.

We recommend practicing exercises for bladder control whether or not you suffer partial or complete urinary incontinence, as a means of strengthening both your central and peripheral nervous systems. You are more likely to achieve good results if you still have some control over your bladder's sphincters.

During the next three weeks, concentrate mainly on a combination of breathing exercises with exercises for your lower back and massage of the abdomen. Use the following exercises to learn how to isolate the movement of your legs from your abdomen and lower back.

23–2 Lie on your back (or in a semi-reclining position, supporting your back with pillows), with both legs outstretched. Now slowly bend one leg, sliding the foot on the floor (see fig 2–30 in the Circulation chapter). Bend the leg as much as you can, and then straighten it as far as you can, while bending the other one. Keep alternating slowly, imagining that your feet are leading the motion. Keep your hands on your abdomen, and tell yourself that the muscles of your abdomen and back have nothing to do with the motion. After bending and straightening the legs ten times, stop and visualize that you are continuing the motion smoothly, with ease. Think that no other muscles but the muscles of the feet are needed for the motion. Now move your legs again. After each ten movements, visualize two or three times that you are bending and straightening the legs. Try to build up to 100 movements, as long as you do not tire yourself.

This exercise is very important for your bladder, because it allows more circulation to the lower abdomen and pelvic floor without exhausting you. Besides, if you do this long enough, your legs will strengthen.

Vary this exercise by pointing your knees outward, each to its own side, rather than upward. This variation will help to reduce the tension in your hips and pelvic floor.

23–3 Lying on your abdomen, bend one leg at the knee and rotate your calf. The movement may feel jerky. Try to draw large, sweeping circles with your calf, and remember to rotate both clockwise and counterclockwise. After a few rotations, stop and visualize that you are moving the calf in rotation, and that the motion is easy and smooth. Alternate between movements and visualization several times, then

rotate only your foot several times. Stop and imagine that your ankle is moving smoothly, in perfect circles. Visualize this rotation in both directions, and now rotate the foot again. Does the movement feel any smoother? Return to rotations of the calf and visualize that the foot is leading the motion. Does that make the calf rotations any easier?

Repeat the whole procedure with your other leg.

Practice also exercise 2–28 of the Circulation chapter; try exercise 4–34 of the Spine chapter – but only if you do not have much of a problem with your legs.

To massage your abdomen, cup your hands by placing each thumb under the first finger, and then move your hands in circular motions on your abdomen, both clockwise and counter-clockwise. Your massage should be gentle but not too soft. Exert more pressure when you massage toward the heart. Refer also to exercise 7–23 in the Massage chapter for massage of the abdomen. Spend ten minutes a day on breathing exercises, twenty minutes working with your back, and twenty minutes massaging your abdomen.

For six weeks, focus mostly on the following exercises. If you see good results with them, continue working with them further, but combine them with the exercises which we will refer to later. Refer to exercises 6–5 and 6–6 in the Nervous System chapter for exercises of the sphincter muscles. Emphasize working with bladder control. After working with exercise 6–6, breathe deeply, cover your eyes with your palms, and imagine that you are seeing total blackness. Alternate these exercises with massage of the abdomen and with exercise 6–2 from the Nervous System chapter.

You may start to feel that you have more control of your bladder, that the area is coming alive. Breathe slowly and deeply, and relax.

Try also exercise 3–15 from the Joints chapter. Work with it only if you can do it with very little effort.

Heat-sensitivity

Another major symptom of systemic weakness is heat-sensitivity.

On one very hot day, Connie came to her session in a wheelchair pushed by a helper. Her arms and legs were immobile. By touching her back, it was obvious that the heat was distributed unevenly in her body. Parts of her back were extremely hot while others were cool. Meir put a towel soaked in cold water on her back, and in no time the towel warmed up – the steaming areas in her back wouldn't cool. For two hours he used cold towels and massage to redistribute the heat in her back. After those two hours, Connie was able to walk without help or braces.

Besides using a cold wet towel and a lot of massage, we recommend avoiding getting overheated. On hot days, take three cold showers, spend time in a cold pool and cool your neck with a cold towel.

If you are sensitive to heat, the next stage of working on your systemic strength is sure to become a favorite of yours.

After spending three months working with all the exercises described so far in this chapter, start working in a pool – where you can work without much resistance of gravity. If you live near a pleasant, sandy beach, have a friend help you walk to the water, and do whichever exercises can be done there; your friend can support you for balance in the water when necessary. Move without strain in any way you like, and make sure you are not tightening your jaw. Here are some suggestions.

23–4 Walk in the water, imagining that your legs are lifting you up.

23–5 At a pool, lean your abdomen and chest against the wall, hold onto a bar or a niche in the wall, bend one leg, and rotate your foot. Do the same with the other leg. Now rotate each leg from the knee.

Standing with your side to the wall, hold it for balance and rotate your whole leg from the hip joint several times. Do the same with the other leg. Remember to do all rotations both clockwise and counterclockwise.

Refer also to exercise 5–44 of the Muscles chapter.

When your legs can move more freely, your balance will improve. When your balance improves, you will be able to build many muscles that have not been in use. One very good way to do this is to walk. Walk before meals rather than after them, to create less of a strain. Try to find an area where you can walk on sand or on grass, where falling will cause you less harm. Otherwise, walk with a friend who is strong enough to prevent you from falling. Refer to the Muscles chapter, the section on Learning to Walk, and remember to breathe deeply as you walk.

Walk backward as much as you can. You do not need instructions to do this right, because you do not have any bad habit to undo – your social position or your emotional state has never influenced the way you walk backward.

An important variation is to walk backward with your feet hip-width apart, rather than close to each other.

Walk sideways. Refer to exercise 9–10 in the Running chapter for two methods of running (or, in this case, of walking) sideways. These exercises are a great way to use muscles you normally don't use.

Remain sensitive to your body's fatigue level. Do not take on stressful tasks if you can help it. This stage of your work on yourself is a stage of building up lost functions, so you need all the energy you can put into it.

The next group of exercises focuses on loosening your jaw and your neck, to create a sense of more space in the occipital area, which is where your skull meets the first vertebra. Because of the tension in the powerful jaw, upper-shoulder and neck muscles, this space is normally narrowed. This narrowing limits the flow of blood and of the cerebrospinal fluid, which nourishes and cushions the central nervous system. Through massage of these areas and movement, you can improve your posture and increase the space between the skull and the uppermost vertebra, and improve the circulation. Refer to exercise 5–40 of the Muscles chapter, and work with the last section – where your head is on the floor (see fig 5–40C). Work also with exercises 5–43 and 5–50 there, with the section on Neck and Shoulders in the Spine chapter, and with exercises 7–12 to 7–15 in the Massage chapter.

You can benefit very much from massage at all stages of your work, and especially from the neurological massage that was described in the Nervous System chapter.

MS and Motor Problems

Motor problems may involve numbness, but more disturbing than that are paralysis and lack of balance. We will describe exercises for some common problems.

Normally we don't expect you to recover all of the function that you may have lost. We estimate that those people who were not confined to a wheelchair when they began to work with us recovered between 60 and 75 percent of what they had lost. Perhaps you would like to have a professional evaluate your progress and help you sense how much you improve.

If You Can Walk but Your Hips are Stiff

23–6 Stand facing a solid table which is at least knee-high. Lift your leg and rest your bent leg on the table. Bring the leg down and repeat with the other leg. You will probably find that you can do this more easily with one leg than with the other. In this case, choose a table that will be a challenge to your stronger leg and continue to alternate between your legs even though you will not reach the table with your weaker leg. Whenever you lift your weaker leg, imagine that it is reaching halfway up between its best achievement so far and what the strong leg can do.

To loosen your hip joints, alternate between exercise 4–13 from the Spine chapter and this next exercise.

23–7 Lie on your back with the soles of your feet together and your knees apart. Lift your left knee off the floor and bring it all the way toward your right knee and then back to where it started. Now move your right knee all the way toward the left knee and then back to where it started. Continue moving each leg in turn.

23–8 Side kicks Holding onto a chair, a table, or anything else for balance, kick each leg in turn sideways, as high as you can. Let your foot be loose, but keep the toes pointing forward, rather than toward the side that you are kicking to (this activates a different set of muscles). Visualize that your foot is leading the motion. Repeat this exercise only a few times so as not to get fatigued.

Kicking sideways is very helpful in improving walking, for two reasons. First of all, some of the muscles which participate in this kicking (the abductors) are normally not exercised enough, but because they assist in flexion of the thigh, and limit the sideways excursion of the hip, they can be of great support for walking. Second, this exercise does strengthen other muscles which normally are used for walking; building them up will improve your balance.

If You Have Problems Writing

Work with the last paragraph of exercise 8–15 in the Vision chapter.

23–9 Sit in front of a table and tap with your fingertips on the table: once with both thumbs, once with both first fingers, once with both second fingers, and so on – going back and forth – to the thirds, to the little fingers, back to third, second, first and thumbs etc.

23–10 At a table, hold a pen in each hand and move both hands in circles – drawing a circle with each one of your hands. Move the hands in opposite directions – one clockwise and one counterclockwise.

If Your Arms Do Not Bend as a Result of Spasm

First, you need massage and passive movement for your arm. Refer to the Massage chapter for massage of the arms, and to the Nervous System chapter for neurological massage. Then do exercise 23–10.

If Your Arm is Very Weak

You will benefit from massage and passive movement of the arm, and also from active or passive rotations of the wrist.

If You Limp

Lie on your back, bend your arms at the elbows, and rotate your forearms. Keep your wrists loose and imagine that your fingertips are leading the motion. Now add to that bending and straightening of the legs, as you did in exercise 23–2. After several months, when you can manage this exercise without much difficulty, try exercise 6–13 of the Nervous System chapter.

If Your Legs are Spastic and You Use a Wheelchair

Have someone rotate your legs passively (refer to exercise 7–26 in the Massage chapter). Your helper should hold your leg very gently and softly. The more you resist, the gentler the leg should be held. Many people tend to think that they should push harder against stronger resistance. The truth is that the less you are pushed against, the more easily your muscles will move. Breathe deeply as your legs are rotated, and just be aware of them.

Never set goals for yourself that are greater than your mind can conceive. Always work toward the next step. Gradually your goals can expand as your mobility increases. Work with the exercises in the Nervous System chapter which you are able to do easily. Try, for example, exercises 6–12 and 6–17 there.

Vision Loss and MS

As a result of multiple sclerosis, you may suffer vision loss or develop double vision or blurring. Work with the Vision chapter and most of all with palming (exercise 8–5), which will allow relaxation of your damaged optic nerve.

After Eighteen Months

Eighteen months is the average time it takes to get to a stage where you don't tend to fatigue from a little exercise, though it may take you six months or it may take two years. When you get to the stage that you can repeat exercises again and again and not get exhausted for the rest of the day, then do so. Return to the exercises which you have done so far and repeat them hundreds of times. Walk for longer periods of time – forward, backward and sideways. Kick sideways (exercise 23–8) up to 200 times a day. Try the more vigorous exercises below.

23–11 Lying on your back with your knees bent, tighten and relax your anal sphincter 100 times.

23–12 To improve your balance, lift your feet alternately up onto a stool. Make sure you have either something to hold onto if you lose your balance or a soft mattress to protect you from hurting yourself if you do fall. Falling may be harmful because it may create a setback.

23–13 Another balancing exercise is to walk on uneven surfaces, such as moderate hills.

CHAPTER 24

Vision Problems

This chapter is for readers who would like some suggestions on what to do for specific eye ailments. Most of the exercises described in the Vision chapter can be done by anyone, with any eye condition. There are some important exceptions, however, in the case of certain severe pathological conditions such as cataract and macular degeneration, and these deserve special attention. We cannot prescribe treatment programs for people we have never seen, and of course each case is unique, so please discuss the suggestions in this chapter with your eye doctor before following them, and use your own judgment about which exercises, and how much of each exercise, you find to be beneficial.

As a general rule, we recommend that anyone who is doing vision-improvement work should be receiving bodywork concurrently. The more pathological the condition – that is, the more it involves harm to actual tissue – the more bodywork is needed, to speed the natural healing process. This should include massage of the face, head, shoulders, chest, back and arms. If you cannot find a good massage therapist, you can do a lot of this massage yourself. Both the Vision chapter and the Massage chapter have instructions on self-massage that will help you. A note for those who are doing bodywork on clients with eye problems: at the Center for Self-Healing we use a massage room which is almost completely dark, providing a rest from all visual stimuli, which our eye clients all appreciate.

Nearsightedness

The majority of people with nearsightedness, or myopia – the inability to see distant things clearly – have acquired the condition, rather than being born with it. If your myopia is acquired, and is not especially severe, then you have an extremely good chance of overcoming it altogether and restoring your former good vision. You should approach vision exercises without any sense of urgency, since trying too hard will automatically counteract the good you do with the exercises. Don't insist on having better vision immediately, but allow the improvement to develop in its own time. With patience, your vision has a good chance of being better than it ever was, and you will also be preventing future deterioration of the eyes.

All of the exercises in the Vision chapter are recommended. If, like many myopic people, you spend a great deal of time reading or doing other close work, you should concentrate at first on palming, to relieve the effects of years of strain on the eyes. You should palm for no less than an hour a day, and do this for two weeks before going on to other exercises. You should then add sunning to your daily regimen. Read the sections on shifting and blinking, and begin to remind yourself to shift and to blink continually throughout the day. When these have become automatic visual habits, go on to the sections entitled Developing Distance Vision and Reading below. While the Stimulating Peripheral Vision exercises in the Vision chapter are good for every eye, they are most important if you have one eye which is stronger than the other.

Some people, especially myopic people, see their vision work as part of a psychological process. In the course of doing the vision exercises, they often experience insights into emotional causes of poor vision, and into the circumstances surrounding them. If emotions and realizations come up for you while practicing vision exercises, talk about them, either with your support group or perhaps with a therapist who can help you to deal with them.

Developing Distance Vision

If your main problem is myopia — which means that you see things better close up and worse far away — you will be pleasantly surprised to discover that your first improvements in clarity will almost certainly be in the realm of distance vision. The reason for this is simple: since you do not see clearly in the far distance, you probably seldom look at things in the far distance, and consequently you do not have so many ingrained, hard-to-change visual habits associated with looking at things in the far distance. Looking into the distance will be a new world to you, so your approach will be more flexible, and your progress will consequently be that much faster.

If you are accustomed to seeing a blur in the distance, that's good — you will be used to the blur and not frustrated by it. It would be nice if you could even enjoy the blur. Think of the soft, overlapping color masses in Impressionist paintings, and appreciate your eyes' ability to create that delicate effect effortlessly. However, even while you are appreciating one of the things your eyes do well, you can inject more clarity into your landscape.

24–1 Find a place that provides you with a genuine vista, preferably one which extends for miles. Remember, how far you can see depends upon the size of the thing you are looking at. If you have ever seen a star, then you know that you can see for billions of miles, which is an encouraging thought in itself. If you have a nice hilltop you can go to, that's wonderful. If not, a window on a second or third story will do just as well.

Look out as far as you can. The 'horizon' is different for everyone. It is basically the farthest distance where your eyes can distinguish anything at all, even if it is only a slight variation in color or shape. Find your own horizon and let your eyes move from point to point along it. Take in every detail, as though you were waiting for something to appear or searching for something you lost. Animals and people with famously good vision, such as hawks, sailors or Australian bushmen, are always scanning their landscape, not necessarily looking for anything specific, just looking for anything at all. This is how your eyes should be looking. Anything that can be seen is of interest to you.

Now move your horizon a little closer, and again move from point to point, from detail to detail. Inevitably you will be able to see more, to distinguish more. For example, distant mountaintops look blue, but those a little closer are clearly not blue; they are instead covered by trees casting bluish shadows. Distant buildings tend to be just blocks in shades of gray, while the closer ones have windows, and those closer still have signs, plants and people in the windows. Each time you bring your horizon a little closer, let your eyes dance from point to point and your mind take in all available details. By the time you have brought your point of focus as close as possible – to your fingertips, to the windowsill, or to the ground at your feet – you will be almost overwhelmed by the variety and clarity of the details you can see. Remember always to blink constantly, to breathe deeply. If your eyes become tired, move your fingers all around your peripheral field and wiggle them rapidly, or stop and palm for a minute.

Now do this exercise in reverse: begin by shifting from point to point on the closest possible object, and gradually move your plane of focus farther and farther away. At each stage, stop for a minute to close your eyes and visualize what you have just seen, calling to mind as many details as you can remember. In this way you will keep a sense of clarity in your vision as you move farther into the distance.

24–2 A similar exercise can be done while walking down a street or a path. Beginning with the point just in front of your feet, allow your eyes to 'sweep' out as far as they can see, to the point at which the line of the sidewalk or the edges of the path converge, and then to sweep back again, blinking continually as you do so. This will keep you continually moving from your farthest horizon back to a point where you can see clearly, and you will have the added benefit of a constant stimulation of your peripheral vision, created by the motion of your walking.

Sometimes you may experience 'flashes' of clear vision, much better than your normal vision. For many myopic people, these flashes will come momentarily, disappear immediately, and recur unexpectedly from time to time. Their great value is that they demonstrate to your mind that your eyes are indeed capable of more than they usually achieve. Vision, as we have said, is partly based on perception, and perception is often based on prior conception. You usually see as well as you expect to see. An experience of good vision, even if temporary, paves the way for further improvement.

Reading

Perhaps more than anything else, our ability to read clearly indicates how well we can see. Usually the first indication of an eye problem will come through noticing at what distance we need to hold a book to read comfortably. At the eye doctor's office, we are asked to look not at pictures to determine our visual acuity, but at rows of printed letters on eye charts which subsequently may become a source of anxiety and frustration.

Reading is one of the most sensitive issues for a nearsighted person, in part because the typical nearsighted person (and there is such a thing) loves to read and would do it until the eyes gave out completely if time and life allowed. What few of us book-lovers remember is that reading is a strenuous physical activity involving a delicately balanced pair of organs. We become so absorbed and entranced by the flow of information from the page to our minds that we forget how hard the eyes are working to create that flow.

There is also the problem of how we connect emotionally with what we are reading, and with the experience of reading itself. If, for example, we are working on a project which is giving us problems, the anxiety surrounding those problems will affect our reading acuity.

Reading can potentially be very harmful for the eyes, as our eyes are biologically designed to change from close to distant focus continually. Reading does not have to be damaging to the eyes, however; in fact, with the help of the reading exercises in this section, you can actually use reading to improve your overall vision. Reading exercises can help us to acquire the habit of shifting, and so are especially helpful for myopia and astigmatism, and can also improve hyperopia, as well as reducing the eyestrain and fatigue which reading can cause.

Just as the other exercises we have learned have been designed to change our visual habits, these exercises are aimed at changing our overall reading habits. Most of us have very poor reading habits, and it is these, not the fact of reading itself, which are responsible for the damage reading can do, by causing

unnecessary strain and stopping the process of shifting, for example. Before we go on to the more specific exercises, here are some general rules that will help make even prolonged reading easier for your eyes:

- Never read in uncomfortable light, whether this means too bright or too dim. The wrong light will tire your eyes faster than anything else. Your eyes will tell you if the light feels wrong to them; all you need to do is pay attention to them. If reading seems to feel difficult, the light is the first thing to check.
- At least every twenty minutes or so, stop and palm for about five minutes. Just as you would naturally take breaks from hard physical labor, your eyes need breaks from the hard labor of reading.
- Remember to blink constantly, to keep your eyes from staring or drying out. If your eyes burn during or after reading, it may be because you become so involved with what you're reading that you forget to blink. Remind yourself as often as you can.
- Try to avoid, as much as possible, anything which is printed in a hard-to-read typeface. We are really surprised sometimes by the total lack of regard for the eyes that is obvious in the design of many publications, which are printed in type so light, so small, so unclear or so elaborate that it would give anyone eyestrain. Try to stay away from these things. And if you have difficulty with necessary things such as documents or phone books, don't strain your eyes trying to read them; read them when your eyes are rested, and in a comfortable light. Make it easy on your eyes.
- Breathe. Even though your mind may be in another world, your body is still in this one, and your eyes need oxygen more than ever,

so keep breathing. There is a tendency to hold one's breath while reading, as in many other concentrated activities, so you will probably have to remind yourself to take deep breaths, as well as to blink.

Nowhere are the principles of shifting as important as they are in reading. The worst thing you can do in reading, from the eyes' point of view anyway, is to try to take in whole sentences, or even whole paragraphs, simultaneously, as most of us avid readers do. When we do this, we are unconsciously imitating the pattern of myopic sight – making large, infrequent jumps and trying to take in a large visual field. Remember that the macula can see only small areas at a time, and that it sees by moving from point to point. If you force your eyes to swallow an entire sentence at one gulp, you make it impossible for the macula to participate fully, and of course the less your macula works the more blurred your sight will be. If you sacrifice clarity for speed, the long-term effects may be a chronic loss of acuity.

Our first goal, therefore, is to reintroduce shifting into the reading process. Train yourself out of looking at whole sentences, or even whole words, or even whole letters. Do you remember learning to write? At that stage you would have been acutely aware of the form of each letter, because you were just learning to reproduce that form in writing. Having learned the Hebrew and Cyrillic alphabets as an adult, Maureen gained a new appreciation for letters as physical forms; in other words, she learned to actually look at them. To read properly, we must learn to look at our own alphabet the same way.

24–3   Take this page, turn it upside down, and read one letter at a time, letting your eyes move from point to point as they slowly and carefully trace the shape of each letter, blinking constantly as you do so. This will automatically make you more aware of the letters, focusing you on the physical act of seeing rather than on the meaning of the words. It will also make you more aware of what your eyes are doing when you read – an awareness we usually lose in our absorption with the contents of a book. If you find this difficult, that means that this is an especially effective exercise for you.

24–4   Make a photocopy of the Snellen eye chart provided on pages 356–7 (or purchase an actual chart from an optical-supply company) and attach it to a wall. Place yourself far enough away from it so that the last several lines are not easy for you to read. You should be able to read the first three or four lines fairly easily, whether this means standing a few yards, a few feet or a few inches away from the chart. Begin by reading the last line which is clearly visible to you – the third, fourth or fifth, for example. Trace all around the outlines of each letter, as if you are drawing the outlines of a block letter with your eyes. You may find that you tense up as soon as you look at the chart, since for many of us that chart represents a test we have repeatedly failed. So relax – breathe, unlock your knees, let go of your abdomen, let your arms hang loose at your sides, and blink. Let your head move slightly and slowly from side to side as you look. Occasionally raise both hands, hold them up by your ears and wiggle the fingers – this will stimulate the peripheral cells and take some of the strain off the central cells.

After you have read each letter in the line, close your eyes and visualize the last letter you have seen. Imagine it as being very large, black and solid on a bright white background. Trace its outlines and move from point to point in your imagination.

When you open your eyes, look at the same letter again and see if it is clearer. Look two or three lines below it and see if you can distinguish between characters and spaces. This will help you to look at smaller areas than you normally tend to look at. Return to the line you started with, and see if it is clearer. If it is, take a look at the line below it. Again move from point to point and sketch the shape of each letter, one by one. If you cannot distinguish the exact letter, then take notice of its general shape and whatever other characteristics — curves, crossbars or whatever — you can distinguish, and at the spaces between the letters. Then close your eyes and repeat your visualization as before. Now return to the first line you read. Blink, breathe, relax your body, and wave your hands at the sides of your face as you shift from point to point on each letter in turn. Do the letters look clearer? Stop the exercise and sun or palm for a few minutes.

Try to repeat this exercise with each of the remaining lines on the chart, even if the last line seems to be no more than a faint black wiggle. Each time you finish with one line, return to your original line. This both rests your eyes and repeatedly gives them the experience of clear sight. If your eyes become tired, stop for a while and palm, imagining blackness.

24–5 Open your eyes, turn your head partially to the left and look at the chart with your right eye, moving from point to point on the letters as before; then turn your head toward the right and look at the chart with your left eye. Then try the opposite process: turn your head to the left, cover your right

eye with your hand, and try to read the chart with your left eye; then repeat to the right. Tilt your head downward, with your chin toward your chest, so that your eyes must look upward to see the chart, and read several letters in this position; then tilt your head back so that your eyes must look down to read. Try reading with your head constantly moving slowly from side to side, so that the eyes must constantly look from different angles to read the letters. These variations may be useful for people with astigmatism, who often find that changing the angle at which they view something improves their clarity immediately. It also helps to break the pattern of staring which often develops when we look at the chart with both eyes for any period of time. The purpose of this particular exercise is mainly to improve your shifting.

In time you may find your original line becoming clearer, sharper and easier to read. When this happens, step backward a foot or so and see whether you can still read the letters in that line easily. If so, then continue the exercise from your new distance. You may also discover that the lower lines become gradually more distinct. If this doesn't happen, don't worry about it — the shifting process by itself is a good exercise for the eyes, even if it doesn't immediately produce noticeable improvements in clarity.

Eye-chart exercises may cause the eyes to feel strained at first. It is important to not allow the eye to strain, so palm or sun before your eyes get tired. We also suggest alternating between eye-chart exercises and those for developing distance vision (24–1 and 24–2).

24–6 Returning to the eye chart, use an eyepatch or your hand to cover one eye,

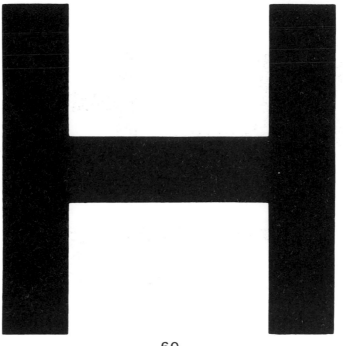

60

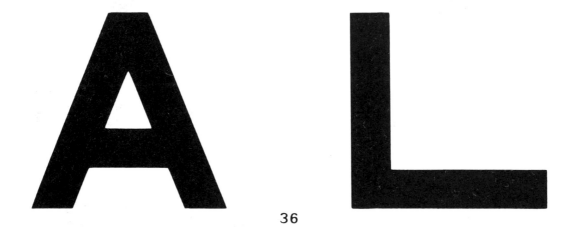

36

24

OLHA
18

ECTNO
12

CLOHNA
9

AENLOHCT
6

HTNELACO
5

AECONHTL
4

The Snellen Eye Chart

preferably your stronger eye if you know which one is stronger. (If you don't know, this is the place to find out. Just cover each eye in turn and look at the line on the chart which is below your 'easy' line; any difference between the two eyes will then be apparent immediately.) This will give the weaker eye a chance to work and the stronger eye a chance to rest. Go through the chart exercises from the beginning, doing each with each eye separately. You may find it a good idea to give your weaker eye extra time with this exercise, since it may need the attention more than the stronger eye.

Most people will find it too strenuous to do all of these chart exercises without a break. We recommend that you try them all, at various times, and in the order we have described, spending no more than ten minutes in total at first on chart exercises, and no more than five minutes on any one exercise. When you have eventually experienced them all, you will be able to choose which ones feel appropriate to you at various times, and to vary them as you please.

24–7   Turn to the page of 'varying print sizes' (page 359) and begin with the largest or next-to-largest print size, whichever is more comfortable for you. Hold the page at a distance which is as far away as you can manage to read clearly. If arm's length is not far enough, you can tape a photocopy to a wall, preferably in sunlight. Now begin to read slowly, one letter at a time, remembering to blink and breathe, to move from point to point on each letter, and to trace the shape of each letter and of the spaces between letters. With your free hand, wiggle your fingers beside one eye to stimulate the peripheral cells, but don't allow your eye to actually look toward the fingers – keep both eyes on the page. Also, be sure to transfer the page to the other hand from time to time, and wiggle the fingers of the other hand beside the other eye. If both your hands are free (and the paper is attached to the wall) wiggle both hands simultaneously. Every minute or so, stop, close your eyes, and try to visualize the very last letter you read – its shape, its details, the shape of the space surrounding it. If you have difficulty visualizing, don't strain to do it – just try as well as you can to remember what the letter looked like. In time, these exercises will help to develop your visual memory.

After you have read several lines in this manner – it will probably take you four or five minutes to do so – move from the word you are reading over to the corresponding word in the block of the next largest print size, without moving the page any closer to you. Follow the letters there without attempting to read them. Even if you cannot read a word, you may have quite a lot of information about it. Can you see how many letters it has, whether the letters go below or above the midline, whether they are rounded or angular? Look at the third-largest type. Can you see the spaces between the words? In order to not strain your eyes, blink, breathe, and wave your hands to the sides of your face. Do not squint. Now turn to the fourth-largest type and look at the spaces between the words. Close your eyes and imagine that the spaces are very distinct, the ink is very black, the page is very white. Open your eyes. Is the white brighter? If so, return to the large print. You may find it much clearer, and seemingly larger. Your mind is now looking at smaller areas than it used to look at before. You are using the central part of your retina, the begin with the largest or next-to-largest print size, whichever is more comfortable for you. Hold the page at a distance which is as far away as you can manage to read clearly. If arm's length is not far enough, you can tape a photocopy to a wall, preferably in sunlight. Now begin to read slowly, one letter at a time, remembering to blink and breathe, to move from point to point on each letter, and to trace the shape of each letter and of the spaces between letters. With your free hand, wiggle your fingers beside one eye to stimulate the peripheral cells, but don't allow your eye to actually look toward the fingers – keep both eyes on the page.

begin with the largest or next-to-largest print size, whichever is more comfortable for you. Hold the page at a distance which is as far away as you can manage to read clearly. If arm's length is not far enough, you can tape a photocopy to a wall, preferably in sunlight. Now begin to read slowly, one letter at a time, remembering to blink and breathe, to move from point to point on each letter, and to trace the shape of each letter and of the spaces between letters. With your free hand, wiggle your fingers beside one eye to stimulate the peripheral cells, but don't allow your eye to actually look toward the fingers – keep both eyes on the page.

begin with the largest or next-to-largest print size, whichever is more comfortable for you. Hold the page at a distance which is as far away as you can manage to read clearly. If arm's length is not far enough, you can tape a photocopy to a wall, preferably in sunlight. Now begin to read slowly, one letter at a time, remembering to blink and breathe, to move from point to point on each letter, and to trace the shape of each letter and of the spaces between letters. With your free hand, wiggle your fingers beside one eye to stimulate the peripheral cells, but don't allow your eye to actually look toward the fingers – keep both eyes on the page.

begin with the largest or next-to-largest print size, whichever is more comfortable for you. Hold the page at a distance which is as far away as you can manage to read clearly. If arm's length is not far enough, you can tape a photocopy to a wall, preferably in sunlight. Now begin to read slowly, one letter at a time, remembering to blink and breathe, to move from point to point on each letter, and to trace the shape of each letter and of the spaces between letters. With your free hand, wiggle your fingers beside one eye to stimulate the peripheral cells, but don't allow your eye to actually look toward the fingers – keep both eyes on the page.

begin with the largest or next-to-largest print size, whichever is more comfortable for you. Hold the page at a distance which is as far away as you can manage to read clearly. If arm's length is not far enough, you can tape a photocopy to a wall, preferably in sunlight. Now begin to read slowly, one letter at a time, remembering to blink and breathe, to move from point to point on each letter, and to trace the shape of each letter and of the spaces between letters. With your free hand, wiggle your fingers beside one eye to stimulate the peripheral cells, but don't allow your eye to actually look toward the fingers – keep both eyes on the page.

Varying Print Sizes

macula. This is one of the best forms of shifting.

Do the same exercise with a black piece of paper between your eyes. Read with your weaker eye, and wave your hand or a piece of paper beside your stronger eye (fig 24–7), but close enough for it to be visible at all times.

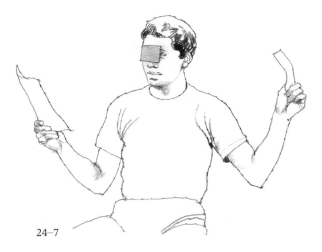

24–7

24–8 Writing, as well as reading, can be either a strain on the eyes or a helpful exercise. The best feature of writing is that your eyes have an opportunity to follow movement, which is a type of exercise that refreshes rather than tires them. Your next exercise is to write out the letters of the alphabet (any alphabet), making the letters very large and clear, and keeping your eyes focused (not staring, but focused) on the movement of your hand as you write, just as you would watch the movement of a bird. After each letter, close your eyes and visualize the pen moving as the letter takes shape. Can you remember the various directions of the pen's movement, and the changes in the letter's shape as you complete it?

You can also do this exercise with very short simple words, still closing your eyes after each letter and visualizing its formation. Even without doing this exercise formally, you can remember, while writing, to watch the movement of your hand and the growth of the letters. This will help your eyes to keep from tiring.

Finding Time for Your Eyes

None of these exercises is actually physically hard to do, and yet many people find it difficult to create an eye-exercise regimen in their lives. The reasons for this are many. One is that the exercises are so simple that it is sometimes hard for people to believe they are really doing anything – even after they have experienced good results from them.

Emotional resistance may also play a big part in keeping us from making a true commitment to improving our vision. This resistance is very normal. We don't like to face the fact of poor vision, and glasses allow us to ignore that fact. When a person with 20/20 vision begins to see a blur, the natural reaction is to want that clear vision back, *as soon as possible*! Seeing clearly is not just perception of details; it also gives a person a sense of being in control, while bad vision can make a person feel helpless. It takes great reserves of patience and trust to do vision exercises instead of just reaching for the glasses.

So you should be prepared for a certain amount of resistance. It may take the form of impatience, emotional disturbance or sometimes sheer boredom. A similar pattern happens in meditation, where the mind will resist our inward searching by putting up an overwhelming screen of boredom. Or you may feel nervous, frustrated or angry. Let yourself feel these things, and, if possible, let them go, but don't make things worse by resisting the resistance. Acknowledge it for what it is, let it come, and let it go. Do not become attached to your negative feelings but concentrate instead on what you are doing, and *just keep doing it*.

The next step is to accept the blurred vision as an appropriate thing to have. In most cases, poor vision is a natural result of how we use our eyes. This does not mean it is your fault — it means that you have the power to change the condition. This can only be done with patience, however. Fighting with yourself, whether you are condemning your eyes, your body or your emotional being, is the least effective thing you can do. You might be surprised to know how many people come to us furious with their eyes at having done this to them. This attitude has to change to something like: 'It's OK that my vision is blurred, for the moment, but I want to do what I can to clarify it, because that will promote the health of my eyes and my body.' In other words, you have to temporarily ask not what your eyes can do for you but what you can do for them.

What will it take for you to make your eye exercises — and your newfound ways of looking at the world — an integrated part of your life? We and our clients have found that one of the most effective ways is to occasionally take an entire day and devote it to your eyes. If this seems like a lot, stop and think about what your eyes do for you. Even the most myopic eyes make life a lot easier and more interesting for their possessor; try to imagine life without them. If any part of you deserves your attention, your eyes do.

If you can get a friend or a group of friends to join you, this will enrich your experience even more — and also make it enough fun that you will want to do it again. For about a year, the two of us used to meet with two other serious vision students and have palming sessions that lasted — with several breaks, of course — for up to six hours. Meir had one legendary session that lasted eleven hours, and believes that this was what enabled him, finally, to earn his California driver's license. Maureen, who has lived in the San Francisco Bay area since childhood, found that the bluish blurs she had seen in the distance for twenty years had resolved themselves into bridges, skylines, shorelines and hilltops with distinct buildings in them. Ylanah, who formerly could see only 20/80 with maximum correction, could now see 20/80 with no correction at all. Ellen had been blinded in one eye by flying glass. After three of these marathon palming sessions she could distinguish between light and shadow with the blind eye, where formerly there had been only darkness; her good eye went from 20/15 to 20/6 — over three times as good as 'normal' 20/20.

During these group sessions, it is very helpful to take turns massaging the shoulders, necks and occasionally the faces of the others. If you do not know how to do massage, you will quickly become proficient, finding that the delicate touch required around the eyes is very different from the powerful kneading that the shoulders usually like. Tell each other what feels good, and let yourself relax completely when your friends work on you. It would be a good idea to refer to the Massage chapter for ideas on upper-body massage techniques. It's also good to do some gentle stretching during your breaks. Try to eat as little as possible, because too much food in your stomach will just put you to sleep.

Your friends can also give you an objective evaluation of how much your vision has actually improved. Of course the ophthalmologist can do the same, but many people — especially those with serious vision problems – find going to the eye doctor so stressful that it adversely affects the test results. People who know you well, on the other hand, have a fairly good notion of how well you can see, and often will notice changes in your vision before you do. The process of gaining vision can be so gradual that an improvement in acuity may become established without our even knowing about it – until an old friend says incredulously, 'You mean you can see that? All the way over there?' On many occasions, friends have begun to describe or to read something for Maureen, only to be told that she can see it for herself. This reminder of how much her vision has changed is a constant encouragement to her.

So, for this purpose, it might be a good idea to follow the palming session with a walk in a park or some other attractive area, and tell each other what you can see. As always, remember that you are not having a competition with yourself – or anyone else. Do not test yourself or demand that you see something better this week than you did last week. Just enjoy putting your eyes through their paces. Concentrate on the exercises, and the results will take care of themselves.

As you walk, practice your distance exercises, letting the eyes sweep out to the horizon and back to you. If you can do so without losing your balance, let your eyes move together in circles as you walk – it may be much easier than it sounds; if not, then just shift constantly and comfortably. It is literally impossible for you to see everything in your environment at once, so take advantage of what your eyes do best and let them move from point to point, enjoying everything they see.

24–9 Find a fairly open spot – a field, a vacant lot, the beach or just a rooftop if that's really the only place you can go to be outdoors. Take an eye chart with you, to hang up on a tree, a fence, or a post. Stand at a distance that allows you easily to read the first four lines on the chart, and sun for a couple of minutes. Then open your eyes and start to swing gently from side to side, blinking and shifting your focus from point to point as you swing. Let your eyes glance very briefly at the chart as it flashes past you, but do not allow your eyes to fix on it. Look at the horizon, look in all directions, look at everything around you, and, incidentally, occasionally look at the chart. Keep this up for as long as ten minutes at a time. Vary what you see by changing your position, by changing directions, by focusing on different points on the horizon. Think of this as an affirmation of all that you *can* see, at this very moment. Don't expect to see the chart more clearly during the exercise itself; you will find that the increased clarity will come gradually, with time. The important thing in this exercise is to become comfortable with the chart, to see it as just another object in the environment, and to make it part of a nice outdoor experience, instead of a grueling ordeal.

When you come to a sunny spot on your vision-improvement day, sit down and sun together. Don't worry about how this looks to other people! No one will call the police to come and take these loonies away. We have been sunning in public for years; we almost always get some kind of response and it's almost always positive. Most people will say something friendly about how nice the sun feels; occasionally some informed person will recognize Dr Bates's exercise and want to know more about it. So, sun with confidence. After all, people are out there doing much sillier things – like tanning.

On your vision-improvement day, try to avoid things which strain your eyes, like reading, television, movies or any sort of work which uses the eyes too much. After your palming, your walk and your sunning, do something nice and relaxing for your body. Get a full massage – you could exchange with your partners for this – take a hot tub, or a sauna, or a swim. Then go out for a light dinner, and finally take a walk again, this time to look at the stars or the city lights, whichever you have more of in your neighborhood. This kind of viewing is very restful and pleasant for your eyes, and the walk will make you ready for a long, restful sleep.

We recommend that you do not discard your glasses immediately. For activities which require acute vision, it is better to use glasses than to return to the old habit of straining the eyes to see better. If after a month of exercising your vision you find that it has improved, we suggest that you have your optometrist fit you with a pair of glasses with a reduced prescription. Those will allow you to drive, or read the blackboard, or any other function for which your eyes need correction, yet will be uncomfortable enough to remind you to continue shifting through your glasses.

Farsightedness

If you have been farsighted since childhood, your condition is called hyperopia, or hypermetropia. Hyperopia results when an eyeball is unusually short from front to back; it can usually be corrected with glasses or contact lenses. If you have become farsighted later in life – the midforties is the most common time for this development – then the condition is called presbyopia, and is believed to result from a stiffening of the lens. This stiffening limits the ability of the eye to change its shape for adjusting from far to near vision. If you find yourself having to hold things farther and farther away to read them, you are probably developing presbyopia. It quite often happens that people suffer from myopia and presbyopia simultaneously, seeing clearly neither at close nor at distant range.

Before you begin with this section, you should read and practice the exercises in the Vision chapter. If you are presbyopic, spend at least two to eight weeks practicing those exercises; if you are hyperopic, you should spend at least two to four months. You will probably notice temporary improvements in your vision very shortly after you begin to practice the exercises. You will know when you are ready to progress when you find these improvements staying with you consistently.

When we work with farsightedness, our main goal is to make the eye more flexible, to give up the sense of stress and strain through which you are trying to see, and to provide the most favorable conditions for the eye, so that no further loss of clarity will occur.

After your initial period of working with the Vision chapter, adopt the following program for two weeks:

- Devote half an hour a day to palming.
- Sun your eyes for no less than forty-five minutes a day; if the sun isn't shining, work with the skying exercise (Vision chapter, exercises 8–6 and 8–7).
- You should also practice reading exercises 24–3, 24–5 and 24–7 (hold the page at a

distance which is as close as you can manage while still able to read clearly). Reading in the sun will be easier for your eyes, since the light contracts your pupils and improves your focus. While you do the reading exercises make sure that the light falls directly onto the page. It is important to give your eyes and your brain plenty of experience with easy, stress-free sight, as this in time will help your brain to stop associating sight with strain.

As you read, notice whether you are straining to see. Do you feel a sense of hardness in the eyes, of tension in your forehead, jaw or neck? Try to let go of it by consciously relaxing the muscles. Closing your eyes for a moment and breathing deeply will help. If you find the light too strong at first, you may begin to squint to shut it out. Don't let yourself do this, as it will only make your eyes and face stiffer and harder. Instead, sun your eyes for a few minutes, blink lightly and continually as you read, and remember to shift continuously from point to point – all of these things will alleviate the glare. You can also massage your forehead and cheekbones while you read, by raking them with your fingers.

After two weeks, you can begin to challenge your eyes a bit more by bringing the page gradually closer to you while you do your reading exercises. As you do this, however, remember that, while you are trying to improve your vision, you are also trying to relax your eyes, so don't overchallenge them. Even if you only move the page a fraction of an inch closer every other day, you are still making progress. You will benefit very much from facial massage at this point. You should massage your own face every day, as described in the Vision chapter (exercise 8–1); it will be helpful if you can get someone else to do it as well.

If you are presbyopic, you will probably see improvement more quickly than will a person who is hyperopic, since the longer you have a condition, the slower it is to change. Presbyopia may improve after about three months; hyperopia can take twice as long.

Retinal Detachment

Extremely severe myopia – a condition which usually starts at a very early age – can be dangerous to your eyes. A myopic eyeball is one which is very long from front to back, and this unusual lengthening may stretch the retina to the point where it may tear or become detached. Severe myopia is, of course, not the only cause of retinal detachment, but it is a leading cause. If you are suffering retinal detachment, you need an ophthalmologist's immediate attention. Retinal-attachment surgery has a very high success rate, and is highly recommended whenever it is possible. Unfortunately, however, the same conditions that caused the original tear may give rise to new tears in other parts of the retina. To prevent this, we recommend starting the vision exercises as soon as the retina has healed, usually two to three months after the surgery. Vision exercises may also be very helpful if your degree of detachment is minimal enough to make surgery unnecessary, or so severe that surgery will not help. Be sure to consult your ophthalmologist about whether these exercises are appropriate for you.

To prevent further detachment, avoid straining your eye excessively and avoid flexing your neck, which means bending it forward. A strong impact on your body is also dangerous to your retinas, so avoid aerobics, riding in cars with poor shock absorbers on bumpy roads, stamping your feet vigorously and any other similar effects.

One of Meir's clients, Liz, has been extremely myopic since childhood; her vision had been corrected to 20/70 at best. In her early twenties she suffered total retinal detachment in one eye and a partial detachment in the other. With the eye whose retina was detached completely, she could see her fingers only if she brought them close to her face and wiggled them; beyond that her vision was a blur. The partially detached retina was reattached and supported with silicone. At the time she came to see Meir, her vision was measured in this eye at 20/200 with contact lenses and glasses combined.

During his first session with Liz, Meir noticed that she almost never blinked. Her ophthalmologist had noticed the same thing and noted it on her chart, but had not discussed it with her. Meir's first instructions to Liz were to do blinking exercises, as well as facial massage to relax the muscles around the eyes which were both inhibiting her blinking *and* growing even stiffer as a result of her not blinking. Liz also learned to use her weak eye, though not for reading or any other strenuous use. She would use it to look only at very large and distinct objects, simply to encourage it to participate in the act of seeing and to balance her vision somewhat. She added distance-vision exercises, a favorite being to watch ocean waves rolling in from the horizon.

Liz spent two hours each day practicing vision exercises. Within one year, her vision in the stronger eye had returned to 20/80 with correction. The acuity in her weaker eye had also increased, and she used it more frequently.

A detached retina naturally weakens the vision in the affected eye, causing an imbalance in the use of the two eyes and a split in the visual field. Even if, like Liz, a person has two detached retinas, very often one eye will be the more severely affected. In such cases you need to encourage the weaker eye to work, but without straining or overchallenging it. You need to provide rest for the stronger eye, which will tend to overwork to compensate for the weaker eye. And you need to try to encourage the two eyes to work together as a unit, in spite of their different acuities.

For this condition, we recommend that you devote as much time as possible to palming, with two and a half hours daily being the minimum. We also suggest that you do twenty minutes of sunning daily. Facial massage will be helpful if it is done VERY GENTLY and NOT IN THE AREA SURROUNDING THE EYES. Limit it to the forehead, jaw and lower cheekbones. While your retina is detached, do not do exercise 8–4 or exercise 4–2 (referred to in the Vision chapter) because they involve neck flexion; wait until long after the recovery period for retinal-attachment surgery has passed, and then discuss them with your ophthalmologist. Peripheral-vision exercises 8–12 to 8–14 and 8–16 to 8–18 are very highly recommended, especially if you have one eye which is weaker than the other, as these exercises help to balance your use of your eyes. Exercise 8–15 and the third stage of 8–19 should be omitted, since they also involve neck flexion.

Work with the section on shifting in the Vision chapter as described, then repeat each exercise while covering your strong eye with your hand. Keep the eye covered for no more than four minutes at a time, four or five times a day; if you find your weaker eye feeling stressed, stop immediately and palm for several minutes before you repeat the shifting.

Fusion

We recommend the following exercise, not only for retinal detachment but for any condition which leaves one eye significantly more active than the other and thus prevents them from fusing. When fusion does not occur, the brain fails to integrate the two separate images it receives from the eyes, either because one eye is much weaker than the other or because the brain is not ready to create bilateral vision. This can happen with virtually any eye disorder. A weaker eye versus a dominant eye can present a real dilemma. If your stronger eye does all the work, it will itself eventually weaken from the strain, while the weaker eye gradually loses whatever acuity it had. If, however, you strain to see with the weaker eye, you can damage it permanently. Ideally, you should encourage both eyes to work, being sensitive to the weaker one and resting it whenever necessary. The following is an excellent exercise to help re-create fusion.

24–10 This exercise requires some equipment. The first thing needed is a pair of plastic glasses with one red and one green lens, such as were used for three-dimensional movies. These glasses are available from the Center for Self-Healing, 1718 Taraval Street, San Francisco, CA 94116, USA, and from some optical-supply companies (which may call them diplopia goggles). In addition, you will need a piece of red plastic acetate (available from hobby and art-supply stores) at least four inches by five inches, a piece of white paper about the same size, a red pen or pencil, some masking-tape, and a pen-light, which is a very thin flashlight and can be bought in any drugstore.

This exercise, like all other vision exercises, should be done without glasses or contact lenses. We suggest that you do some palming before and after.

Sit at a table, without putting the red-and-green glasses on as yet, and use the red pen to draw on the white paper a circle one to two inches in diameter and a cross with vertical and horizontal lines both about two inches long. Place the paper over the sheet of red acetate, and put the red-and-green glasses on. Hold the paper and acetate together in one hand, and look at your drawing. You should be able to see your circle and lines only with your 'green' eye, since the red lens will cancel out the red lines of your drawing. If your 'red' eye can see the lines, you may need to sit in a dimmer light or to use a lighter shade of pencil or pen. Usually, however, your 'red' eye will see only a blank page.

Now turn your pen-light on, and hold it under the acetate and paper so that its light is directed through them, toward your eyes (fig 24–10). You should be able to see the light only with your 'red' eye, since the combination of the red acetate and the green lens will cancel out the light. If your 'green' eye can see the light, then the pen-light may be too

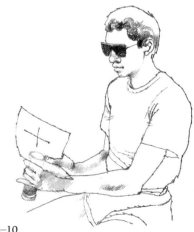

24–10

strong, and a coat of masking-tape over it will solve that problem.

This is not one of our simpler exercises. Now that you have gone through the manual part of this intelligence test, let's get to the vision part of it. Remember, you have one eye which cannot see the drawing you made and another eye which cannot see the light under the page. What you will be trying to do in this exercise is to trace the outlines of your drawings with the pen-light. In order to do this, obviously you need to see both the lines and the light, and to see them simultaneously. With one eye seeing only light and the other seeing only lines, the only way they can do this is to work together. Each eye will be sending the brain different information, and the brain will integrate this information into a single image — that of the light tracing along the lines.

It may appear to you that you are following the lines with the light when this is not actually happening. To know whether you are succeeding, it is probably best to do this exercise with someone else watching. If this is not possible, you can simply look over the top of the glasses every minute or so, to see whether the light is indeed where it appears to be under the line. You may be surprised to find, for example, that you can follow a vertical line perfectly, but perhaps miss a horizontal line by an inch.

If you find yourself unable to do this exercise at all, it means that one of your eyes is not only weak but is being repressed — its information is being ignored by the brain. In this case, palm for a minute or two, imagining that you can follow the lines with the light; push the glasses up on your head and, without the glasses, trace the lines with the light. Keeping this visual image in your mind's eye, put the glasses back and try again.

Never work with this exercise for more than fifteen minutes, as it can be exhausting for your eyes. Always palm after doing it.

It does make a difference which eye looks through the red side and which looks through the green, as the brain is more attracted to the light than to the lines. It is best, therefore, to spend more time with the weak eye looking through the red (which means looking at the light), because it then gets the chance to be dominant for the duration of the exercise.

Macular Degeneration

Macular degeneration is now the leading cause of blindness in the West. It is most common among the elderly, but its incidence among middle-aged people is increasing. The macula is the place on the retina where vision is most acute, so, when the macula begins to deteriorate, visual acuity is gradually lost, and partial or total blindness can be the ultimate result. We believe that several factors may contribute to macular degeneration: overuse of near vision and underuse of distance vision; staring; and using glasses, which narrow your active visual field and limit the use of your peripheral vision. All three of these put undue stress on your central vision, and may cause it to weaken.

We are not suggesting that you should not use your eyes — a healthy use of the eyes stimulates them and keeps them strong. What we are saying is that using them in ways which oppose their natural mode of function will weaken and eventually damage them. The natural functions of the eye include constant change from near to distant focus, use of both the central and the peripheral field, and, most especially, the constant moving from point to

367

point which we call shifting – the direct opposite of staring.

The function and nature of the macula are described in detail in the Vision chapter, in the section on shifting. Please read the entire Vision chapter, paying special attention to this section. The exercises which will benefit you most, however, are palming, to relieve and prevent strain to your eyes; sunning, because the majority of your light-sensitive cone cells are in your macula, and sunlight stimulates and strengthens them; and shifting exercises 8–20 to 8–23, to strengthen your macula. Emphasize also exercises 24–1 and 24–2 in this chapter, which combine shifting with distance vision. This is important, as the majority of people suffering from macular degeneration use their eyes mostly for close work, and have let their distance vision deteriorate. Peripheral exercises (Vision chapter 8–13 to 8–19) can also be helpful, by taking the stress off your central vision and by balancing the use of your eyes.

You may have been offered laser therapy as a treatment for macular degeneration. In the experience of our clients, this treatment can sometimes be helpful, though in a limited way, so this is a possibility you may want to discuss seriously with your ophthalmologist.

Don't let your age deter you from seeking improvement in your vision: some of our most successful clients have begun their fight against macular degeneration in their seventies. One of these, Joseph, was seventy-three, with distance vision measured at 20/400 and near vision which was so minimal it could not even be measured. He also saw multiple images as a result of astigmatism. As a pharmacist, he had been using his eyes almost exclusively from a near distance for many years, mainly indoors in poor light, and had been completely

dependent on his glasses, using them even when it was not strictly necessary. Since Joseph's near vision was the most damaged, Meir began by teaching him the distance-vision exercises, along with sunning and palming. When his eyes became comfortable with shifting on objects in the distance, Joseph was ready to go on to the closer shifting exercises, and eventually even to reading exercises. Joseph also did exercises and received massage to alleviate the tension in his shoulders and upper back, which had produced a hunched-over posture and deterioration in his cervical spine. The bodywork seemed to speed the progress of his eye improvement, probably by allowing better circulation of blood to his head. His distance vision eventually improved to 20/25, and he was able to read easily with glasses.

As with any other condition, the degree of improvement in macular degeneration will vary from person to person, and will depend to some degree not just upon the condition of the eyes but on the overall physical condition.

Retinitis Pigmentosa

In this condition, vision loss first appears in the peripheral field, spreading to the central field usually only after years. Tunnel vision is the result. Since the peripheral field contains most of the rod cells which function in dim light, night vision is severely affected – sometimes being lost altogether.

We have worked successfully with several people with retinitis pigmentosa. One was Barbara, whose vision had been normal until the age of eight, at which time it began to deteriorate rapidly due to retinitis pigmentosa.

By the age of twenty-two, when she began her work with Meir, she had no significant vision left. All she retained was a limited sense of color variation and one memory of being able, during a train ride, to distinguish some details such as place and dimension. Meir felt that the apparent movement of the scenery past the windows of the train might have stimulated activity in her peripheral field, as movement does in healthy eyes.

During the course of her Self-Healing work, it became evident that Barbara still had several tiny healthy patches on each retina. Most of her work was done outdoors, during movement, as she and Meir walked in the mountains outside the city. She found that she could sense the difference between light and shadow, and used this to distinguish shapes. This led, in time, to her being able to trace with her eyes the shapes of very large printed letters – in fact, to read.

Barbara was triumphant. She was now able to write her college papers and exams with felt pens, rather than with Braille. She could read large signs. One day at a market with her guide dog, she chose a carton of yogurt from a shelf so naturally that a woman standing nearby accused her of faking blindness to get the financial benefits – which delighted Barbara.

We have worked with other clients with much less severe cases of retinitis pigmentosa than Barbara's. Naturally, each person's needs are different, and will respond to different exercises. One client, though definitely diagnosed with retinitis pigmentosa, responded more strongly to deep-tissue bodywork on her neck and jaw, where her tension was so extreme that it was evidently interfering with her eyes. All of the exercises in the Vision chapter can be helpful with retinitis pig

mentosa. We have found the Peripheral Vision exercises, 8–13 to 8-19, to be exceptionally helpful. We have both had a number of clients who experienced a temporary increase in their peripheral range after only one session of peripheral work.

We also recommend that you work with flashing or blinking lights. The equipment for these exercises can be bought in almost any hardware store. You need colored light-bulbs, in as many different colors as you can find; a light-socket attached to a light-cord (electric cord), and an adaptor called a 'flasher' which is inserted between the socket and the bulb and causes the bulb to flash on and off at regular intervals. Flashers may be hard to find outside the United States. If you cannot find one, any other device that can make the light-bulb blink every one or two seconds will do. If all else fails, you can order flashers from us, at the Center for Self-Healing (see Final Note for our address).

24–11 The blinking lights help to stimulate those areas of the periphery where vision has been lost. To use them, first sit in a room which has been made as dark as possible, and palm for five minutes to relax your eyes. Start with the red bulb, as this is the color most people find easiest to see and are most comfortable with. Cover your better eye completely by holding a piece of cloth over it with one hand. Let the red light blink. Hold it about a foot away from your face and move it around the whole visual field that the eye may have. Can you tell when it is on and when it is off? Can you distinguish its color? If you can tell that it is blinking, you have something to work with.

Be aware that your retinal cells may tire very quickly. If you can only notice the blinking for half a minute before you lose it, practice half a minute at a time, and then palm your eyes for five minutes. If you do not lose it quickly, watch the blinking for three minutes at a time between the short palming sessions.

When you can identify the red light – even if it sometimes seems pink, and sometimes just white – you have come to a stage where the little vision you have in your damaged eye can already support the better vision you have in your other eye. Without allowing your head to move or following it with your eyes, hold the light-socket, and move it up and down and from side to side, to determine at what distance you can see it and where your range of vision ends. Find out how far up, how far down, how far to the left and how far to the right you can move the bulb and still see it, without moving your head or your eyes. Try to find the area where the bulb becomes blurred or indistinct; perhaps you can see only the color, or can see the blinking only occasionally. Hold the light in this blurry area and move it up and down, back and forth and in circles, all within that small range where you can just barely see it. Close your eyes and imagine that you see it clearly, then open your eyes and move the light again. Notice whether your image of the bulb is becoming any clearer or brighter. If so, move the bulb just a little further away, so that it once again becomes barely discernible, and repeat the whole process. If not, move the bulb back to where you saw it quite clearly, and simply move it in as many directions as possible within that clear range of vision – and then try again from the beginning.

If your problem is with your outermost periphery, then begin by holding the light so that it stimulates first your central field, and then very gradually move it out to stimulate the outer periphery. If you have a 'ring of blindness' – that is, your central vision and outer periphery are active, but the inner periphery is damaged – then exercise in an alternating fashion, moving both from the center out toward the blind ring and from the far periphery inwards toward the blind ring. If your blindness is in patches, then work from any area where you see well toward the area where vision is lost.

Try all of the colors, but spend the greatest amount of time working with the colors that you see best. Stop every five minutes to palm for five minutes, to avoid straining the newly stimulated cells. You may choose to work with one eye at a time, or have two lights and work with both simultaneously or alternately. If you use two, it's best to use the same color light-bulbs at any one time.

Ideally, you should have someone else holding the light-socket for you (fig 24–11), since then there will be no question about the range of vision, or exactly how far the bulb

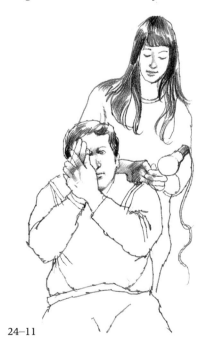

24–11

was moved before your perception of it changed etc. If your condition is severe enough to have impaired your color sense, ask your partner to change the color of the light-bulb without telling you what color is in the socket, so that you can try to determine for yourself what color you are seeing.

Some ophthalmologists are of the opinion that sunlight speeds the deterioration process in retinitis pigmentosa. We don't want to oppose any advice your physician may give you, so any decision to practice or not to practice the sunning exercise must be left entirely to you. We have found, however, that this exercise has been beneficial to people with retinitis pigmentosa. If, and only if, your ophthalmologist does not oppose the practice of sunning, try it and judge for yourself whether it is helpful for you. You may want to show your doctor the Sunning section in the Vision chapter, and to discuss it thoroughly together. In any case, if you decide to do this exercise, read the section very carefully, and follow the instructions exactly, so that you will not damage your eyes.

Palming is to damaged eyes what bed rest is to a damaged body. For the first six months of your exercise regimen, you should palm for two hours every day. The results of this deep rest will astonish you.

Shifting exercises will be most helpful if you do them with the more functional areas of your eye covered, concentrating on the less functional area. Imagine as you do them that the weaker area of the eye is all you have to see with, and use shifting to take in every detail that you can.

If you can read at all, whether it is easy or difficult, then you may practice any of the reading exercises that you find suitable.

Glaucoma

Glaucoma, or hypertension of the eyes, is a stressor that at lower levels may not be a problem in itself but can lead to other problems such as peripheral-vision loss and optic-nerve damage. At higher levels, glaucoma can cause blindness.

If you have had an increase in eye pressure and your ophthalmologist has suggested the use of drugs, you may want to get a second and a third opinion before you begin the drugs. Consult specialists who have worked extensively with glaucoma. Once drugs are introduced, the body becomes dependent on them and it becomes very difficult to do without them, as they weaken whatever capacity the eye has to deal with the increased pressure. This is why many of the better ophthalmologists are not in a hurry to get their patients started on drugs. Drugs may be needed when the eye pressure is unstable. For example, if the pressure in your eye jumps suddenly from 18 mm Hg to 26, this could cause blindness. If the pressure had risen to 26 gradually and stabilized there, the body would have adjusted to it and the danger of being blinded would lessen. So be sure that you have a doctor you trust, so that you can follow his or her directions with the utmost confidence. Do not do any of the exercises in this book without first having your doctor approve them.

Your first goal in working with glaucoma will be to work with the symptoms, to improve your peripheral vision and strengthen the activity of your optic nerve. **Reducing the pressure in your eyes will take a long time, and you will need to practice the exercises faithfully during that time. You cannot**

expect the pressure to return to its pre-glaucoma level, as this generally does not happen. If it stabilizes somewhere in between the normal level and the danger level, you have achieved a great success.

We believe that glaucoma, whatever patho-physiological symptoms it presents, develops initially as a result of incorrect use of the eyes: both from an imbalanced use of the two eyes, in which one works hard and the other is repressed or unused, and from an imbalanced use of different parts of the eye, usually straining the central field while neglecting the periphery.

We therefore recommend that you work extensively with the peripheral-vision exercises in the Vision chapter, exercises 8–13 to 8–19, to correct peripheral-vision loss and balance the use of the two eyes. Many of the cells in the peripheral field are rod cells, which are active in dim light. The peripheral cells are also stimulated by movement. You can use both of these attributes to stimulate and so to strengthen the peripheral cells by taking walks under the moonlight or starlight, as far away from artificial light as possible. Both the dim light and the movement will wake up the periphery, in a very gentle, non-stressful way, using cells that normally do not get a chance to function. If you have experienced a great deal of periphery loss, work with the other peripheral exercises for several weeks before doing this one, and it would probably be best to ask a companion to go with you.

Your work should not, however, be limited to the peripheral field. Shifting exercises 8–20 to 8–24 are strongly recommended, to improve the functioning of your central field of vision. If you have one eye which is significantly stronger than the other, you should work with the fusion exercise, 24–10.

The following exercises should be done only after at least three months of practice of the basic exercises suggested above – when your eyes are comfortable and relaxed, and you have already begun to notice some improvement in your vision. They are exercises designed *eventually* to either reduce or stabilize eye pressure. They must be approached with the utmost patience. If you don't do them in a relaxed manner, if you are in too much of a rush to get results, then your anxiety may even produce an increase in eye pressure. And remember that even stability can be a sign of progress, as it is in any condition that involves deterioration. We have seen clients rush to their doctors after one eye session, hoping to find their pressure lowered, and disappointed to find it only stabilized. Try to make your expectations realistic, to appreciate every improvement you are able to make, including stabilization.

If you have already started using eye drops, ask your ophthalmologist whether there is any possibility of reducing their use. Explain what you are doing, and ask for his or her support. Your progress should be monitored very carefully by your doctor during this stage. And, of course, your doctor must approve of these exercises.

The first exercise is facial massage, as described in exercise 8–1 in the Vision chapter. We believe that tension in the facial muscles creates pressure which can add to the pressure within the eyes themselves. It will be best if you practice this massage on yourself first, before you ask anyone else to massage you, so that you can establish what level of pressure on the face seems comfortable and safe to you. You should spend no less than ten minutes twice daily massaging your face, beginning very gently and only increasing pressure gradually, at a comfortable pace.

The second exercise is palming. Normally we recommend palming, and a lot of it, as a matter of course; it is the most basic of all healing exercises for the eyes. However, in the case of glaucoma there is a difficulty involved, in that being in darkness tends to increase eye pressure somewhat. We find, however, that this is counterbalanced by the extremely relaxing effect that palming has, both upon the optic nerve – which can tend to become damaged in glaucoma – and upon the eye and face muscles. The reduction in tension in these muscles helps ultimately to reduce eye pressure. We recommend that you practice palming in short sessions of ten minutes, as often daily as you can manage.

For the third exercise, a visualization exercise, you will need a partner – someone who does not have glaucoma. Sit in a room which is pleasantly but not completely darkened. Close your eyes, relax your eyes and face as you do before palming, and barely touch your fingertips to your closed eyelids. Do not put any pressure on the eyes, as this can hurt them, especially the retinas. Keep the fingertips barely touching the closed lids as you visualize that they are slowly penetrating the eyeballs. Imagine that the eyeballs are completely soft, and that they grow softer as you touch them. Now touch one eyelid of your partner. Sense the degree of softness of that eye, and compare it to how your eyes feel. Imagine your eyes feeling as soft as your partner's eye. The light touch may actually help your eyes to relax enough so that they do soften slightly; in any case, the visualization is relaxing to the eyes and mind. After a minute or so, stop and massage very gently around the eyes. Visualize

your fingers softening the areas they touch, even the bones of the eye socket.

Whenever you do your vision exercises from now on, stop intermittently to close the eyes, touch the lids, and imagine the eyes softening.

Keratoconus

Keratoconus is a slowly progressive condition in which the cornea of the eye gradually assumes a conical shape. Besides changes in the eye's refractive action, redness and a feeling of tension, this condition brings with it the danger of thinning and scarring of the cornea. In such cases the cornea may need to be surgically replaced.

There are two ways to approach keratoconus, short of surgery. One is the use of contact lenses designed to place pressure on the cornea and help it to keep its normal shape. The other is with vision exercises.

Leonard, a man in his forties who suffered from keratoconus, came to work with Meir after his condition had progressed to the point where he could not wear contact lenses. He was afraid that a cornea transplant was the only thing that could help him. He had become dependent on the now useless lenses, especially in his weaker right eye. As with many who have keratoconus, strong light troubled his eyes, giving a sense of glare, to which he responded by squinting to shut out the light. Along with massage to relax his facial muscles from the effects of this constant squinting, Leonard found sunning, in all of its varieties, to be the exercise which helped him most. It reduced his sensitivity to light and eliminated the sense of glare he had suffered, making it unnecessary to squint. He also improved greatly through doing blinking exercise 8–10 and peripheral-vision exercise 8–15. Rather than doing exercise 8–10 in the dark, however, as it is usually done, Leonard did it in strong light, while massaging his forehead, and found that it augmented his sunning exercises. Leonard also benefited from daily palming sessions and from facial and upper-body massage.

Because his tension had built up over many years, Leonard needed about four months of weekly sessions of both eye-work and body-work before he noticed a significant change in his condition. At about that time, he found that his ability to tolerate light had increased dramatically, and also that he was now able to wear his contact lenses in comfort, with no ill effects. He has been able to postpone corneal surgery indefinitely. He still needs occasional sessions to support his progress. His vision, which when he began his exercise program was 20/200 in the strong eye and 20/400 in the weak one, now measures at 20/80 and 20/200. (His ophthalmologist was surprised, but not curious, at this improvement.)

During the first three months of working with keratoconus, spend forty minutes to one hour daily sunning or skying – exercises 8–6 and 8–7 – and spend about one hour each day with shifting, blinking and peripheral exercises, particularly those described in Leonard's story.

Get as much facial massage as you can, both self-massage and massage from others. If you have a support group, they can do this for you. This type of massage is described in the Vision chapter, under exercise 8–1. To the techniques there, add the following: while your eyes are closed, ask your partner to press down slightly with all fingertips on your forehead and then shake the fingers – without lifting them – so as to vibrate the forehead muscles.

After three months you can reduce by half the sunning and palming, and facial massage can decrease to once a week.

Crossed Eyes (Strabismus) and Lazy Eye (Amblyopia)

In strabismus, the visual problems can originate from imbalance of the external muscles of the eyes, but in many cases this imbalance is a result of the brain poorly integrating the visual information from the two eyes. Therefore, to work with this condition, we need to engage the brain in consciously seeing with both eyes. Working with a lazy eye is similar. Many people with a lazy eye tend not to use that eye at all, and whatever information it does send to the brain may be unconsciously suppressed. Sometimes a lazy eye may actually have good acuity. In such a case, your main concern is to help the two eyes to work together as a unit, or to 'fuse'. If the lazy eye also has poor acuity, then you need to work on that as well as on fusion.

Whether you have strabismus or amblyopia, you should begin your program by working with the Vision chapter for two weeks, doing all of the exercises as described with no special emphasis. You will naturally find some which seem more helpful than others, and some you enjoy more, but try all of them. Even if you are not myopic, you may benefit from the distance-vision or reading exercises given earlier in this present chapter – we have seen people improve 20/20 vision to 20/6 through shifting exercises.

Amblyopia

If your weaker eye is myopic or farsighted, refer to the sections on those problems and follow the instructions there. Whether your acuity is poor or good, however, you should emphasize shifting exercises, both from near distance and from far. Shifting is used in exercises under different titles: as 'Shifting', 8–20 to 8 24 in the Vision chapter; 'Distance Vision', 24–1 and 24–2 in this chapter; and 'Reading', 24–5 to 24–9. During any of these exercises, and at other times during the day, you can patch or cover your stronger eye for no more than five minutes at a time and do the exercise – or any other activity – solely with the weaker eye. Doing this for extended periods of time may strain the weaker eye and so cancel out any benefits, but doing it regularly and frequently for short periods will accustom the weaker eye to working without stressing it. While working with the patch, stimulate your peripheral cells by waving or wiggling your fingers about eight inches to the side of the working eye – this too helps to relieve strain on it.

Now that you have captured the attention of the amblyopic eye, you should emphasize relaxation of the eyes; again, your goal is to avoid straining the newly active eye. Read the section on palming (exercise 8–5), and palm for two hours per day for at least a week, or until you feel that your eyes have genuinely relaxed. You can break the two hours to several twenty-minute sessions if you like, but the longer each session is, the deeper its effect.

After this preparation – not before – begin working intensively with the 'peripheral-vision' exercises, 8–13 to 8–19 in the Vision chapter. If you tried to do these exercises initially, you would probably wind up doing them with only your stronger eye, so it is very important that you work with shifting and with relaxation before going on to these. Though they are designed to be done with both eyes simultaneously, you should make a point of doing each exercise as described, and then *repeating it using only the weaker eye*. Practice these exercises faithfully for one month.

Last, practice the fusion exercise, 24–10, to gain coordination of the two eyes.

Strabismus

You will be working to use and strengthen your eyes' external muscles, to make them strong and flexible and able to allow any movement that may be needed for full use of your eyes. Begin with exercise 8–2 in the Vision chapter and go on to blinking exercises 8–9 to 8–11. All of these will help to give your external muscles more strength and control, as will the following additional exercises. (You may find it more relaxing to do the next two exercises while lying down.)

24–12   Cover one eye with your hand, and move the other eye in circles, several times in each direction. You can do this throughout the day, any time you have a moment.

24–13   Look with both eyes as far as you can upward, downward, left and right. Then combine the movements by looking first upward, then – while still looking up – moving both eyes slightly to the right, so that they are now looking at an upward diagonal. Keep your eyes in this position for the space of three deep breaths – in and out – blink several times, and then move your eyes – still looking upward – to the left. Hold them there for three breaths, blink several times, and look downward. While looking down, repeat the whole process. Look to the left and, while doing so, move both eyes up and down; look to the right and in that position move the eyes up and down, as described. If you feel any aching or sense of strain, stop and palm for several minutes before continuing.

Then move both eyes together in slow, full circles. When you move the eyes in circles, first focus on something directly ahead of you and close to you, and rotate your point of focus around it, so that the circle your eyes make covers only a small field. Then gradually expand the size of your circle, until the circle takes in the farthest points in your peripheral field. For example, you might begin simply by looking at your nose in a mirror, and your circle would cover only the middle of your face; you would end, however, with a circle that took in the floor, the ceiling and the farthest corners of the room.

You can also try doing this exercise with your eyes closed, concentrating on the feeling of the movement rather than on what you are seeing; this may be a challenge at first but it will help to create more movement within your eyes.

These exercises are not easy, and you will probably want to take frequent breaks during your practice. During these breaks you will gain a lot of relief by palming, by massage of the face and around the eyes, and by applying warm compresses to the closed eyes. Many people use a compress soaked in a tea of eyebright, a herb available from health-food stores. Be careful with this tea, however, as it stains. If none of these things helps, dis-continue the exercises for the day, do a long palming session instead, and try again the following day. You may find that the initial discomfort disappears very quickly. Practice these exercises for two months before going on to the following, which focus on the role of the brain.

Perhaps you have double vision. If you do not, be aware that these exercises may temporarily produce double vision, and that this may be a good sign, since it means that the brain is receiving hitherto-suppressed information from the weaker eye. We recommend that you do some palming both before and after these exercises.

Refer to fusion exercise 24–10 in this chapter.

24–14 You will need a large piece of paper and a pencil. Very slowly, draw a line that extends from the middle of the paper all the way upward – away from you – and, as you do so, focus not on the line itself but on the pencil, letting your eyes travel up and down the length of the pencil slowly and continuously. Now draw another line, this time beginning at the top of the page and bringing it toward the middle, closer to you, and again let your eyes travel continuously and repeatedly up and down the length of the pencil. Then take a break for a minute or two, and look away from the paper into the distance, out of a window if possible, or just close your eyes and imagine that you are looking at a distant horizon. Continue with this exercise for eight to ten minutes, taking frequent breaks to look into the distance, and then palm for ten minutes.

Practice exercise 8–18 from the Vision chapter, then return to exercise 24–13 in this section, this time doing it only with your weaker eye, while the stronger eye is patched or simply covered with one hand.

Initially, spend only a month working with these fusion exercises daily. Working too long or too hard on them will only cause strain and hamper your progress toward fusion. After this month, return to more basic exercises such as palming, sunning, shifting and blinking. You may also want to work with the rest of your body – doing vision exercises often increases your awareness of your body in general. If you have discovered an area that needs attention, such as your back, then refer to the chapter or chapters in this book with information about that area. You may even find it helpful to forget about your eyes altogether for a month and concentrate on your body. After this period, return to the fusion exercises and see if your results with them have improved.

You may notice that, even though you make progress, your strabismus may return when you are tired or stressed.

If you have a cross-eyed infant, get a diagnosis from an ophthalmologist as soon as possible. Is one eye blind or partially blind? In this case, you should begin working with exercises as soon as possible. Vision develops early in the brain, and you want to prevent the baby from developing a lazy eye. You may also find that a two-month-old baby is more cooperative than an eighteen-month-old.

Your doctor may suggest patching. This is fine, but only for short periods of five minutes or so. The problem with patching is that, while it does force the weak eye to work, it also sends a message to the brain that you can see only with one eye or the other, not with both together. To strengthen both eyes at once, use a small piece of masking-tape to attach a piece of paper about one-inch square between the baby's eyes, just above the nose. A very young baby won't mind this, and can keep it on for hours. While the paper is attached, you can attract the baby's attention to various moving objects or blinking lights, keeping them moving as the baby's eyes follow them. Even without the paper, encouraging the baby to watch moving objects is a good idea, and this includes mobiles hanging over the crib.

Waving or wiggling your fingers in the baby's peripheral field also helps in keeping both eyes active. Children have a short attention span, so doing this frequently but for short periods of time will probably be easier on both of you.

Be cautious about surgery.

Cataracts

A cataract is an opacity of the lens, or of part of the lens, of the eye. It is thought to be caused by a change in the structure of the proteins of which the lens is made. Once a cataract appears, it tends to increase in size, gradually spreading over the lens and blurring vision. If you have a cataract, your ophthalmologist will probably recommend that it be surgically removed. Most ophthalmologists prefer to operate only after the cataract has become 'mature' – that is, not until it is relatively large and dense and causing a substantial loss of vision. At that time the entire lens can be removed, and sometimes replaced with an artificial-lens implant. Cataracts were once the leading cause of adult blindness. Today, cataract surgery is one of ophthalmology's greatest success stories.

Any surgery has its risks, and cataract surgery is no exception. Through our work we have met some for whom the operation has not been fully successful, as well as some for whom the operation is not an option. Some people simply prefer to avoid surgery of any kind. It is our experience that surgery may be delayed or avoided altogether by improving vision through relaxation and exercises.

This is an important personal choice, and should be made with an open mind and on the basis of as much information as possible. We know one woman who has been blinded by cataracts for ten years, yet refuses cataract surgery because of her unshakable faith in natural healing. In our opinion, this type of faith borders on fanaticism, and is not in her best interests. However, if your vision is deteriorating due to cataracts, you may want to consider the amount of vision you still have and weigh it against the possible bad effects of surgery. If your vision is weak but still functional, it may be worthwhile for you to work to improve it naturally. Our general rule is that, if your vision is still better than 20/200, vision exercises may help. After that point, surgery may be your best option.

Many people have a combination of cataracts and macular degeneration. If this is the case with you, you can try the exercises for these conditions for two or three months, and see whether your vision improves. If it does not and your ophthalmologist has recommended surgery, you should consider it very seriously. The surgery will allow more light into the eye, which the macula needs in order to avoid further degeneration. Therefore the operation will help with both conditions.

You may be inclined to choose surgery rather than vision exercises if you know that your cataract is very dense. Don't let this factor put you off. It has been documented that the density of a cataract does not necessarily correlate with the amount of vision available. In other words, you might have a very dense cataract and yet see more and better than another person with a lighter cataract.

Cataracts sometimes appear in conjunction with other illnesses. Lucy, one of our clients with multiple sclerosis, also found herself developing cataracts. We suggested that she relax her eyes through palming, and so she added two hours of palming daily to her other exercises. Because of her multiple sclerosis, she had lost strength and balance in her walking, and so was doing exercises for her legs and back. Apparently, some combination of improvements in her circulation, neurological functioning and other factors caused her cataracts to disappear within four months.

When you start to work on improving your vision, be aware that you can only gain. You may be able to improve your vision despite the cataracts, like more than half of the people we have worked with. You may even be able to eliminate the cataracts altogether, though this is rare. But, even if you don't succeed in increasing your vision, you still will have learned better visual habits, relaxed your eyes, released them from strain, and improved your circulation. In short, you will have given yourself a better chance of coming through surgery successfully. You will not waste any time through working on yourself. If you can take two weeks to work intensively on your eyes, you are likely to benefit greatly.

The location of your cataract has a greater impact on your vision than does its size. A central cataract will generally cause more blurring of vision than a peripheral one. The most important question, however, is: what is the quality of your vision? To what extent has it become blurred, or dimmed? Cataracts hamper the penetration of light into your retina. You will probably find yourself straining to see because of lack of light.

We suggest that your first essential exercise should be palming – exercise 8–5 in the Vision chapter. We cannot stress enough how important relaxation is in the healing of cataracts. Practice palming for at least twenty minutes at a time, several times a day.

The next exercise which we find helpful – but which is considered controversial – is sunning, and lots of it. Many people believe that sunlight actually causes cataracts, and therefore try to avoid it at all costs. We believe that it is not sunlight but one's reaction to it that is harmful: eyes that have not become accustomed to strong sunlight wear a squint or a frown. It is this tensing of the eyes to shut out the glare that is harmful. This is discussed at greater length in the Vision chapter in the section on sunning, exercise 8–6. Unfortunately, most people with cataracts tend to tense against the light even more than the average person, when in fact light is what they need most.

Please read the section on sunning, and then discuss this exercise with your ophthalmologist; don't experiment with it if he or she is opposed to it. If your doctor approves, then follow the Vision chapter's instructions on both sunning and skying, exercise 8–7. During sunning, always massage your face: around your eyes, at your temples, cheekbones and forehead, and behind your ears. You may also want to have a member of your support group watch you while you are sunning, to make sure that you are not squinting against the sun. Relaxing the muscles around your eyes allows more light to penetrate and conse-

quently helps your vision tremendously. To really see the difference, sun for a minute and note the color that you see with your eyes closed. Is it yellow? orange? red? Now tighten the muscles around your eyes, squeezing them as tightly shut as possible. Does this make everything appear darker, even though your eyes were closed to start with? Now relax those muscles – without opening your eyes – and notice the color you see now. Is it brighter? This means that more light is penetrating, because your facial muscles are allowing it to do so. You may not be aware of it, but the chances are good that you are unconsciously tightening your eye muscles all the time. Sunning can make your eyes so comfortable with light that you can gradually lose that unconscious squint.

Probably, one of your eyes is more functional than the other. If so, even if you have cataracts in both eyes, you will benefit from exercises 8–13 to 8–19, which work to balance the use of your eyes and to limit the stronger eye's dominance while strengthening the weaker eye. Exercise 8–12, patching of the stronger eye, may be done occasionally as well. Read also the sections on shifting and on distance-vision exercises in this chapter, and practice these exercises to see which seem most helpful to you. These may then be added to your exercise regimen. Expect to work on your eyes for about two hours daily – the condition you are seeking to remedy is not just functional but organic, and changing it requires dedication.

Visual strain imposes stress not only on the eyes but on the entire body. Because of this, we suggest that you receive a body massage, which should include some facial massage, twice weekly. You may want to exchange massages with members of your support group, or get the help of a professional massage therapist.

Congenital Cataracts

Congenital cataracts may result from illness, from genetic factors or from unknown causes. A child with normal vision can, by the age of about eight weeks, see a person's face from a distance of two to three feet. The infant's brain is programmed to expect to see this well at this time. If something, such as a cataract, is blocking the vision at this stage, then normal visual development does not happen. Visual development depends upon both the eyes and the brain, and if the brain does not receive the expected stimuli from the eyes then a visual pattern develops which can result in poor vision for life. The resultant stress upon the optic nerve can also cause nystagmus, or involuntary eye movement. (Nystagmus, by the way, is unique to humans. However, other animals also develop poor vision if deprived of the proper stimuli at the critical stage.)

If the congenital cataract is dense and centrally located, the general practice is to remove the lens surgically within the first several weeks of the infant's life, and to fit the child with contact lenses immediately. This allows the brain to receive the information it needs from the eyes, at the time when it needs it. If no complications result from the surgery, the child may in time have normal or near-normal vision. Since it is completely unrealistic to expect an infant to benefit from vision exercises in such a short time – less than eight weeks – the surgery is highly recommended.

However, your child may benefit very much from vision exercises after recovering from the surgery. An eye without a lens, depending upon powerful contact lenses almost from birth, is certainly more vulnerable than a normal eye, and can use the support that vision exercises provide. Glaucoma or retinal detachment may also result from the surgery, and here also preventive measures may help. It is never too early to begin to strengthen your child's eyes. Your first goal is to provide as much relaxation for the eyes as possible. Your second goal is to develop the eye's ability to accommodate – that is, to change from near to distance vision while maintaining clarity – despite the lack of the natural lens. If this is done, the prescription of the contact lenses may eventually be reduced.

Read the Vision chapter carefully, not so much to learn specific exercises as to understand the concepts behind them. You can help your baby's eyes to relax by palming them while he sleeps, and by massaging his face gently. You can help him learn to shift by getting him to look at things which are moving, such as waves, clouds, kites, birds, dogs, mobiles, people running or dancing, or even just your fingers moving. You can usually get your child's interest and attention just by being interested in something yourself, so pay attention to moving things and draw your baby's attention to them too. When he is a little older, you can roll or toss a ball toward him, and have him toss it back to you. You can point out details in his picture-books, such as tails or ears or spots on a dog.

Keep the contact lenses in the child's eyes during vision exercises until he is about five years old. At that age the child's visual and mental development will be advanced enough to allow him to participate in and benefit from exercises without the lenses. With the lenses out, you can do sunning and palming, but concentrate mainly on shifting, encouraging your child to follow moving objects with his eyes, to look at the details of both large objects, such as trees and houses, and small ones, such as flowers, toys, pictures, rocks or whatever interests him. You can also encourage him to look at distant objects, even if he cannot see them clearly. You should be prepared to spend from two to four hours daily working with your child's vision, but fortunately much of this can be done in the course of taking walks, playing, reading stories or even watching television. From time to time, you should have the child's eyes examined to see whether his contact-lens prescription might be reduced. Some eye doctors are more helpful about this than others, so you may wish to get a second opinion before giving up on a lowered prescription.

Strabismus and nystagmus can both occur as side effects of the cataract. If your child suffers from either of these, please consult the appropriate sections in this chapter.

If cataracts develop later in childhood, the surgery can be postponed for a longer period than in infancy, since the necessary early brain–eye development has already taken place. With your ophthalmologist's approval, you can spend about three months working intensively with the exercises we have suggested. If you see that your child's vision improves as a result, then ask your doctor whether the surgery may be postponed indefinitely while the child continues instead with the exercises. Remember, these exercises address more than just the cataract: they strengthen the eye as a whole and train your child in visual habits which will improve vision for life.

Unsuccessful Surgery

Surgery may sometimes result in scarring, retinal detachment or glaucoma. Please see the sections on retinal detachment and glaucoma in this chapter if you have either of these problems. The exercise we recommend most highly for recuperation is palming, whether the damage is small or great. As soon after surgery as possible, begin palming for three hours a day, in sessions of at least twenty minutes each. After two weeks, add exercises from the Vision chapter, particularly exercises 8–13 to 8–19, to stimulate and strengthen the weaker eye. Massage of your upper body will also help to promote healing.

Learn from your experiences. If you suffered retinal detachment as a result of cataract surgery in one eye, then be cautious about proceeding with surgery in the other eye.

Astigmatism

Astigmatism results from an irregularly shaped cornea. We believe that it is caused and perpetuated mainly by stress, like many eye problems. There are several exercises which are especially helpful for astigmatism.

Begin by testing your vision with a standard eye chart, and note which is the lowest line you can see clearly. Then practice all of the exercises in the Vision chapter; there are none which are not useful for you. If you are farsighted, you can then go on to practice the regimen recommended in the Farsightedness section of this chapter. Do these basic exercises until you can read at least two lines further down on the eye chart than you could initially.

People who have succeeded in reducing their myopia often find that their astigmatism becomes more apparent to them. Instead of seeing a general blur, they now see double or even multiple images. This does not mean that the astigmatism has worsened, only that the mind is more able to sort out what the eyes have been seeing all along.

At this stage, you should emphasize sunning. Eyes which are too sensitive to light tense to avoid it, putting pressure on the muscles around the eyes and intensifying the distortion of the cornea.

24–15 We have found this exercise effective with astigmatism, although often there may be no progress for a while, followed by a sudden significant improvement. You will need an eye chart and a small page with very large print on it – anywhere between half an inch to an inch in size. Place the eye chart at a distance where you can read several lines while the others are blurred, and read the letters there, one by one, practicing your shifting as in exercise 24–4. Occasionally flash the page with the large print in front of you. Do not look at it, but do not make an effort not to look at it. Once in a while your brain may choose to focus on it and perhaps recognize a letter even though it moved fast. As we said, it may take several sessions before that happens. Astigmatism creates a sense of blur. Flashing the page in front of your eyes creates an artificial blur, and your brain may find a way to focus through it.

Nystagmus

Both of the authors, as well as many others with nystagmus, or involuntary eye movement, have been able to reduce this condition dramatically. A decrease in nystagmus automatically produces an improvement in acuity as well. We have not, however, known anyone who has eliminated nystagmus altogether by using exercises. We would like to hear about it if anyone has done so.

People who have had nystagmus since birth or infancy normally have poor vision, with myopia, astigmatism and double vision being common. Vision development was hampered at this early, critical stage, making nystagmus difficult to correct – but it can be done, with a lot of work. Maureen, whose nystagmus was a genetic condition, reduced it by about 60 percent. Meir, whose nystagmus was a secondary condition resulting from cataracts, has reduced it by more than 80 percent.

You should begin with long palming sessions. You have probably noticed that your nystagmus worsens when you are tired or upset; this condition is closely linked to the nervous system. Perhaps more for someone with nystagmus than for anyone else, palming relaxes not just the eyes but the mind too, serving almost as a meditation. Both of us have had our most dramatic leaps of improvement in vision after very long (six-hour) palming sessions. Because of the strong connection between the eyes and the nervous system in nystagmus, we also very strongly suggest that you work simultaneously with the exercises in the Nervous System chapter. These will be challenging but rewarding; they will give you the combination of relaxation and control which is essential to relieving nystagmus.

All of the exercises in the Vision chapter are essential, but none more so than sunning (exercise 8–6). Nystagmus is usually linked with hypersensitivity to light, so it is crucial that you train your eyes to become comfortable with light. Both sunning and skying (exercise 8–7) are extremely useful. Choose hours when the sunlight is not overly strong, take frequent small palming breaks during the sunning session, and massage your forehead frequently – if you don't, you will simply add to your sense of discomfort and strain with light and the nystagmus will worsen; if you do, you will find this exercise more helpful than any other.

We also recommend that you spend time working with the exercises listed in the Strabismus section of this chapter.

Most people with nystagmus would not be aware of the problem if other people had not told them they had it. The brain learns very early to ignore the movement in the visual images relayed by the eyes. In most – not all – cases, the person with nystagmus does not sense the eye movement, does not see the environment as moving, and often cannot see the nystagmus when looking into a mirror – even when someone else standing behind and looking into the mirror at the same time sees it very clearly. For Maureen, the first time she had any sense of what her nystagmus looked like was when she asked a friend to look into her eyes and to follow their movement. As she watched her friend's eyes begin to swing back and forth, she knew for the first time what her own had been doing for nineteen years.

How, then, can you control a condition that on some level seems almost mythical? First, you have to become physically aware of it. The more you are aware of it, the more you

can control it. This has been demonstrated with biofeedback machines, but you don't need one of these when you have your own eyes, hands and nerves.

24–16 Close your eyes, breathe deeply, and touch your closed eyelids very gently with your index and middle fingers. Feel whether your eyes are moving or are still. The lighter your touch, the more you will be able to feel, as too much pressure can interfere with the accustomed movement. Even if your eyes are completely still, you have begun to attract the attention of your conscious mind to the nystagmus – an important first step.

24–17 Next, look into a mirror – another cheap biofeedback device. If you must look from very close, that's fine; otherwise, stand about eight inches away. Instead of trying to watch your eyeballs, look at the bridge of your nose, just between and above the eyes. If you concentrate on this area, you will become able to see the movement of your eyes. Now you can concentrate on trying to control them. Breathe deeply, drop your shoulders, relax your body. We have found that it sometimes helps to do hip rotations – moving the lower body, from the hips down, in circles like a belly dance, keeping the upper body still   all the while continuing to look at the bridge of the nose in the mirror. This exercise is good for balance, for posture, for the spine and for the central nervous system. Follow the movements of your eyes, and try to slow them down, to direct them, to still them. Some people have been able to do this, for very short periods, on the first attempt; others take much longer. Ultimately, however, this is a dramatically effective exercise. Even if you are successful, however, do not keep this up for more than a few minutes. Rest from it, then return to it frequently throughout the day.

Maureen can recommend the mirror exercise from the heart. When she came for her first session with Meir, she was more than a little worried that he might be some sort of charlatan, and this wasn't helped by his being half an hour late for her session. Nervous and irritated, she said to him, 'Please, I need to believe in you – there are people who think you might be a quack.' To which Meir replied, 'If anyone is going to be the quack it is you, because you are going to do all the work!' – a good thing to remember for anyone involved or interested in Self-Healing. At that, Maureen began to suspect that she had come to the right place. The very first exercise – the mirror exercise – confirmed this. For the first time in her life, she was able to see her own eyes moving. More, she could see that they slowed somewhat when she consciously directed them to do so. The effects lasted for the rest of that day and into the next. They have not stopped improving since that day. The partnership in Self-Healing with Meir has lasted just as long.

Final Note

The book you have just read is different from any other exercise book. We believe it will give you a lifetime's useful service. It has programs for many different needs: for ailments as diverse as muscular dystrophy and macular degeneration; for improving skills from running to playing the harp.

You have begun with the sections that address your own problem or goal. Probably, in working with the exercises in those sections, you have begun to experience a subtle – or perhaps dramatic – change in how you relate to your own body. The book can help you enhance that change. As you become more in touch with your own local awareness, you may find yourself picking up the book to work on your breathing, to learn how to improve the circulation in your cold feet or to do a back bend, just because you never did it before. You will return to the book in times of crisis and in moments of personal growth. At such times, exercises which once seemed irrelevant will become exactly what you need.

The best way to approach the book is in stages. Start with the sections that relate to your present goal, and work very thoroughly with those exercises. Then work your way through the entire book from beginning to end, selecting the exercises that feel most helpful to you. Your developing kinesthetic awareness – a sense of where and how your body needs to move – will guide you. Write down your exercise program and do the exercises consistently. Avoid doing them mechanically or unconsciously. Every movement in your program can deepen your local awareness.

The third stage in your Self Healing journey is to go through the book again from beginning to end. You will have a completely different experience. By now you will have been doing Self-Healing for a year or two, and you will have a very different body. Your understanding of your body's needs will be deeper, more holistic. Kinesthetic awareness will again tell you what your next step should be: if you cultivate it, your Self-Healing practice will never become stale. Perhaps your next step is to discover that the vision exercises ease your chronic low-back pain or that the back exercises heal your wrist. Connections that seemed strange may start to make sense.

The last stage is to develop your own exercises. You will now have a large fund of knowledge from which to draw. You will simply move spontaneously, letting go of your thoughts and just feeling, listening and responding. When Meir, as a teenager, reached this stage, he let the motions come freely, experienced the results, then realized what the new exercises were 'for'. Every exercise in this book was discovered by someone in this fashion. Such moments of experimentation and discovery will teach your mind what your body needs. They will free you from the self-limiting patterns of movement you acquired from experience, habit and culture – patterns that contribute to dysfunction and sickness.

When you have such moments, feel free to share them with us. We would be delighted to hear from you. We will be glad to listen and learn, or to answer questions. You can write or call us at the Center for Self-Healing (1718 Taraval Street, San Francisco, CA 94116, USA (415) 665–9574, fax (415) 665–1318), or quite possibly you can tell Meir about it in person. He travels extensively. If you instruct us to put you on our mailing-list, we can keep you informed about projected workshops, lectures and classes in your area. Possibly there is a practitioner in your area we can refer you to.

Your Self-Healing work is one of the most important things you will ever do. Please give it the time and attention it requires. It is a lifetime process, a continual transformation in which you change yourself and the world of which you are a part. The energy that you create in movement transforms the matter that is your body. Increasingly, you become more in tune with the ceaseless movement of nature, the earth, the universe. To move anew is to be reborn, at any age, time and again.

The exercises in this book that were most helpful immediately are:

The exercises in this book that were most helpful six months to one year after I began working with it are:

Exercises that I invented, inspired by this method, are:

Index

Note: references in bold figures denote main entries.

Index

Index

Index

Index

Index